Institute of Cancer Research Library

Colorectal Cancer

CLINICAL SURGERY INTERNATIONAL

Editorial Advisory Board

D. C. Carter MD FRCS
(Chairman) Regius Professor of Clinical Surgery, University of Edinburgh, Edinburgh, UK.

John Cameron MD
Alfred Blaclock Professor and Chairman of Department of Surgery, The Johns Hopkins University School of Medicine, Baltimore, Maryland, USA.

Glyn G. Jamieson MB BS MS FRACS FACS
Dorothy Mortlock Professor of Surgery, University of Adelaide; Chairman, Division of Surgery, Royal Adelaide Hospital, Adelaide, Australia.

Volumes published

Vol. 1 **Large Bowel Cancer**
    J. J. DeCosse

Vol. 2 **Nutrition and the Surgical Patient**
    G. L. Hill

Vol. 3 **Tissue Transplantation**
    P. J. Morris

Vol. 4 **Infection and the Surgical Patient**
    H. C. Polk

Vol. 5 **The Biliary Tract**
    L. H. Blumgart

Vol. 6 **Surgery of the Thyroid and Parathyroid Glands**
    E. L. Kaplan

Vol. 7 **Peptic Ulcer**
    D. C. Carter

Vol. 8 **Arterial Surgery**
    J. J. Bergan

Vol. 9 **Shock and Related Problems**
    G. T. Shires

Vol. 10 **Breast Disease**
    J. F. Forbes

Vol. 11 **Gastrointestinal Haemorrhage**
    P. S. Hunt

Vol. 12 **Liver Surgery**
    S. Bengmark and L. H. Blumgart

Vol. 13 **Intestinal Obstruction**
    L. P. Fielding and J. P. Welch

Vol. 14 **Surgery of Inflammatory Bowel Disorders**
    E. C. G. Lee and D. J. Nolan

Vol. 15 **Anorectal Surgery**
    J. J. DeCosse and I. P. Todd

Vol. 16 **Pancreatitis**
    D. C. Carter and W. Warshaw

Vol. 17 **Emergency Abdominal Surgery**
    R. C. N. Williamson and M. J. Cooper

Vol. 18 **Modern Operative Techniques in Liver Surgery**
    B. Launois and G. G. Jamieson

Vol. 19 **Laparoscopic Digestive Surgery**
    P. L. Testas and B. J. Delaitre

CLINICAL SURGERY INTERNATIONAL

Colorectal Cancer

EDITED BY

NORMAN S. WILLIAMS

Professor of Surgery, The Royal London Trust, Academic Surgical Unit,
The Royal London Hospital, Whitechapel, London

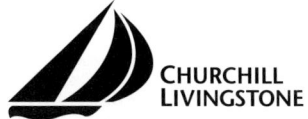

NEW YORK EDINBURGH LONDON MADRID MELBOURNE SAN FRANCISCO AND TOKYO 1996

CHURCHILL LIVINGSTONE
Medical Division of Pearson Professional Limited

Distributed in the United States of America by Churchill Livingstone Inc., 650 Avenue of the Americas, New York, N.Y. 10011, and by associated companies, branches and representatives throughout the world.

© Pearson Professional Limited 1996

All rights reserved. No part of this publication may be reproduced, stored in a retrieval system, or transmitted in any form or by any means, electronic, mechanical, photocopying, recording or otherwise, without either the prior permission of the publishers (Churchill Livingstone, Robert Stevenson House, 1–3 Baxter's Place, Leith Walk, Edinburgh, EH1 3AF), or a licence permitting restricted copying in the United Kingdom issued by the Copyright Licensing Agency Ltd, 90 Tottenham Court Road, London, W1P 9HE.

First published 1996

ISBN 0443 05133 X

British Library Cataloguing in Publication Data
A catalogue record for this book is available from the British Library.

Library of Congress Cataloging in Publication Data
A catalog record for this book is available from the Library of Congress.

For Churchill Livingstone
Commissioning Editor: Miranda Bromage
Copy Editor: Holly Regan-Jones
Project Controller: Anita Sekhri
Design Direction: Erik Bigland

Produced by Longman Singapore Publishers (Pte) Ltd.
Printed in Singapore

The publisher's policy is to use paper manufactured from sustainable forests

Contents

Introduction   vii

Contributors   ix

1. The molecular biology and genetics of colorectal cancer   1
   L. Cawkwell and P. Quirke

2. Early diagnosis and screening   21
   D. H. Bennett and J. D. Hardcastle

3. Colorectal polyps and their management   39
   S. Nivatvongs and S. Dorudi

4. Clinicopathological staging   55
   R. C. Newland, P. H. Chapuis and O. F. Dent

5. Sphincter saving resection and total reconstruction for low rectal cancer   69
   N. S. Williams

6. Local procedures, including endoscopic resection   93
   G. F. Buess

7. Laparoscopic surgery in colorectal cancer   103
   T.-A Teoh and S. D. Wexner

8. Obstruction and perforation   123
   D. A. Rothenberger, J. Mayoral and K. Deen

9. Adjuvant radiotherapy   135
   R. D. James

10. Adjuvant chemotherapy and immunotherapy for colorectal cancer   151
    D. J. Kerr

11. Surveillance and recurrence   159
    L. Pahlman

12. Treatment of colorectal liver metastases   173
    T. J. Babineau and G. Steele, Jr

Index   185

Introduction

Colorectal cancer remains the second most common malignant neoplasm in the Western World. Whereas in the past there has been much pessimism with regard to prognosis, in recent years optimism has abounded. This is due to a variety of factors which include greater specialization, breakthroughs in the understanding of basic oncological processes and involvement of other specialists apart from surgeons. This book examines some of the latest developments, and in addition explores some of the more contentious issues. It is not meant to be fully comprehensive, but attempts to highlight the areas which in the 1990s are likely to influence clinical management. The explosion in molecular biology has had a great impact in understanding the disease, and Lynn Cawkwell and Phillip Quirke review the area and provide insight into the ramifications of this knowledge. There is little doubt in most clinicians' minds that early diagnosis and screening will improve prognosis, and Jack Hardcastle and D. H. Bennett, who are involved in the Nottingham faecal occult blood study, are in a unique position to assess current progress. The adenoma-carcinoma sequence is now established, and the management of polyps is thus crucial in preventing cancer. Santhat Nivatvongs and Sina Dorudi review recent developments. It is becoming clearer that radical surgery and adjuvant therapy should be targeted at patients who have a high risk of recurrence. It is essential, therefore, to identify such patients as early as possible. Professor Newland, Pierre Chapuis and Owen Dent attempt to rationalize the complicated subject of staging. Chapters 5, 6 and 7, written by myself, Gerhard Buess and Steven Wexner, respectively, address advances in surgical techniques designed primarily to improve quality of life. I have concentrated on reconstructive procedures after radical surgery for rectal cancer, which eliminate the need for a permanent colostomy. Gerhard Buess, on the other hand, reviews local techniques and concentrates on his ingenious minimally invasive method of removing rectal cancer by the endo-anal route. Finally, Steven Wexner and Tiong-Ann Teoh explore the contentious issue of laparoscopic surgery for colorectal cancer.

Unfortunately, approximately 25% of patients with colorectal cancer present with obstruction or perforation. These are life-threatening conditions which need skilled therapy by a team of specialists. David Rothenburger reviews this important area, and highlights the progress that has occurred. Adjuvant therapy is perhaps the key to improving prognosis in established cases. Roger James demonstrates the important role radiotherapy can play, and David Kerr not only outlines the ever-increasing place of chemotherapy, but also highlights how immunotherapy and gene therapy are likely to be important future modalities.

There has been considerable debate as to whether it is necessary to follow up patients after their surgery for colorectal cancer. Lars Pahlman addresses this issue, and in the light of present knowledge indicates how this is best achieved. Once the tumour has metastasised, most clinicians throw up their hands in despair, but Glen Steele sees this as a challenge, and indicates that for selected patients there should be more optimism.

All in all, I hope this book illustrates why many individuals involved in managing patients with colorectal cancer feel optimistic about the future. I am grateful to all the expert contributors who have brought this work to fruition, and hope it will inspire others to carry the torch and improve the lot of patients with this disease.

Norman S. Williams

Contributors

T. J. Babineau MD
Assistant Professor, Department of Surgery, Harvard Medical School, Boston, Massachusetts, USA

D. H. Bennett Bsc MB BS FRCS
Ann Hunter Research Fellow, Department of Surgery, Queens Medical Centre, University Hospital, Nottingham, UK

G. F. Buess MD FRCS(Edin)
Director, Section for Minimally Invasive Surgery at the Department of General Surgery, Eberhard-Karls-Universitat, Tubingen, Germany

L. Cawkwell Bsc(Hons)
Research Assistant, Algernon Firth Institute of Pathology, Research School of Medicine, University of Leeds, Leeds, UK

P. H. Chapuis DS(Q'LD) FRACS
Clinical Associate Professor of Surgery, Department of Colon and Rectal Surgery, The University of Sydney, Concord Repatriation General Hospital, Sydney, Australia

K. Deen MD MS FRCS
Post Doctoral Associate, Division of Colon and Rectal Surgery, University of Minnesota Medical School, Minneapolis, Minnesota, USA

O. F. Dent MA PhD
Visiting Professor, Department of Surgery, Faculty of Medicine, University of Sydney, Sydney, Australia

S. Dorudi Bsc PhD FRCS
Lecturer/Senior Registrar in Surgery, Academic Surgical Unit, The Royal London Hospital, Whitechapel, London, UK

J. D. Hardcastle MA Mchir FRCS FRCP
Professor of Surgery, Department of Surgery, Queens Medical Centre, Nottingham, UK

R. D. James MRCP FRCR
Consultant in Clinical Oncology, The Christie Hospital, Manchester, UK

D. J. Kerr Bsc MB ChB MRCP MD Msc PhD
Professor of Clinical Oncology, Birmingham Institute for Cancer Studies, Queen Elizabeth Hospital, Edgbaston, Birmingham, UK

J. Mayoral MD
University Texas Health Sciences, San Antonio, Texas USA

R. C. Newland MB BS BSc(Med) DCP FRCPA
Clinical Associate Professor of Pathology, Concord Repatriation General Hospital, University of Sydney, Sydney, Australia

S. Nivatvongs MD
Consultant in Colon and Rectal Surgery, Mayo Clinic, Rochester, Minnesota, USA

L. Pahlman MD FACS
Associate Professor, Department of Surgery, Uppsala University, Uppsala, Sweden

P. Quirke BM PhD MRCPath
Head of Histopathology and Senior Lecturer in Pathology, United Leeds Teaching Hospital, NHS Trust, Leeds. Reader in Molecular Pathology, University of Leeds

D. A. Rothenberger MD FACS
Clinical Professor of Surgery, Department of Colon and Rectal Surgery, University of Minnesota Medical School, Minneapolis, Minnesota, USA

G. Steel Jr MD PhD
Chairman, Department of Surgery, New England Deaconess Hospital, Boston, Massachusetts, USA

T.-A. Teoh MB BS M MED (Surgery) FRCS(Edin)
Registrar, Department of General Surgery, Tan Tock Seng Hospital, Singapore

S. D. Wexner MD FACS FASCRS
Chairman and Presidency Program Director, Department of Colorectal Surgery, Cleveland Clinic, Florida, Fort Lauderdale, Florida, USA

N. S. Williams MB MS FRCS
Professor of Surgery, Director Academic Surgical Unit, The Royal London Hospital, London, UK

1 The molecular biology and genetics of colorectal cancer

L. CAWKWELL   P. QUIRKE

Introduction

Colorectal cancer (CRC) is primarily a genetic disease with lesions being either somatically induced by environmental agents or inherited through the germline. Familial adenomatous polyposis (FAP) and hereditary non-polyposis colorectal cancer (HNPCC) are the main types of inherited CRC. Sporadic CRC is thought to involve several genes in a multistep pathway. Oncogenes, tumour suppressor genes and DNA repair genes are involved. Some of these genes are also involved in FAP and HNPCC.

We will first look at the different forms of CRC and then we will take a detailed look at normal cell regulatory pathways. Next we will explain what can go wrong with these pathways and how this can lead to malignancy. Finally we will review the evidence for gene involvement in each type of CRC including how these genes are altered and what effect these alterations would have on normal cell regulatory pathways.

Types of colorectal cancer

Sporadic CRC is well dealt with elsewhere in this book; however, a proportion of CRC cases have an inherited component which leads to a predisposition to CRC at an earlier age.

Familial adenomatous polyposis (FAP)

FAP is an autosomal, dominantly inherited condition where the affected individual develops thousands of adenomas in their colorectum at an early age. If the colon is not surgically removed, then in most cases at least one of these adenomas will develop into a malignant tumour by the age of 40. FAP is thought to account for about 1% of total CRC cases and there are several variant forms. These include Gardner's syndrome, where extracolonic lesions occur, and Turcot syndrome, where tumours of the nervous system occur, in addition to colonic polyposis.

Hereditary non-polyposis colorectal cancer (HNPCC)

HNPCC (reviewed in Lynch et al 1993) is a dominantly inherited condition which predisposes the individual to CRC at an early age and is thought to account for up to 6% of total CRC cases. Unlike FAP, however, HNPCC does not have a clear phenotype such as polyposis. HNPCC families are distinguished by a strong family history of CRC. The 'Amsterdam' criteria (Vasen et al 1991) for determining HNPCC families require that there should be at least three individuals in two generations with CRC and that there should be one CRC diagnosis before the age of 50.

There are two forms of HNPCC. Lynch type 1 predisposes to CRC only, whereas Lynch type 2 predisposes to CRC as well as extracolonic lesions, especially endometrial carcinoma. The CRC tumours in HNPCC form from adenomas and are located predominantly on the right (proximal) side of the colon, but the reason for this is not clear. Variants of HNPCC include

Muir–Torre syndrome which predisposes to internal malignancies (often CRC) with a high frequency of sebaceous gland tumours.

Progression of CRC

There are two pathways for progression to CRC.

Adenoma–carcinoma pathway

The most common path is the adenoma–carcinoma sequence. Here the colonic crypt undergoes abnormal proliferation eventually leading to the formation of a dysplastic polypoid structure called an adenoma. The size and degree of dysplasia of the adenoma can increase and eventually may progress to a malignant tumour.

Ulcerative colitis (UC)-associated cancer and the dysplasia–carcinoma pathway

The second pathway is the dysplasia–carcinoma sequence as seen in UC-associated CRC. Hyperproliferation of the crypt is induced by UC and this can result in low-grade dysplasia which may progress to high-grade dysplasia and subsequently to carcinoma. Patients with UC are at increased risk of developing CRC (Gyde et al 1988, Isbell & Levin 1988).

Genes involved in normal cell regulatory pathways

This section explains what is known so far about how normal cells control proliferation, differentiation, communication, adhesion, death and DNA repair. All of the known cancer genes are involved in some way in these pathways, as we will see later. There is still much to be learnt about these pathways and their interactions and thus the pathways and the protein activities described are partially based on models inferred from evidence of in vitro protein interactions. There may be tissue-specific differences in these pathways and the particular proteins involved may be different in different organs. We do not yet know the specific details for the colorectum.

Adenomatous polyposis coli gene (APC)

Little is known about the function of the APC gene product but it is known to be associated with a complex of proteins that make up the adherens junctions in the plasma membrane (Su et al 1993a). Adherens junctions maintain the epithelial cell layers and thus probably are involved in cell adhesion, cell-to-cell communication and may also anchor the actin cytoskeleton, which is the cytoplasmic structure that gives a cell its shape.

The adherens junctions are made up of a transmembrane protein, epithelial (E) cadherin, which has an extracellular and an intracellular domain. The intracellular domain associates with three catenin proteins, α, β, and γ. Anchorage of the actin cytoskeleton may be mediated through α-catenin. There is evidence that β-catenin is bound to E-cadherin, α-catenin and also to the APC protein (Rubinfeld et al 1993, Su et al 1993a). Transmission of cell adhesion signals and contact inhibition signals could be mediated through this APC/β-catenin subunit.

Mutated in colorectal cancer gene (MCC)

Both the function and importance of the MCC protein are unknown. The MCC gene is located close to the APC gene and their sequences show short regions of similarity (Kinzler et al 1991). This led to the suggestion that their proteins could physically interact, but as yet this has not been demonstrated. The MCC protein could have a signal transduction function since it shows homology to the signal transduction activation region of the G protein coupled m3 muscarinic acetylcholine receptor (Kinzler et al 1991).

Ras

The ras gene family includes H-, N- and K-ras (for review see Barbacid 1987). Ras codes for a membrane-bound protein called ras-p21. When a growth factor receptor receives a growth signal from an extracellular growth factor (GF) this activates a chain of signal transmission that involves the ras-p21 protein (reviewed in Khosravi-Far & Der 1994).

Ras-p21 is controlled by a molecular switch involving the exchange of guanosine diphosphate (GDP) and guanosine triphosphate (GTP). Normal ras-p21 is held in an inactive state, bound to GDP whilst the cell is in a resting state. To transduce signals ras-p21 must be activated (Fig. 1.1) and this involves its binding to GTP. The signal is then passed to a cascade of downstream molecules eventually leading to transcription of genes required for cell growth or differentiation. After the signal has been transmitted active ras-p21 has to be deactivated. Ras-p21 has intrinsic GTPase activity which hydrolyses GTP to GDP, but a GTPase activating protein (GAP) is required to increase the efficiency of this reaction.

The ras signal transduction pathway has been widely studied and some of the molecules up and

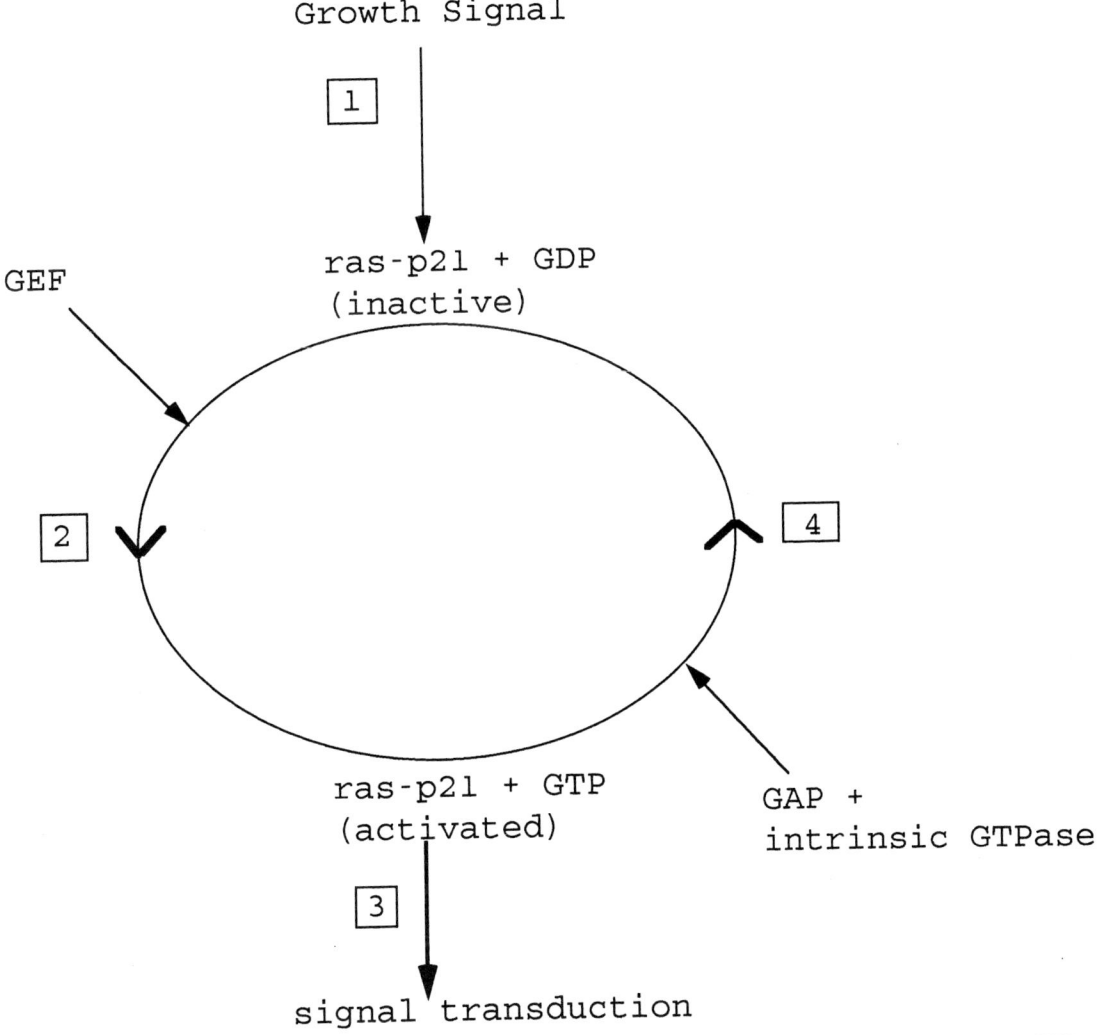

Fig. 1.1 Ras-p21 activation and deactivation. (1) A growth signal is received. (2) GDP is released by action of the GEF (guanine nucleotide exchange factor) protein and is replaced by GTP. (3) Activated ras-p21 bound to GTP transduces the growth signal to downstream molecules. (4) ras-p21 is deactivated by hydrolysis of GTP to GDP carried out by its intrinsic GTPase activity. This process is accelerated by GAP (GTPase activating protein). See text for further details and references.

downstream of ras in the pathway are now known. Studies on the epidermal growth factor receptor pathway show that when a signal is received by this receptor, a cytoplasmic protein complex including an adaptor protein (GRB2), which binds to the receptor, and a guanine nucleotide exchange factor (GEF) (Feig 1994) is brought into contact with the membrane-bound ras-p21. In this pathway the GEF protein involved is the SOS protein (Chardin et al 1993). The SOS protein promotes the release of GDP from ras-p21. GEFs are thought to initiate ras-p21 activation by stabilizing the p21 protein in a nucleotide-free state. This allows the more prevalent cytosolic GTP to take its place and this activates ras-p21. There are several GEFs which could be associated with different types of GF receptors or which could have tissue specificity.

Two GAPs are known that are able to deactivate ras-p21. The first is known as p120 (Trahey et al 1988) and the second is the product of the neurofibromatosis type 1 gene (NF1) (Ballester et al 1990, Martin et al 1990, Xu et al 1990). These GAPs are ubiquitous but distinct proteins and could possibly show tissue-specific differences in their deactivation of ras-p21. Ras is thus controlled through the balance of activating GEFs and deactivating GAPs. There is also a third type of regulatory protein involved. The ras guanine nucleotide dissociation inhibitor (GDI) (Bollag & McCormick 1993) has a potent ability in preventing the dissociation of GDP from ras-p21, possibly caused by inhibiting GEFs.

The molecules downstream of ras-p21 in the signalling pathway include Rho (Ridley et al 1992) and Raf1 (Finney et al 1993, Zhang et al 1993). The Rho pathway is believed to act in the regulation of actin cytoskeleton organization (Ridley & Hall 1992). The Raf1 pathway has been studied in some depth and it is known that Raf1 transduces the growth signal to the mitogen-activated protein kinase (MAPK) cascade (Leevers & Marshall 1992). These kinases transmit the signal through protein phosphorylation. MAPKs can activate nuclear transcription factors such as myc and jun (see below).

Myc

The product of the myc gene, myc-p62, is a nuclear protein that can activate the transcription of genes required for growth promotion by allowing entry into the cell cycle. The myc-p62 protein can only bind DNA when it is dimerized with the max protein (Amati et al 1993). The max protein is present at constant levels in the cell and in the absence of myc-p62 it forms max protein homodimers that bind the DNA sites that the myc/max protein dimer would bind (Fig. 1.2). Max/max protein dimers, however, cannot activate transcription and thus block cell proliferation. When the myc gene is activated the max/max protein dimers are removed from the DNA by phosphorylation by casein kinase II (ckII) (Berberich & Cole 1992). When max/max protein homodimers are not bound to DNA they are relatively unstable and since max proteins preferentially associate with myc-p62, the formation of stable myc/max protein heterodimers occurs, which can activate transcription.

Jun and fos

The products of the jun and fos genes (jun-p39 and fos-p62) are nuclear proteins which associate to form the fos/jun protein complex (reviewed in Curran & Franza 1988). This complex can bind to AP1 binding sites located in the promoter region of certain genes and thereby activate their transcription. The products of the genes which have AP1 binding sites are required for progression through the cell cycle.

Retinoblastoma 1 (RB1)

The nucleus-localized protein product of the RB1 gene is involved in cell cycle regulation (reviewed in Sherr 1994). The unphosphorylated form of the RB1 protein maintains cells in a resting state (Fig. 1.3). Phosphorylation of the protein accompanies the transition of cells from G1 to S phase of the cell cycle (Buchkovich et al

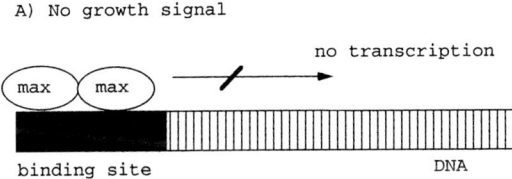

Fig. 1.2 Model for myc and max. (A) In the absence of a growth signal the max protein forms homodimers which bind to DNA and block transcription of genes required for proliferation. (B) When a growth signal is received the myc gene is transcribed to produce the myc-p62 protein and the max/max dimers are removed from the DNA by phosphorylation by casein kinase II (ckII). The max/max proteins dissociate from each other and bind to myc-p62. The myc-p62/max dimers then bind to the DNA and activate transcription of the genes required for proliferation. For further details and references see text.

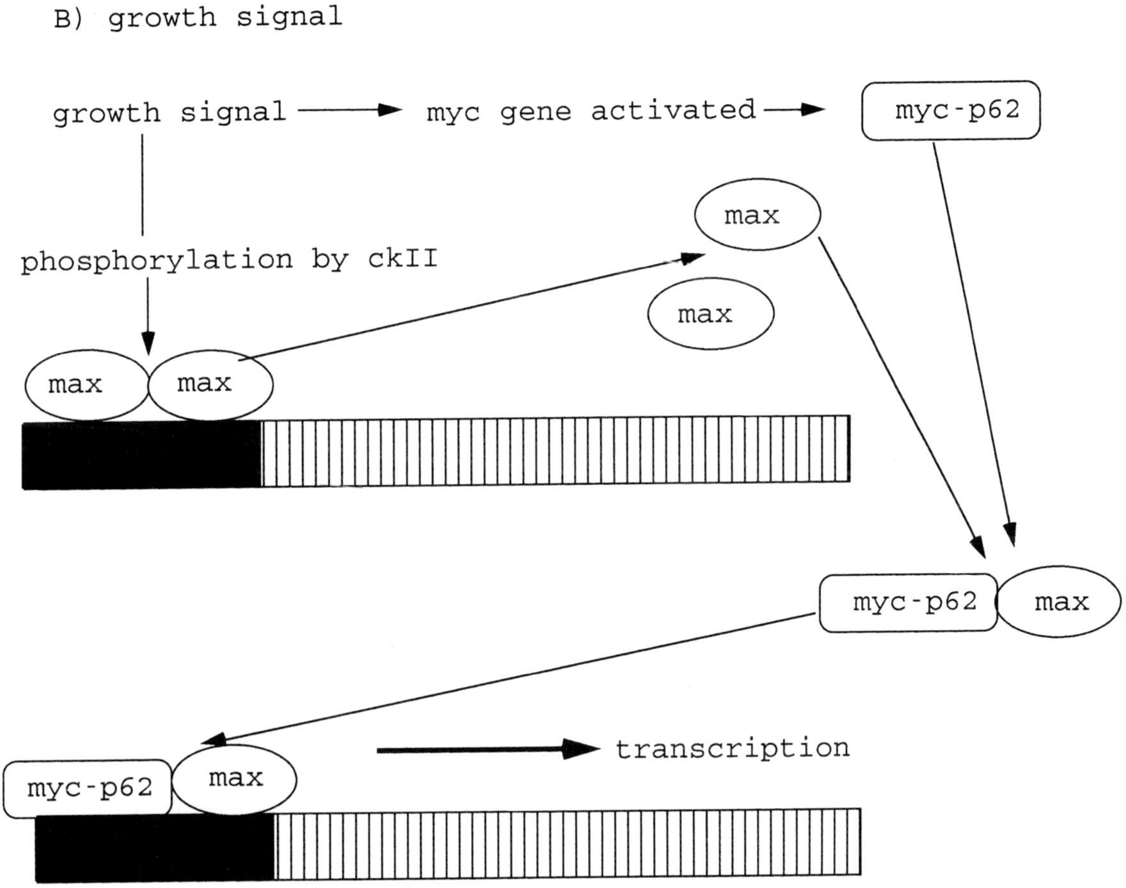

1989, Chen et al 1989, DeCaprio et al 1989, Mihara et al 1989).

Unphosphorylated RB1 protein can bind to transcription factors, including E2F and SP1 (Horowitz 1993). This prevents the transcription factors from binding to their DNA targets and thus blocks transcription. When the RB1 protein becomes phosphorylated it can no longer bind to these transcription factors and so they are released and can then initiate the expression of the genes that are required for the cell to enter S phase. Putative E2F binding sites have been found in the promoter region of some of the genes involved in cell proliferation, e.g. myc and fos (Horowitz 1993).

RB1 protein phosphorylation is regulated by

A) no growth signal

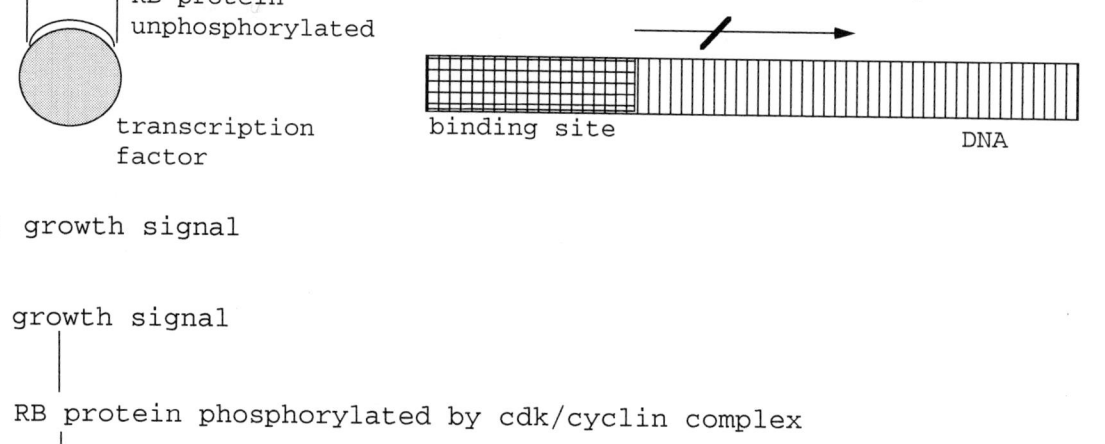

B) growth signal

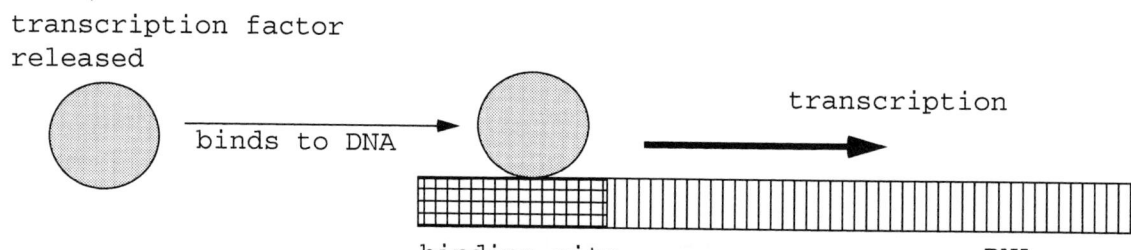

Fig. 1.3 Model for RB1 protein activity. (A) In the absence of a growth signal the RB1 protein is unphosphorylated and sequesters the transcription factors required to activate the genes required for proliferation. (B) When a growth signal is received the RB1 protein becomes phosphorylated by a cdk/cyclin complex. This causes the RB1 protein to release the transcription factor which can then bind to DNA and activate gene transcription. See text for further details and references.

G1 cyclin dependent kinases (cdks) (for review see Sherr 1994). In the normal cell cdks are responsible for the phosphorylation of the RB1 protein when growth stimulation is required. The activity of cdks is controlled by positive and negative extracellular growth signals. In order for the RB1 protein to activate the genes required for growth it must become phosphorylated so that the transcription factors it has sequestered are released. The pathway to phosphorylation of the RB1 protein initially requires that cdk4 activates cdk2. cdk2 then forms a complex with cyclin E. This complex has to be activated by threonine phosphorylation, catalysed by a cyclin-activating kinase (CAK) and it is thought that it then phosphorylates the RB1 protein.

During the resting stage phosphorylation of the RB1 protein can be blocked by other proteins including p16. The p16 protein (the product of the MTS1 gene) is known to inhibit the activity of cdk4 (Kamb et al 1994). RB1 protein phosphorylation is also blocked as a result of signals from transforming growth factor β1 (TGFβ1). TGFβ1 is an extracellular protein which can inhibit cell growth in some cells and stimulate it in others. The TGFβ1 molecule binds to a cell surface receptor complex which then transmits the signal. If the signal is for growth inhibition then synthesis of cdk4 is inhibited which in turn means that cdk2 would not be activated and thus there would be no cdk2/cyclin E complexes available to phosphorylate and activate the RB1 protein (Koff et al 1993).

p53

The p53 protein appears to act as a tetramer and seems to have a major role as a cell cycle checkpoint protein. It is known that DNA-damaging agents induce a rise in p53 levels, which in turn blocks the cell cycle in G1 (Kastan et al 1991). This would allow the cells time to correct any DNA damage before the DNA is replicated and thus prevent the perpetuation of errors and mutations. It is also known that p53 has the ability to induce apoptosis (programmed cell death) (Shaw et al 1992, Yonish-Rouach et al 1991) which it may do if the DNA damage is not successfully repaired.

It is not yet known how DNA damage leads to p53 induction but three genes that p53 activates following DNA damage are known. The first is the GADD45 gene which is turned on by p53 in response to DNA damage (Kastan et al 1992). The second is the WAF1/CIP1 gene (El-Deiry et al 1994). The WAF1/CIP1-p21 protein is a potent inhibitor of the activity of the cyclin-dependent protein kinases (cdks) which, as described earlier, are responsible for activating the RB1 protein by phosphorylation. The WAF1/CIP1 protein appears to bind to cdk/cyclin complexes rendering the complex inactive (El-Deiry et al 1994). Whilst the cdk/cyclin complex required for RB1 protein activation is inactive the cells would be held in G1. Wild type p53 protein can also inhibit transcription of the RB1 gene directly (Shiio et al 1992).

The third gene activated by p53 following DNA damage is the MDM2 gene (Price & Park 1994). The p53 gene appears to control its own regulation since the p53 protein can activate transcription of the MDM2 gene (Barak et al 1993) whose product can bind to the p53 protein and blocks its transcription activation function (Momand et al 1992), possibly by concealing its activation domain (Oliner et al 1993). This reversal of the G1 block would be required to get the cells back into cycle after the DNA damage has been repaired.

Deleted in colorectal cancer gene (DCC)

Little is known about the DCC gene product (Fearon et al 1990). It is a cell surface glycoprotein which may be involved in cell–cell or cell–matrix interactions on the basis of its similarity to neural cell adhesion molecules (NCAMs) (Fearon et al 1990).

NM23

There are two NM23 genes (H1 and H2) (Steeg et al 1988), which are 18 kilobases apart (Chandrasekharappa et al 1993), both localized at 17q21.3 (Backer et al 1993). Each gene produces a separate protein. These proteins exhibit nucleoside diphosphate kinase (NDPK) activity (Backer et al 1993) which converts nucleoside diphosphates into nucleoside triphosphates and may have a role in signal transduction. The actual role of the NM23 proteins is not known (Royds et al 1994a) but it has been suggested that an array of different NDPKs could be produced by varying both the ratios of different NM23 subunits and the type of bonds used that make up a functional NDPK complex (Backer et al 1993). A role for NM23 and its NDPK activity in the polymerization of microtubules has also been proposed (Lakshmi et al 1993).

hMSH2 and hMLH1

The proteins encoded by these genes act in a pathway which repairs mismatched DNA base pairs. Errors which occur during DNA replication must be repaired so that mutations are not introduced. Incorporation of the wrong base by DNA polymerase can occur (Loeb & Cheng 1990) but also repeated sequences, such as tracts of cytosine-adenine, can cause pairing problems during replication (Krawczak & Cooper 1991, Richards & Sutherland 1994) which have to be corrected by the mismatch repair system.

During replication it is possible that the template strand can become dissociated from the strand being synthesized. If the region that has become dissociated contains a repeated DNA sequence then when the strands reassociate, they may slip and pair incorrectly in the repeat region (so-called slipped mispairing), causing loops to be formed. Such loops could lead to the addition or deletion of bases, depending on whether the loop forms in the template strand or in the strand that is being synthesized. Mismatched loops would be corrected by the mismatch repair system.

What can go wrong with cell regulation?

Oncogenes

Protooncogenes are normal cellular genes which function in a positive manner in cell growth and differentiation. They act in the pathways that involve extracellular signals, transmitted via cell surface receptors, that trigger changes in gene expression which determines the growth and differentiation status of the cell. If these genes become mutated or altered in some way they are then known as activated oncogenes and these can disrupt normal cell growth and behaviour. Activated oncogenes have a positive effect on moving the cell towards malignancy (a simple analogy is that the 'accelerator pedal' driving cell growth has become 'stuck'). Alterations of protooncogenes can lead to a change in the normal activity or increased production of the gene product. Mutation, structural alteration and amplification can give rise to the activation of a protooncogene.

Protooncogenes encode growth factors, growth factor receptors, signal transducers and nuclear proteins.

Growth factors

Growth factors (GFs), such as the epidermal growth factor, give the initial signal which is transduced to the nucleus causing the cell to begin replication by entering the cell cycle. Alteration of protooncogenes that leads to the increased production of a GF or to the production of a GF at an inappropriate time or place will have an effect on cell growth.

Growth factor receptors

Growth factor receptors, such as the epidermal growth factor receptor, span the cell membrane and usually consist of an extracellular ligand-binding domain to bind GFs and an intracellular domain that transduces the mitogenic signal from the GF. Signal transducers usually have tyrosine kinase activity. Alterations or amplification of protooncogenes which encode GF receptors can lead to an increased number of receptors or to abnormal receptors which do not require GF stimulation.

Signal transducers

Signal transducers, such as ras, act as messengers generally carrying the growth signal from the GF receptor to the nucleus. Alteration of protooncogenes that encode signal transducers can lead to an increased level of signal transmission.

Nuclear factors

The products of protooncogenes which act in the nucleus, such as fos, myc and jun, function in cell cycle control and gene transcription. Products which control gene expression act on the DNA itself and this is the final site of action for messages sent from GFs. Nuclear factors are involved in DNA replication and gene transcription and thus overexpression or inopportune expression of a protooncogene product encoding a nuclear factor may have a deleterious effect on the control of cell growth.

Tumour suppressor genes

Some tumour suppressor (TS) gene products are involved in the negative control of cell growth and differentiation, e.g. RB1, p53 and NF1. This entails a complex pathway including cell cycle and cell differentiation controls. Deletion or mutational inactivation of these TS genes is thought to lead to loss of the normal regulation of cell growth since the cell will have lost the function of its cell growth 'brakes'. Other TS genes, such as APC, MCC and DCC, could have a role in cell–cell or cell–matrix communication which ensures that the correct adhesion and contact inhibition signals are maintained.

For most TS genes it seems that only a single functional copy of the gene is required to maintain normal development. Thus a germline TS gene mutation will be harmless but inactivation of the second allele may induce malignant growth. Classically, following Knudson's 'two-hit' hypothesis (Knudson 1987) based on the retinoblastoma gene (RB1), one copy of a TS gene is inactivated through mutation and this is followed by a second somatic alteration (deletion or mutation) in the homologous allele leading to total inactivation of the gene product.

In inherited disease all cells of the body carry one copy of the inactivated TS gene. The chance of a second somatic 'hit' affecting that gene in any cell, and thus leading to total inactivation of the protein, is relatively high since all cells carry the initial germline defect. The frequency of disease in such individuals is high and usually develops at an earlier age. If the lesion is not carried in the germline the chance of accumulating two 'hits' in the same gene in the same cell is much lower and thus disease onset in these sporadic cases is usually late.

Mutation can lead to the abolition of function of the TS gene product, most commonly by causing a truncation of the protein. However, there is evidence that some mutations in some TS genes, e.g. APC and p53, can lead to the production of a mutant protein which can associate with and possibly inhibit or inactivate the wild type protein. Such mutations would thus have a dominant effect.

The second alteration of TS genes is often loss of heterozygosity (LOH; allele loss) (Ponder 1988) which results in deletion of a copy of the TS gene. This can be mediated through loss of a whole normal chromosome by non-dysjunction, through deletion of a region of the normal chromosome containing the homologous TS gene allele or by recombination where a copy of the mutant allele replaces the normal homologous allele. LOH at TS gene loci appears to occur in a non-random manner since sites of TS genes are deleted with a high and consistent frequency. This implies that there is selection for the uncovering of the recessive mutation in the first allele; however, the mechanism for this is unknown.

Mutation of TS genes is difficult to study since most TS genes are large and mutations can be spread over large regions of the gene. However, screening techniques such as single strand conformation polymorphism (SSCP) assays (Orita et al 1989) can be used to detect the presence of a mutation before the DNA is sequenced to determine the actual type of mutation. If the types of gene mutation that occur most commonly are those which result in an alteration of the size of the protein product then in vitro transcription–translation assays can be used for screening to determine the size of the protein produced (Powell et al 1993). For example, a shorter length protein with a lower molecular weight will be produced if a gene mutation creates a premature termination codon.

Allele loss assays can be used to rapidly assess the deletion of TS gene alleles. A polymorphic marker close to or within the TS gene of interest is used to distinguish the maternal and paternal chromosomes. There are two types of polymorphic markers used. Restriction fragment length polymorphisms (RFLPs) are based on sequence polymorphisms which affect the sequence of a restriction enzyme recognition site. Thus one allele may have the correct sequence for the restriction enzyme to cut but the second allele may have a different sequence which the enzyme does not cleave.

The second type of marker are microsatellites, which are short repeated DNA sequences that exhibit length polymorphisms (Weber & May 1989). One allele may have, for example, 10 repeats of a short DNA sequence motif but the second allele could have 20 repeats, giving an overall difference in length between the two alleles. Individuals who are heterozygous for the marker (i.e. have a different type of allele on each chromosome) can then be assessed for allele loss at that site. Samples of tumour DNA along with corresponding normal tissue DNA are assayed and the relative amounts of each allele are compared between the normal and tumour (Fig. 1.4). Allele loss can be quantitated by assessing the change in the ratio of the two alleles between the normal and tumour DNA sample (Cawkwell et al 1993, MacGrogan et al 1994, Solomon et al 1987).

DNA repair genes

DNA repair genes, such as hMSH2 and hMLH1, act to repair both spontaneous and induced mutations in DNA. Spontaneous mutations and errors in DNA replication occur and these are corrected by the cell's array of repair enzymes. Lesions induced by chemical or physical (e.g. radiation) agents must be repaired by the appropriate repair enzymes. If critically positioned mutations or errors are left uncorrected then malignancy can be induced. Thus if DNA repair genes are altered or mutated in some way the repair pathways can be compromised.

Metastasis genes

Metastasis is a complex process believed to involve multiple genes. A role for metastasis genes in late stages of cancer progression has been implicated. The NM23 gene is a putative metastasis suppressor gene (reviewed in Royds et al 1994a).

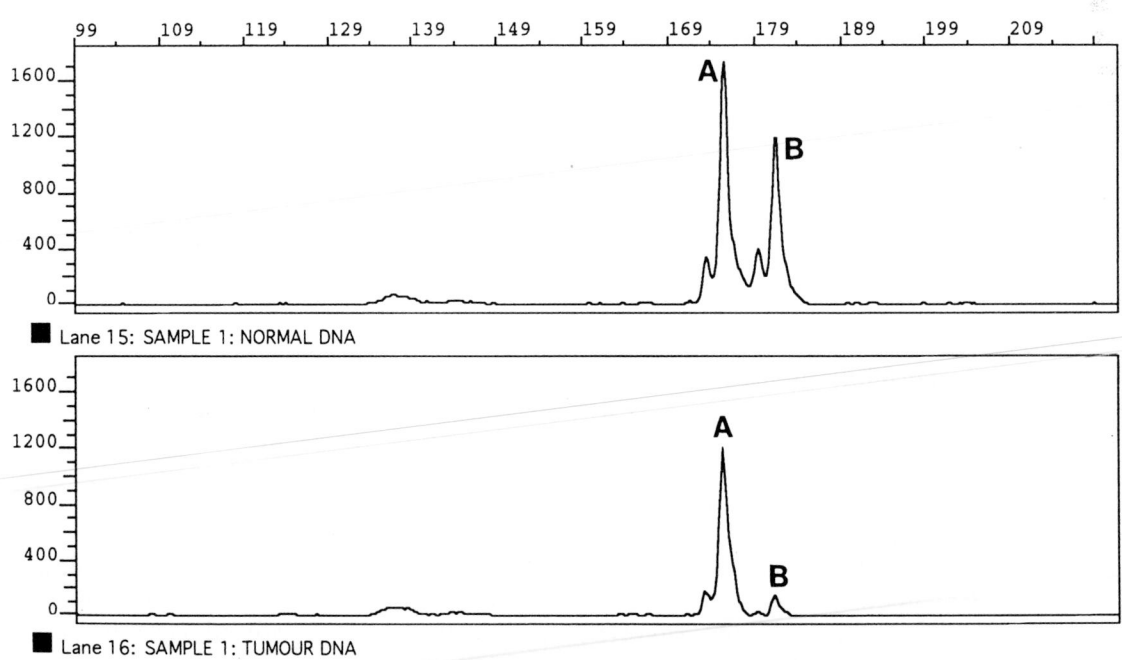

Fig. 1.4 Detection of allele loss in tumour DNA using fluorescently labelled microsatellites and an automated DNA sequencer. The values along the top show the size of the DNA in base pairs and the values along the side are arbitrary height values. The upper trace shows the normal DNA sample. Alleles A and B of a tumour suppressor gene are distinguished by their length due to a difference in the number of repeats of a cytosine-adenine (CA) motif in a non-transcribed region of their DNA sequences. The lower trace, showing the corresponding tumour sample from the same patient, indicates that almost all of allele B has been lost from the tumour. This is inferred by the significant (and quantifiable) reduction in height of this allele in the tumour trace as compared to the normal trace. A total loss of an allele is rarely seen due to the small amount of normal cells which contaminate the tumour specimen. For further details see Cawkwell et al (1993).

Gross DNA changes

DNA ploidy

Changes in cell DNA content as measured by flow cytometry are a classic feature of tumour cells. Diploid cells can become aneuploid through the gain or loss of individual chromosomes at mitosis, resulting in an abnormal number of chromosomes. Duplication of the entire chromosome set through mitotic non-dysjunction can lead to a tetraploid clone which can then also subsequently gain or lose chromosomes. The detection of aneuploid clones is thought to reflect gross chromosomal changes.

DNA methylation

Substantial DNA hypomethylation (loss of methyl groups) is generally related to gene activation. The role of hypomethylation in tumourigenesis is unclear but it may contribute to genome instability and aneuploidy as it may inhibit chromosome condensation at mitosis, causing problems in chromosome pairing and dysjunction (Goelz et al 1985). Abnormal hypermethylation can also occur, possibly caused by an increase in the activity of DNA methyltransferase (El-Deiry et al 1991), which could silence the transcription of important genes (Ohtani-Fujita et al 1993).

Genetic alterations in CRC

In this section we will describe the evidence regarding which genes are involved in the various types of CRC. The ways in which these genes are altered in CRC will be described and then the possible effects that such gene alterations could have on normal cell regulation will be discussed. These normal cell regulatory pathways were described earlier in this chapter.

FAP

Germline mutations of the APC gene are responsible for FAP and Gardner's syndrome (Nishisho et al 1991). A cytogenetically visible deletion of the long arm of chromosome 5 (5q) (Herrara et al 1986) led to the subsequent cloning of the APC gene located at 5q21 (Groden et al 1991, Joslyn et al 1991, Kinzler et al 1991, Nishisho et al 1991).

More than 60 different germline mutations have so far been identified in FAP patients, the majority of whom have a mutation in the APC gene (Powell et al 1993), and almost all of these mutations lead to the truncation of the protein product (Miyoshi et al 1992a, Powell et al 1993). It is known that some forms of the truncated APC protein can associate with the normal APC protein (Su et al 1993b) and thus possibly inhibit its normal function. The normal function of the APC protein is not known but, as described earlier, its possible role in regulating contact inhibition and adhesion signals would mean that a loss of APC function could interrupt these signalling pathways.

HNPCC

HNPCC appears to be caused by mutations in a DNA mismatch repair gene. Through family linkage studies it seems that about 60% of HNPCC cases are caused by the hMSH2 gene on chromosome 2p (Fishel et al 1993, Leach et al 1993, Peltomäki et al 1993) and a further 30% of cases are caused by the hMLH1 gene on chromosome 3p (Bronner et al 1994, Lindblom et al 1993, Papadopoulos et al 1994). Germline mutations in HNPCC tumours have been found in the hMSH2 and hMLH1 genes (Bronner et al 1994, Leach et al 1993, Papadopoulos et al 1994).

The mismatch repair enzymes hMSH2 and hMLH1 act in the same pathway (reviewed in Lindahl 1994) and if one of these enzymes is defective then mismatched bases will not be repaired. This will lead to genome-wide mutations, the amount of which will presumably be increased with every round of replication. Mutations in these mismatch repair genes lead to the appearance of a clear genetic marker known as microsatellite instability (Aaltonen et al 1993). Microsatellites are short repeated DNA sequences which exhibit length polymorphisms. As explained earlier, repeated sequences can cause special problems during replication by slipped mispairing (Krawczak & Cooper 1991, Richards & Sutherland 1994) and these errors have to be corrected by the mismatch repair enzymes. If the errors are not corrected then novel alleles appear in the tumour DNA (Fig. 1.5), which are not represented in the normal DNA, due to insertions and deletions in the repeat sequences caused by uncorrected mismatched loops. These novel allele bands are easily detected by amplifying regions of DNA that contain microsatellites.

Microsatellite instability is also seen in Muir–Torre syndrome (Honchel et al 1994).

Genetic changes in sporadic colorectal adenocarcinomas

Colorectal adenocarcinoma has been widely studied because of its well-defined progression from normal epithelium to a premalignant adenoma and then to carcinoma.

A multistep model for genetic events in colorectal cancer progression has been proposed (Fearon & Vogelstein 1990, Vogelstein et al 1988). This model suggests that there is mutational activation of oncogenes coupled with inactivation of tumour suppressor genes, by mutation or deletion, and that mutations in at least four or five genes are required to produce a malignant tumour. It appears that the total accumulation is what determines tumour behaviour, rather than the order of events. There is a large range of genetic alterations that have been found in sporadic colorectal tumours but as yet no single alteration has been seen in every tumour.

Oncogenes in sporadic CRC

Mutations of codon 12 of the K-ras gene occur in sporadic colorectal cancers with a frequency of about 40% (Bell et al 1991, Laurent-Puig et al 1991). There is a much higher incidence of these

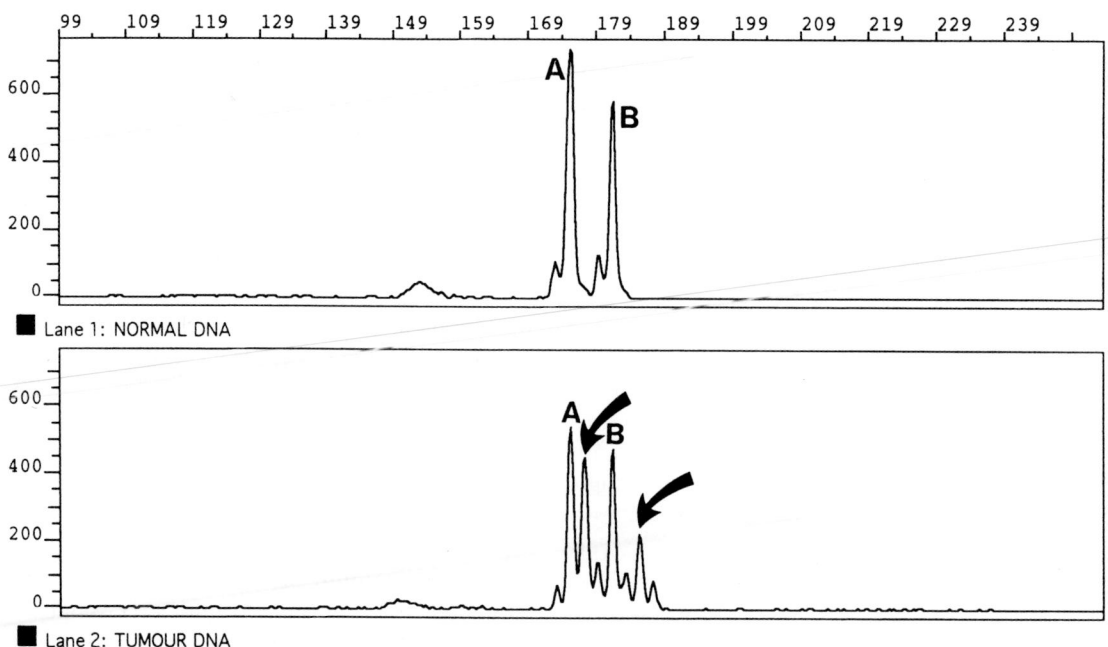

Fig. 1.5 Detection of microsatellite instability using fluorescently labelled microsatellites and an automated DNA sequencer. As described in Figure 1.4, the upper trace shows two alleles (A and B) in the normal DNA sample. However, in the corresponding tumour DNA sample from the same patient (lower trace) there are four alleles. The constitutional alleles A and B are still apparent but two additional alleles (arrowed) are also seen. This represents microsatellite instability. For full explanation of this, see text.

mutations in the rectum than in the colon (Bell et al 1991). K-ras mutations are seen at similar frequencies in large adenomas and carcinomas but K-ras mutation is an infrequent event in small adenomas (Scott et al 1993, Vogelstein et al 1988). This indicates that K-ras mutation may be involved in the transition from a small to a large adenoma or may be an initiating event in a small proportion of adenomas which then progress more rapidly to larger adenomas (Fearon & Vogelstein 1990). Mutant ras-p21 may not deactivate by the hydrolysis of GTP, either by escaping the effects of GAP or by an enhanced ability to bind GTP. This could stabilize ras-p21 in the active, signal transmitting state, allowing a continuous flow of mitogenic signals to the nucleus and leading to malignant transformation due to unscheduled cell proliferation. A mutated ras-p21 upstream of Rho could also hypothetically have a profound effect on regulation of cell shape and motility and also on cell–cell interactions.

In normal colonic mucosa myc protein is restricted to the nuclei of cells in the proliferating zones of the crypts. Increased expression of myc in colorectal tumours has been reported (Erisman et al 1985, Nagai et al 1992) but in most cases this did not appear to be due to either amplification or gross rearrangement of the gene but could be due to hypomethylation (Sharrard et al 1992). Normal myc protein is down-regulated when cells are in a resting state. If myc becomes activated then inappropriate or excessive production of the myc protein could prevent cells leaving the proliferative stage.

Tumour suppressor genes in sporadic CRC

Mutations of the APC gene occur early since it has been reported that over 60% of sporadic adenomas carry an APC gene mutation (Powell et al 1992). Even adenomas as small as 0.5cm in diameter were found that contained an APC mutation (Powell et al 1992). A similar frequency of APC mutations was found in colorectal cancers. Somatic mutations of APC give rise to a truncated gene product in the majority of cases (Miyoshi et al 1992b) and some truncated APC proteins are known to have the ability to associate with normal APC molecules, possibly inhibiting their normal function (Su et al 1993b). Over 60% of the somatic APC mutations were found to cluster in a small region (equivalent to less than 10% of the coding region) (Miyoshi et al 1992b). Allele loss of the APC gene region has been reported in up to 35% of adenomas (Vogelstein et al 1988) and in up to 45% of CRC tumours (Ashton-Rickardt et al 1989).

Since APC mutations have been found in the smallest adenomas it has been suggested that loss or mutation of one APC allele is an early event that could somehow initiate epithelial hyper-proliferation (Powell et al 1992). The recent finding of APC association with the adherens junctions suggests that APC may have a role in cell adhesion and contact inhibition signalling pathways.

The 'mutated in colorectal cancer' (MCC) gene is a candidate tumour suppressor gene located close to APC at 5q21. Allele loss of the MCC gene has been observed (Ashton-Rickardt et al 1991, Iacopetta et al 1994) at frequencies similar to that of APC. However, since MCC and APC are less than 500 kilobases apart, it has been suggested that MCC deletion only occurs concomitantly with APC loss and that APC is the target for deletion on 5q21 (Curtis et al 1994). Mutation of MCC is uncommon (Curtis et al 1994) which also suggests that MCC is not an independent tumour suppressor gene in CRC.

Mutations of the p53 gene, located at 17p13, occur frequently in colorectal tumours but infrequently in adenomas (Kikuchi-Yanoshita et al 1992) and is thus a late, rather than an initiating, event which may accompany the progression from adenoma to carcinoma. The majority of mutations are point mutations and occur in the most conserved regions of the gene (Hamelin et al 1994, Lothe et al 1992). Allele loss of the p53 gene is also seen frequently (up to 75% of cases) in colorectal tumours (Campo et al 1991, Cawkwell et al 1994, Iacopetta et al 1994), but infrequently in adenomas (Kikuchi-Yanoshita et al 1992). Kikuchi-Yanoshita et al (1992) reported that most of the tumours with p53 allele loss also had a p53 mutation. Unlike APC mutations, mutations of p53 do not frequently result in truncation of the protein. Mutations of the p53 gene frequently produce a mutant protein that is more stable than the wild-type protein and can accumulate to high levels in the cell (Kikuchi-Yanoshita et al 1992). Some p53 gene mutations are known to result in the production of a mutant protein which in some instances can bind to normal p53 proteins in an oligomeric complex, inactivating the transcriptional activation activity of the whole complex (Kern et al 1992). As we described earlier in the chapter, the normal p53 protein has an important role as a cell cycle checkpoint protein. If the normal function of p53 is abolished it could be envisaged that DNA mutations would accumulate since the cell cycle would not be interrupted to allow sufficient time for DNA repair to be completed before DNA containing errors is replicated.

In some studies, p53 mutation (Hamelin et al 1994) and overexpression detected by immunohistochemistry (which detects stabilized, i.e. mutant, p53) (Auvinen et al 1994, Sun et al 1992) have been found to correlate with poor survival in sporadic CRC.

The RB1 gene region appears to play a role in some sporadic CRC tumours (Wildrick & Boman 1994). Allele loss of the RB1 gene at 13q14.2 has been detected in colorectal tumours (Meling et al 1991), but more frequently increased RB1 gene copy number and expression have been noted (Lothe et al 1992, Meling et al 1991). This may be due to an increase in the copy number of part or all of chromosome 13 (Lothe et al 1992, Wildrick & Boman 1994). No gross structural alterations of the RB1 gene (Wildrick & Boman 1994) or RB1 protein size alterations (Gope et al 1990) have been reported in CRC. However, an intensive search for point mutations in the RB1 gene has not been reported. The effect that increased RB1 gene copy number would have in colon cancer cells is not clear as yet.

The DCC gene at 18q21 is a candidate tumour suppressor gene identified due to a high frequency of allele loss on 18q in CRC (Fearon et al 1990). Deletions, insertions and point mutations of the DCC gene were also noted (Fearon et al 1990). Allele loss involving the DCC gene region in CRC was originally reported to be as frequent as 71% (Fearon et al 1990); however, using intragenic DCC markers this frequency was found to be substantially lower (29–33%) (Cawkwell et al 1994, Huang et al 1993). Allele loss of the DCC gene appears to be a late event in CRC progression since Ookawa et al (1993) found that the highest frequencies of allele loss were in late stage tumours and metastases. The DCC protein is expressed in most normal tissues but its expression is decreased or absent in the majority of colorectal tumours (Fearon et al 1990, Itoh et al 1993), which may cause disruption of normal cell–cell contacts and cell adhesion.

The NF1 GAP protein is the product of a tumour suppressor gene and loss of functional NF1 GAP can in some tumours lead to an increase in active GTP-bound ras-p21 (Basu et al 1992). Allele loss of NF1 was found to occur in only 14% of sporadic colorectal tumours (Cawkwell et al 1994) and therefore does not appear to play a major role.

Loss on chromosomes 1p (Laurent-Puig et al 1992), 2p (Meling et al 1991), 8p (Fujiwara et al 1994, Yaremko et al 1994), 11q (Keldysh et al 1993) and 14q (Young et al 1993) has been observed and there may thus be further tumour suppressor genes involved in colorectal cancer.

DNA repair genes in sporadic CRC

Microsatellite instability has also been described in sporadic adenocarcinomas (Ionov et al 1993, Thibodeau et al 1993) and in a few adenomas (Shibata et al 1994). It is not known as yet whether this is due to mutations in the same mismatch repair genes that cause HNPCC or indeed whether these sporadic cases could in fact be HNPCC cases that were not identified due to insufficient family data. This idea is supported by the finding that sporadic CRC tumours with microsatellite instability tend to be found on the right side of the colon (Lothe et al 1993, Thibodeau et al 1993) which is a feature of HNPCC.

Microsatellite instability also appears to confer a better prognosis (Lothe et al 1993, Thibodeau et al 1993) although the reasons for this are not clear.

Metastasis genes in sporadic CRC

The role of the putative metastasis suppressor gene NM23 (Steeg et al 1988) in colorectal cancer is not clear since both allele loss (Cohn et al 1991) and increased levels of NM23 RNA (Haut et al 1991, Myeroff & Markowitz 1993) or protein (Royds et al 1994b) have been described. Other studies on mainly Dukes B and C stage cancers failed to detect either mutations (Bafico et al 1993) or significant levels of allele loss (Cawkwell et al 1994, Iacopetta et al 1994).

However, there is evidence that allele loss, mutation and a relative lowering of RNA and protein expression (in relation to non-metastatic tumours which show increased expression) are only evident in late-stage tumours associated with metastases (Cohn et al 1991, Wang et al 1993, Yamaguchi et al 1993). A role for NM23 in colorectal tumour metastasis is therefore not confirmed and the mechanisms causing increased expression in CRC tumours, and the effects this would have on NDPK activity, are also unclear.

Gross DNA changes in sporadic CRC

Substantial DNA hypomethylation is seen in adenomas (and is therefore an early event) and tumours in comparison to normal mucosa (Goelz et al 1985). This could lead to a release of the constraints on gene expression imposed by methylation or could cause problems at mitosis. Regional hypermethylation also occurs in colorectal tumours (Baylin et al 1991), which may play a key role in loss of tumour suppressor gene function by silencing gene transcription or by somehow marking targets for allele loss (Baylin et al 1991).

A substantial proportion (up to 78%) of colorectal tumours exhibit DNA aneuploidy (Meling et al 1991, Offerhaus et al 1992, Quirke et al 1987) which reflects genetic instability of the tumour cells and may be linked to gene losses (Offerhaus et al 1992). There is evidence that p53 alterations may play a role in the generation of aneuploid subclones in colorectal tumours (Carder et al 1993).

Genetic changes in UC-associated CRC

The genes involved in UC-cancer appear to be the same as those involved in sporadic colorectal adenocarcinomas; however, there seem to be differences in the frequency, site distribution and timing of the alterations.

Mutations at codon 12 of K-ras were seen in 22–24% of UC-associated carcinomas (Bell et al 1991, Chaubert et al 1994), which is a lower frequency than that seen in sporadic adenocarcinomas, and the site distribution of these mutations also differed (Bell et al 1991). In the UC-associated rectal cancers only 9% showed a K-ras mutation (as compared to 72% of sporadic rectal cancers). K-ras mutation has also been found in dysplastic regions (Chaubert et al 1994).

Allele loss of the p53 gene has been described in 33% of low-grade dysplasias, 63% of high-grade dysplasias and in 85% of UC-cancers (Burmer et al 1992). This same study also found that p53 loss only occurred in the tumours which were DNA aneuploid and not in diploid tumours, which suggests that aneuploidization may precede p53 allele loss. Mutation of the p53 gene is also seen in dysplastic regions (Yin et al 1993) and these findings suggest that inactivation of p53 occurs at an early non-invasive stage in the dysplasia–carcinoma pathway of UC, which is in contrast to the later inactivation of p53 in sporadic adenocarcinomas.

Allele loss of the APC/MCC region (33%) and the RB1 gene (33%) has also been described (Greenwald et al 1992) and there is evidence for the involvement of a gene on chromosome 8p since this region undergoes allele loss in 50% of UC carcinomas with loss also occurring in dysplastic regions (Chang et al 1994).

Conclusions

Knowledge of the genetic events which take place in colorectal carcinogenesis could be of importance in screening, diagnosis, prognosis and also in gene therapy (Sikora 1994).

The genetic bases for FAP and HNPCC are now clear; however, the causes of UC-associated

CRC and sporadic colorectal adenocarcinoma appear to be more complex. Several genes have already been implicated and there are further genomic loci which warrant investigation. There are several studies underway to assess the relative importance, in terms of tumour characteristics and patient survival, of the genes that are already implicated but as yet their roles are not fully known. Diagnostic tests are already being developed (Cawkwell et al 1994, Sidransky et al 1992) to take advantage of the genetic basis of CRC as soon as the genes of importance have been determined.

Knowledge of the genetic basis of FAP has meant that presymptomatic testing using non-invasive molecular techniques is now possible (reviewed in Petersen 1994). Individuals at risk can thus be identified and kept under close clinical surveillance.

For HNPCC, the use of microsatellite instability as a molecular diagnostic tool is being assessed. HNPCC has no clear phenotype such as polyposis, with diagnosis relying on family history at present, and thus a molecular marker would be a valuable tool for identifying individuals and families at risk.

Since the genes responsible for FAP and HNPCC are now known it may also be possible to develop gene therapy strategies to correct the defects in these genes when their full function is determined.

Acknowledgements
The authors' research work on colorectal cancer is supported by the Yorkshire Cancer Research Campaign.

References

Aaltonen LA, Peltomäki P, Leach FS et al 1993 Clues to the pathogenesis of familial colorectal cancer. Science 260: 812–816

Amati B, Brooks MW, Levy N et al 1993 Oncogenic activity of the c-myc protein requires dimerization with max. Cell 72: 233–245

Ashton-Rickardt PG, Dunlop MG, Nakamura Y et al 1989 High frequency of APC loss in sporadic colorectal carcinoma due to breaks clustered in 5q21–22. Oncogene 4: 1169–1174

Ashton-Rickardt PG, Wyllie AH, Bird CC et al 1991 MCC, a candidate familial polyposis gene in 5q.21, shows frequent allele loss in colorectal and lung cancer. Oncogene 6: 1881–1886

Auvinen A, Isola J, Visakorpi T, Koivula T, Virtanen S, Hakama M 1994 Overexpression of p53 and long-term survival in colon carcinoma. British Journal of Cancer 70: 293–296

Backer JM, Mendola CE, Kovesdi I et al 1993 Chromosomal localization and nucleoside diphosphate kinase activity of human metastasis-suppressor genes NM23-1 and NM23-2. Oncogene 8: 497–502

Bafico A, Varesco L, de Benedetti L et al 1993 Genomic PCR-SSCP analysis of the metastasis associated NM23-H1 (NME1) gene: a study on colorectal cancer. Anticancer Research 13: 2149–2154

Ballester R, Marchuk D, Boguski M et al 1990 The NF1 locus encodes a protein functionally related to mammalian GAP and yeast IRA proteins. Cell 63: 851–859

Barak Y, Juven T, Hafner R, Oren M 1993 MDM2 expression is induced by wild type p53 activity. EMBO Journal 12: 461–468

Barbacid M 1987 Ras genes. Annual Review of Biochemistry 56: 779–827

Basu TN, Gutmann DH, Fletcher JA, Glover TW, Collins FS, Downward J 1992 Aberrant regulation of ras proteins in malignant tumour cells from type 1 neurofibromatosis patients. Nature 356: 713–715

Baylin SB, Makos M, Wu J et al 1991 Abnormal patterns of DNA methylation in human neoplasia: potential consequences for tumour progression. Cancer Cells 3: 383–390

Bell SM, Kelly SA, Hoyle JA et al 1991 c-Ki-ras gene mutations in dysplasia and carcinomas complicating ulcerative colitis. British Journal of Cancer 64: 174–178

Berberich SJ, Cole MD 1992 Casein kinase II inhibits the DNA-binding activity of max homodimers but not myc/max heterodimers. Genes and Development 6: 166–176

Bollag G, McCormick F 1993 Identification of a novel ras regulator: a guanine nucleotide dissociation inhibitor. FASEB Journal 7: A1125

Bronner CE, Baker SM, Morrison PT et al 1994 Mutation in the DNA mismatch repair gene homologue hMLH1 is associated with hereditary non-polyposis colon cancer. Nature 368: 258–261

Buchkovich K, Duffy LA, Harlow E 1989 The retinoblastoma protein is phosphorylated during specific phases of the cell cycle. Cell 58: 1097–1105

Burmer GC, Rabinovitch PS, Haggitt RC et al 1992 Neoplastic progression in ulcerative colitis: histology, DNA content, and loss of a p53 allele. Gastroenterology 103: 1602–1610

Campo E, de la Calle-Martin O, Miquel R et al 1991 Loss of heterozygosity of p53 gene and p53 protein expression in human colorectal carcinomas. Cancer Research 51: 4436–4442

Carder P, Wyllie AH, Purdie CA et al 1993 Stabilised p53 facilitates aneuploid clonal divergence in colorectal cancer. Oncogene 8: 1397–1401

Cawkwell L, Bell SM, Lewis FA, Dixon MF, Taylor GR, Quirke P 1993 Rapid detection of allele loss in colorectal tumours using microsatellites and fluorescent DNA technology. British Journal of Cancer 67: 1262–1267

Cawkwell L, Lewis FA, Quirke P 1994 Frequency of allele loss of DCC, p53, RB1, WT1, NF1, NM23 & APC/MCC in colorectal cancer assayed by fluorescent multiplex polymerase chain reaction. British Journal of Cancer 70: 813–818

Chandrasekharappa SC, Gross LA, King SE, Collins FS 1993 The human NME2 gene lies within 18kb of NME1 in chromosome 17. Genes, Chromosomes and Cancer 6: 245–248

Chang M, Tsuchiya K, Batchelor RH et al 1994 Deletion mapping of chromosome 8p in colorectal carcinoma and dysplasia arising in ulcerative colitis, prostatic carcinoma, and malignant fibrous histiocytomas. American Journal of Pathology 144: 1–6

Chardin P, Camonis JH, Gale NW et al 1993 Human sos1: a guanine nucleotide exchange factor for ras that binds to GRB2. Science 260: 1338–1343

Chaubert P, Benhattar J, Saraga E, Costa J 1994 K-ras mutations and p53 alterations in neoplastic and nonneoplastic lesions associated with longstanding ulcerative colitis. American Journal of Pathology 144: 767–775

Chen P-L, Scully P, Shew J-Y, Wang JYJ, Lee W-H 1989 Phosphorylation of the retinoblastoma gene product is modified during the cell cycle and cellular differentiation. Cell 58: 1193–1198

Cohn KH, Wang F, Desoto-Lapaix F et al 1991 Association of nm23-H1 allelic deletions with distant metastases in colorectal carcinoma. Lancet 338: 722–724

Curran T, Franza BR 1988 Fos and jun: the AP-1 connection. Cell 55: 395–397

Curtis LJ, Bubb VJ, Gledhill S, Morris RG, Bird CC, Wyllie AH 1994 Loss of heterozygosity of MCC is not associated with mutation of the retained allele in sporadic colorectal cancer. Human Molecular Genetics 3: 443–446

DeCaprio JA, Ludlow JW, Lynch D et al 1989 The product of the retinoblastoma susceptibility gene has properties of a cell cycle regulatory element. Cell 58: 1085–1095

El-Deiry WS, Nelkin BD, Celano P et al 1991 High expression of the DNA methyltransferase gene characterises human neoplastic cells and progression stages of colon cancer. Proceedings of the National Academy of Sciences USA 88: 3470–3474

El-Deiry WS, Harper JW, O'Connor PM et al 1994 WAF1/CIP1 is induced in p53-mediated G1 arrest and apoptosis. Cancer Research 54: 1169–1174

Erisman MD, Rothberg PG, Diehl RE, Morse CC, Spandorfer JM, Astrin SM 1985 Deregulation of c-myc gene expression in human colon carcinoma is not accompanied by amplification or rearrangement of the gene. Molecular and Cellular Biology 5: 1969–1976

Fearon ER, Vogelstein B 1990 A genetic model for colorectal tumorigenesis. Cell 61: 759–767

Fearon ER, Cho KR, Nigro JM et al 1990 Identification of a chromosome 18q gene that is altered in colorectal cancers. Science 247: 49–56

Feig LA 1994 Guanine-nucleotide exchange factors: a family of positive regulators of ras and related GTPases. Current Opinion in Cell Biology 6: 204–211

Finney RE, Robbins SM, Bishop JM 1993 Association of pRas and pRaf-1 in a complex correlates with activation of a signal transduction pathway. Current Biology 3: 805–812

Fishel R, Lescoe MK, Rao MRS et al 1993 The human mutator gene homolog MSH2 and its association with hereditary nonpolyposis colon cancer. Cell 75: 1027–1038

Fujiwara Y, Ohata H, Emi M et al 1994 A 3-Mb physical map of the chromosome region 8p21.3-p22, including a 600-kb region commonly deleted in human hepatocellular carcinoma, colorectal cancer, and non-small cell lung cancer. Genes, Chromosomes and Cancer 10: 7–14

Goelz SE, Vogelstein B, Hamilton SR et al 1985 Hypomethylation of DNA from benign and malignant human colon neoplasms. Science 228: 187–190

Gope R, Christensen MA, Thorson A et al 1990 Increased expression of the retinoblastoma gene in human colorectal carcinomas relative to normal colonic mucosa. Journal of the National Cancer Institute 82: 310–314

Greenwald BD, Harpaz N, Yin J et al 1992 Loss of heterozygosity affecting the p53, Rb, and MCC/APC tumor suppressor gene loci in dysplastic and cancerous ulcerative colitis. Cancer Research 52: 741–745

Groden J, Thliveris A, Samowitz W et al 1991 Identification and characterization of the familial adenomatous polyposis coli gene. Cell 66: 589–600

Gyde SN, Prior P, Allan RN et al 1988 Colorectal cancer in ulcerative colitis: a cohort study of primary referrals from three centres. Gut 29: 209–217

Hamelin R, Laurent-Puig P, Olschwang S et al 1994 Association of p53 mutations with short survival in colorectal cancer. Gastroenterology 106: 42–48

Haut M, Steeg PS, Willson JKV, Markowitz SD 1991 Induction of nm23 gene expression in human colonic neoplasms and equal expression in colon tumors of high and low metastatic potential. Journal of the National Cancer Institute 83: 712–716

Herrara L, Kakati S, Gibas L, Pietrzak E, Sandberg A 1986 Brief clinical report: Gardner syndrome in a man with an interstitial deletion of 5q. American Journal of Medical Genetics 25: 473–476

Honchel R, Halling KC, Schaid DJ, Pittelkow M, Thibodeau SN 1994 Microsatellite instability in Muir–Torre syndrome. Cancer Research 54: 1159–1163

Horowitz JM 1993 Regulation of transcription by the retinoblastoma protein. Genes, Chromosomes and Cancer 6: 124–131

Huang TH-M, Quesenberry JT, Martin MB, Loy S, Diaz-Arias AA 1993 Loss of heterozygosity detected in formalin-fixed, paraffin embedded tissue of colorectal carcinoma using a microsatellite located within the deleted in colorectal carcinoma gene. Diagnostic Molecular Pathology 2: 90–93

Iacopetta B, DiGrandi S, Dix B, Haig C, Soong R, House A 1994 Loss of heterozygosity of tumour suppressor gene loci in human colorectal carcinoma. European Journal of Cancer 30A: 664–670

Ionov Y, Peinado MA, Malkhosyan S, Shibata D, Perucho M 1993 Ubiquitous somatic mutations in simple repeated sequences reveal a new mechanism for colonic carcinogenesis. Nature 363: 558–561

Isbell G, Levin B 1988 Ulcerative colitis and colon cancer. Clinical Gastroenterology 17: 773–791

Itoh F, Hinoda Y, Ohe M et al 1993 Decreased expression of DCC mRNA in human colorectal cancers. International Journal of Cancer 53: 260–263

Joslyn G, Carlson M, Thliveris A et al 1991 Identification of deletion mutations and three new genes at the familial polyposis locus. Cell 66: 601–613

Kamb A, Gruis NA, Weaver-Feldhaus et al 1994 A cell cycle regulator potentially involved in genesis of many tumour types. Science 264: 436–440

Kastan MB, Onyekwere O, Sidransky D et al 1991 Participation of p53 protein in the cellular response to DNA damage. Cancer Research 51: 6304–6311

Kastan MB, Zhan Q, El-Deiry WS et al 1992 A mammalian cell cycle checkpoint pathway utilizing p53 and gadd45 is defective in ataxia telangiectasia. Cell 71: 587–597

Keldysh PL, Dragani TA, Fleischman EW et al 1993 11q deletions in human colorectal carcinomas: cytogenetics and restriction fragment length polymorphism analysis. Genes, Chromosomes and Cancer 6: 45–50

Kern SE, Pietenpol JA, Thiagalingam S, Seymour A, Kinzler KW, Vogelstein B 1992 Oncogenic forms of p53 inhibit p53-regulated gene expression. Science 256: 827–830

Khosravi-Far R, Der CJ 1994 The ras signal transduction pathway. Cancer and Metastasis Reviews 13: 67–89

Kikuchi-Yanoshita R, Konishi M, Ito S et al 1992 Genetic changes of both p53 alleles associated with the conversion from colorectal adenoma to early carcinoma in familial adenomatous polyposis and non-familial adenomatous polyposis patients. Cancer Research 52: 3965–3971

Kinzler KW, Nilbert MC, Su L et al 1991 Identification of FAP locus genes from chromosome 5q21. Science 253: 661–665

Knudson AG 1987 A two-mutation model for human cancer. Advances in Viral Oncology 7: 1–17

Koff A, Ohtsuki M, Polyak K, Roberts JM, Massagué J 1993 Negative regulation of G1 in mammalian cells: inhibition of cyclin E-dependent kinase by TGF-β. Science 260: 536–539

Krawczak M, Cooper DN 1991 Gene deletions causing human genetic disease: mechanisms of mutagenesis and the role of the local DNA sequence environment. Human Genetics 86: 425–441

Lakshmi MS, Parker C, Sherbet GV 1993 Metastasis associated MTS1 and NM23 genes affect tubulin polymerisation in B16 melanomas: a possible mechanism of their regulation of metastatic behaviour of tumours. Anticancer Research 13: 299–304

Laurent-Puig P, Olschwang S, Delattre O et al 1991 Association of Ki-ras mutation with differentiation and tumor-formation pathways in colorectal carcinoma. International Journal of Cancer 49: 220–223

Laurent-Puig P, Olschwang S, Delattre O et al 1992 Survival and acquired genetic alterations in colorectal cancer. Gastroenterology 102: 1136–1141

Leach FS, Nicolaides NC, Papadopoulos N et al 1993 Mutations of a mutS homolog in hereditary nonpolyposis colorectal cancer. Cell 75: 1215–1225

Leevers SJ, Marshall CJ 1992 MAP kinase regulation – the oncogene connection. Trends in Cell Biology 2: 283–286

Lindahl 1994 DNA surveillance defect in cancer cells. Current Biology 4: 249–251

Lindblom A, Tannergård P, Werelius B, Nordenskjöld 1993 Genetic mapping of a second locus predisposing to hereditary non-polyposis colon cancer. Nature Genetics 5: 279–282

Loeb LA, Cheng KC 1990 Errors in DNA synthesis: a source of spontaneous mutations. Mutation Research 238: 297–304

Lothe RA, Fossli T, Danielsen HE et al 1992 Molecular genetic studies of tumor suppressor gene regions on chromosomes 13 and 17 in colorectal tumours. Journal of the National Cancer Institute 84: 1100–1108

Lothe RA, Peltomäki P, Meling GI et al 1993 Genomic instability in colorectal cancer: relationship to clinicopathological variables and family history. Cancer Research 53: 5849–5852

Lynch HT, Smyrk TC, Watson P et al 1993 Genetics, natural history, tumor spectrum, and pathology of hereditary nonpolyposis colorectal cancer: an updated review. Gastroenterology 104: 1535–1549

MacGrogan D, Levy A, Bostwick D, Wagner M, Wells D, Bookstein R 1994 Loss of chromosome 8p loci in prostate cancer: mapping by quantitative allelic imbalance. Genes, Chromosomes and Cancer 10: 151–159

Martin GA, Viskochil D, Bollag D et al 1990 The GAP-related domain of the neurofibromatosis type 1 gene product interacts with ras p21. Cell 63: 843–849

Meling GI, Lothe RA, Borresen AL et al 1991 Genetic alterations within the retinoblastoma locus in colorectal carcinomas. Relation to DNA ploidy pattern studied by flow cytometric analysis. British Journal of Cancer 64: 475–480

Mihara K, Cao X-R, Yen A et al 1989 Cell-cycle dependent regulation of phosphorylation of the human retinoblastoma gene product. Science 246: 1300–1303

Miyoshi Y, Ando H, Nagase H et al 1992a Germ-line mutations of the APC gene in 53 familial adenomatous polyposis patients. Proceedings of the National Academy of Sciences USA 89: 4452–4456

Miyoshi Y, Nagase H, Ando H et al 1992b Somatic mutations of the APC gene in colorectal tumors: mutation cluster region in the APC gene. Human Molecular Genetics 1: 229–233

Momand J, Zambetti GP, Olson DC et al 1992 The mdm-2 oncogene product forms a complex with the p53 protein and inhibits p53-mediated transactivation. Cell 69: 1237–1245

Myeroff LL, Markowitz SD 1993 Increased nm23-H1 and nm23-H2 messenger RNA expression and absence of mutations in colon carcinomas of low and high metastatic potential. Journal of the National Cancer Institute 85: 147–152

Nagai MA, Habr-Gama A, Oshima CTF, Brentani MM 1992 Association of genetic alterations of c-myc, c-fos, and c-Ha-ras protooncogenes in colorectal tumours. Diseases of the Colon and Rectum 35: 444–451

Nishisho I, Nakamura Y, Miyoshi Y et al 1991 Mutations of chromosome 5q21 genes in FAP and colorectal cancer patients. Science 253: 665–669

Offerhaus GJA, de Feyter EP, Cornelisse CJ et al 1992 The relationship of DNA aneuploidy to molecular genetic alterations in colorectal carcinoma. Gastroenterology 102: 1612–1619

Ohtani-Fujita N, Fujita T, Aoike A et al 1993 CpG methylation inactivates the promoter activity of the human retinoblastoma tumor-suppressor gene. Oncogene 8: 1063–1067

Oliner JD, Pietenpol JA, Thiagalingam S, Gyuris J, Kinzler KW, Vogelstein B 1993 Oncoprotein MDM2 conceals the activation domain of tumor suppressor p53. Nature 362: 857–860

Ookawa K, Sakamoto M, Hirohashi S et al 1993 Concordant p53 and DCC alterations and allelic losses on chromosomes 13q and 14q associated with liver metastases of colorectal carcinoma. International Journal of Cancer 53: 382–387

Orita M, Suzuki Y, Sekiya T, Hayashi K 1989 Rapid and sensitive detection of point mutations and DNA polymorphisms using the polymerase chain reaction. Genomics 5: 874–879

Papadopoulos N, Nicolaides NC, Wei Y-F et al 1994 Mutation of a mutL homolog in hereditary colon cancer. Science 263: 1625–1629

Peltomäki P, Aaltonen LA, Sistonen P et al 1993 Genetic mapping of a locus predisposing to human colorectal cancer. Science 260: 810–812

Petersen GM 1994 Knowledge of the adenomatous polyposis coli gene and its clinical application. Annals of Medicine 26: 205–208

Ponder B 1988 Gene losses in human tumours. Nature 335: 400–402

Powell SM, Zilz N, Beazer-Barclay Y et al 1992 APC mutations occur early during colorectal tumorigenesis. Nature 359: 235–237

Powell SM, Petersen GM, Krush AJ et al 1993 Molecular diagnosis of familial adenomatous polyposis. New England Journal of Medicine 329: 1982–1987

Price BD, Park SJ 1994 DNA damage increases the levels of MDM2 messenger RNA in wtp53 human cells. Cancer Research 54: 896–899

Quirke P, Dixon MF, Clayden AD et al 1987 Prognostic significance of DNA aneuploidy and cell proliferation in rectal adenocarcinomas. Journal of Pathology 151: 285–291

Richards RI, Sutherland GR 1994 Simple repeat DNA is not replicated simply. Nature Genetics 6: 114–116

Ridley AJ, Hall A 1992 The small GTP-binding protein Rho regulates the assembly of focal adhesions and actin stress fibers in response to growth factors. Cell 70: 389–399

Ridley AJ, Paterson HF, Johnston CL, Diekmann D, Hall A 1992 The small GTP-binding protein rac regulates growth factor-induced membrane ruffling. Cell 70: 401–410

Royds JA, Rees RC, Stephenson TJ 1994a NM23 – a metastasis suppressor gene? Journal of Pathology 173: 211–212

Royds JA, Cross SS, Silcocks PB, Scholefield JH, Rees RC, Stephenson TJ 1994b NM23 'anti-metastatic' gene product expression in colorectal carcinoma. Journal of Pathology 172: 261–266

Rubinfeld B, Souza B, Albert I et al 1993 Association of the APC gene product with B-catenin. Science 262: 1731–1734

Scott N, Bell SM, Sagar P, Blair GE, Dixon MF, Quirke P 1993 p53 expression and K-ras mutation in colorectal adenomas. Gut 34: 621–624

Sharrard RM, Royds JA, Rogers S, Shorthouse AJ 1992 Patterns of methylation of the c-myc gene in human colorectal cancer progression. British Journal of Cancer 65: 667–672

Shaw P, Bovey R, Tardy S, Sahli R, Sordat B, Costa J 1992 Induction of apoptosis by wild-type p53 in a human colon tumor-derived cell line. Proceedings of the National Academy of Sciences USA 89: 4495–4499

Sherr CJ 1994 The ins and outs of RB: coupling gene expression to the cell cycle clock. Trends in Cell Biology 4: 15–18

Shibata D, Peinado MA, Ionov Y, Malkhosyan S, Perucho M 1994 Genomic instability in repeated sequences is an early somatic event in colorectal tumorigenesis that persists after transformation. Nature Genetics 6: 273–281

Shiio Y, Yamamoto T, Yamaguchi N 1992 Negative regulation of Rb expression by the p53 gene product. Proceedings of the National Academy of Sciences USA 89: 5206–5210

Sidransky D, Tokino T, Hamilton SR et al 1992 Identification of ras oncogene mutations in the stool of patients with curable colorectal tumours. Science 256: 102–105

Sikora K 1994 Genes, dreams, and cancer. British Medical Journal 308: 1217–1221

Solomon E, Voss R, Hall V et al 1987 Chromosome 5 allele loss in human colorectal carcinomas. Nature 328: 616–619

Steeg PS, Bevilacqua G, Kopper L et al 1988 Evidence for a novel gene associated with low tumor metastatic potential. Journal of the National Cancer Institute 80: 200–204

Su L-K, Vogelstein B, Kinzler KW 1993a Association of the APC tumor suppressor protein with catenins. Science 262: 1734–1737

Su L-K, Johnson KA, Smith KJ, Hill DE, Vogelstein B, Kinzler KW 1993b Association between wild type and mutant APC gene products. Cancer Research. 53: 2728–2731

Sun X-F, Carstensen JM, Zhang H et al 1992 Prognostic significance of cytoplasmic p53 oncoprotein in colorectal adenocarcinoma. Lancet 340: 1369–1373

Thibodeau SN, Bren G, Schaid D 1993 Microsatellite instability in cancer of the proximal colon. Science 260: 816–819

Trahey M, Wong G, Halenbeck R et al 1988 Molecular cloning of two types of GAP complementary DNA from human placenta. Science 242: 1697–1700

Vasen HFA, Mecklin J-P, Meera Khan P, Lynch HT 1991 The International Collaborative Group on Hereditary Non-polyposis Colorectal Cancer. Diseases of the Colon and Rectum 34: 424–425

Vogelstein B, Fearon ER, Hamilton SR et al 1988 Genetic alterations during colorectal-tumor development. New England Journal of Medicine 319: 525–532

Wang L, Patel U, Ghosh L, Chen H-C, Banerjee S 1993 Mutation in the nm23 gene is associated with metastasis in colorectal cancer. Cancer Research 53: 717–720

Weber JL, May PE 1989 Abundant class of human DNA polymorphisms which can be typed using the polymerase chain reaction. American Journal of Human Genetics 44: 388–396

Wildrick DM, Boman BM 1994 Does the human retinoblastoma gene have a role in colon cancer? Molecular Carcinogenesis 10: 1–7

Xu G, Lin B, Tanaka K et al 1990 The catalytic domain of the neurofibromatosis type 1 gene product stimulates ras GTPase and complements ira mutants of S. cerevisiae. Cell 63: 835–841

Yamaguchi A, Urano T, Fushida S et al 1993 Inverse association of nm23-H1 expression by colorectal cancer with liver metastasis. British Journal of Cancer 68: 1020–1024

Yaremko ML, Wasylyshyn ML, Paulus KL, Michelassi F, Westbrook CA 1994 Deletion mapping reveals two regions of chromosome 8 allele loss in colorectal carcinomas. Genes, Chromosomes and Cancer 10: 1–6

Yin J, Harpaz N, Tong Y et al 1993 p53 point mutations in dysplastic and cancerous ulcerative colitis lesions. Gastroenterology 104: 1633–1639

Yonish-Rouach E, Resnitzky D, Lotem J, Sachs L, Kim-Chi A, Oren M 1991 Wild-type p53 induces apoptosis of myeloid leukaemic cells that is inhibited by interleukin-6. Nature 352: 345–347

Young J, Leggett B, Ward M et al 1993 Frequent loss of heterozygosity on chromosome 14 occurs in advanced colorectal carcinomas. Oncogene 8: 671–675

Zhang X, Settleman J, Kyriakis JM et al 1993 Normal and oncogenic p21^{ras} proteins bind to the amino-terminal regulatory domain of c-Raf-1. Nature 364: 308–313

2 Early diagnosis and screening

D. H. BENNETT J. D. HARDCASTLE

Introduction

The aim of screening is to detect neoplasia of the colon and rectum before it reaches an advanced stage, survival being directly related to the stage at presentation (Deans et al 1994). Diagnosis when the tumour is at a less advanced stage currently offers the best hope of reducing mortality.

The philosophy of screening for colorectal cancer is based on the premise that the disease is common, the natural history and biology are partially understood and, if detected at a less advanced stage, the condition is curable.

Colorectal cancer is now the second commonest malignancy in the Western World. In England and Wales, it accounts for over 13% of all registered malignancies. Table 2.1 indicates how the incidence of and mortality from colorectal cancer have changed over the last 20 years. While there has been a steady increase in the number of cases reported, the mortality has remained fairly constant, resulting in an improvement in 5-year relative survival from 22% to 37% over the last 20 years (Cancer Research Campaign Handbook 1993, OPCS 1980).

Table 2.1 Registrations of and deaths from colorectal cancer for England and Wales (reproduced with permission from OPCS, Cancer statistics: registrations 1972–1992)

Year	Registrations of new cases of colorectal cancer	Deaths recorded
1992	Not available	17 186
1987	25 042	17 053
1982	23 961	16 008
1977	23 171	16 462
1972	19 561	16 306

For a screening programme to be effective, several variables have to be considered. Feasibility factors include patient compliance, test safety and performance (sensitivity, specificity and predictive value), test positivity rates and cost. The compliance of the general population with the recommendations of screening for colorectal cancer is a significant determinant of feasibility and it is important to distinguish between efficacy (results under ideal conditions) and effectiveness (results under real conditions). One method of incorporating compliance into detection is to calculate cancer detection rates, comparing the number of cancers detected in the total population offered screening (effectiveness) with the number of cancers detected in the group which completes the trial protocol (efficacy). It should also be remembered that case-control studies do not take compliance into account as each case is matched to one or more controls (100% compliance).

Sensitivity reflects the proportion of persons with colorectal neoplasia who are correctly identified by the test. Ideally, the sensitivity of the test should be high (>90%); once the sensitivity falls to 50%, the screening procedure is likely to miss as many cancers as it detects.

Specificity reflects the proportion of persons with no colorectal neoplasia whose screening test is negative. Although it need not be as high as sensitivity, the lower the specificity, the greater the number of unnecessary investigations, increasing both the frequency of adverse effects and the cost of screening. For example, a test with a specificity of 90% will result in around 5000 individuals undergoing unnecessary investigation

Colorectal cancer

because of a false-positive result when a population of 50 000 asymptomatic individuals is screened.

Uncertainty about the effectiveness of screening for colorectal cancer is reflected by the absence of a national screening policy. The effectiveness of a screening programme can be demonstrated both directly and indirectly. Only studies that show a benefit in the screened population, regardless of the individual results of detection and therapies instituted, provide direct evidence of effectiveness. For colorectal cancer screening, the definitive verification of effectiveness is an improved survival rate in the screened population.

Additional evidence for the effectiveness of screening comes from indirect or inferential studies. Examples include the detection of a greater number of early stage tumours by screening, few cancers being missed by the screening test and improved survival by the treatment of early cancers and adenomas. If indirect evidence of this kind is pooled, an inference can be made that screening for colorectal cancer may be beneficial. However, using such 'surrogate outcomes' on their own is misleading as bias is introduced with each assumption and a false conclusion may be inferred.

It must also be remembered that people undergoing screening are asymptomatic and have not sought medical help. Therefore, any adverse effects of screening must be quantitated and balanced against the possible beneficial effects of improved survival (Feldman 1990). False-positives, false-negatives and even true-positive diagnoses may produce adverse effects. Patients are exposed to the complications of diagnostic investigation (usually colonoscopy) following a false-positive test while a false-negative test may give a false sense of security, with a possible delay in investigating subsequent symptoms. A true-positive test both exposes the person with incurable disease to the consequences of earlier knowledge of his or her impending doom and may also shorten their lifespan by the complications of further diagnostic and therapeutic interventions.

When reviewing the data available, the published outcome is extremely important. It should reflect the primary goal of screening, which is improved survival. If the question of survival benefit remains unanswered, the effectiveness of screening remains unproven. Whether it is the cancer-specific or the overall mortality rate which is the more important outcome remains controversial. Patients who die from colorectal cancer that had not been diagnosed prior to death and patients who die as a result of the screening procedure itself are included in overall mortality figures. When the disease has a low prevalence, uncommon adverse reactions become more important. For example, if screening detects one cancer per 1000 individuals screened and colonic perforations occur at a rate of one per 1000 performed, the number of false-positive test results (sensitivity) becomes important in assessing the relative merits of screening.

Finally, having established the effectiveness of a screening programme, the burden of illness, likely compliance of the population requiring screening and cost-effectiveness of the programme become integral considerations.

Target population

It is clear that for screening to be effective, an 'at-risk' population needs to be identified. The general population can be divided into two groups, those at average risk and those at high risk. The incidence of colorectal cancer increases exponentially with age (Fig. 2.1), 90% of cases

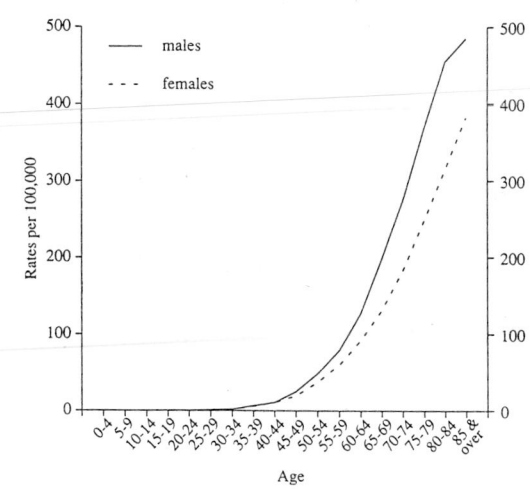

Fig. 2.1 Incidence of colorectal Cancer by age. (Reproduced with permission from Cancer statistics: registrations 1988, series MB1, no. 21.)

arising in those over 50 years old. The condition is therefore too rare before this age to make screening cost-effective and most studies have taken 50 as the age of entry. This older age group constitutes the population at average risk for colorectal cancer unless other risk factors apply.

High-risk groups

Table 2.2 lists those conditions conferring a high risk of developing colorectal cancer. The inherited susceptibilities to colorectal cancer are usually divided into the polyposis and non-polyposis syndromes. Familial adenomatous polyposis (FAP) is associated with the presence of large numbers of adenomatous polyps throughout the colon whereas a smaller number of adenomas are present in the non-polyposis syndromes and these are predominantly sited within the proximal colon.

FAP, an autosomal dominant condition with a high penetrance, has a population frequency of between one in 7000 and one in 30 000 (Alma & Lieznerski 1973). Progression to colorectal cancer occurs in approximately 90% of untreated patients by their 50s (Burt and Samowitz 1988) and probably accounts for 1% of observed colorectal cancer cases (Jarvinen 1992). The gene responsible for FAP, the adenomatous polyposis coli (APC) gene, has been identified on chromosome 5q21 (Groden et al 1991) and codes for a protein believed to be attached to E-cadherin which may be involved in cell–cell interactions. The precise manner in which germline mutation in the APC gene leads to adenoma formation and subsequently to carcinoma is not yet understood. However, the length of the truncated APC protein appears to be important: APC truncated around codon 1300 may have little suppressor activity, leading to the development of multiple adenomas (>5000), whereas APC truncated in other locations may have more suppressor activity, hence fewer adenomas (<2000) (Nagase et al 1992).

Prior to the localization of the APC gene, screening affected relatives had entailed annual sigmoidoscopy from puberty to at least 40 years of age before a family member could be considered unaffected. Subjects at increased risk of developing FAP were also screened for additional phenotypic markers such as congenital hypertrophy of the retinal pigment epithelium and mandibular osteomas which are also common in this condition. However, the identification of the gene has allowed the development of genetic probes and genetic screening (Powell et al 1993) can now exclude the presence of a mutated allele in the majority of family members.

An attenuated variant of FAP has also been described (Lynch et al 1990). It is characterized by flat adenomas numbering in the dozens to hundreds in the right colon, a risk of colorectal and extracolonic malignancies and late onset of adenomas and carcinomas. Germline mutation in the FAP gene results in a truncated, partially functional APC protein although other modifier genes are also believed to be involved (Eng & Ponder 1993).

The non-polyposis syndromes are dominantly inherited predispositions to colorectal cancer and are divided into two subcategories: hereditary site-specific colon cancer (Lynch syndrome I), which predisposes specifically to colorectal cancer, and cancer family syndrome (Lynch syndrome II), in which there is a predisposition to colorectal cancer, endometrial cancer, ovarian cancer or stomach cancer (Lynch et al 1985). Combined, they are estimated to account for 5–6% of all colorectal cancers (Lynch et al 1993a). The gene believed to be responsible for HNPCC has been identified as hMSH2 (Leach et al 1993), a

Table 2.2 Risk factors for the development of colorectal cancer

Polyposis syndromes
Familial adenomatous polyposis syndromes
   Familial adenomatous polyposis
   Gardner's syndrome
   Turcot's syndrome
   Attenuated FAP

Non-polyposis colon cancer syndromes
Hereditary non-polyposis colon cancer (HNPCC)
   Hereditary site-specific colon cancer (Lynch syndrome I)
   Cancer family syndrome (Lynch syndrome II)

Non-syndrome familial colon cancer
   Family history – colorectal adenomas
                    – colorectal cancer
   Personal history – colorectal adenomas
                     – colorectal cancer

Chronic inflammatory bowel disease

mismatch repair gene on chromosome 2p16, although detailed linkage analysis studies have identified additional candidate genes such as hMLH-1 (Lindblom et al 1993), PMS-1 and PMS-2 (Papadopoulos et al 1994). Until the underlying genetic mutations are characterized and genetic tests developed, screening HNPCC kindreds involves colonoscopy of all first-degree relatives at 2–3 yearly intervals (Lynch et al 1993a). If adenomas are detected, the screening interval is reduced to annually.

Family history

First-degree relatives of colorectal cancer cases are also at an increased risk of developing colorectal cancer (Winawer et al 1991), estimates ranging from a 2–4-fold (Stephenson et al 1991) to an eight-fold increase in risk (Duncan & Kyle 1982). In a recent case-controlled study, St John et al (1993a) concluded that first-degree relatives have a modest (two-fold) increase in risk which increases if more than one first-degree relative is affected or if diagnosis of the index case was at an early age (before 45 years). Relatives of patients with colorectal adenomas or carcinoma also have a three-fold increased risk of developing adenomas (Cannon-Albright et al 1988).

It is therefore important when recommending screening strategies to consider absolute risk as well as the test performance. The current family history screening strategy employed in Nottingham is shown in Table 2.3. Similar recommendations have been adopted by the American Society for Gastrointestinal Endoscopy and the Gastroenterological Association (Bond 1993). Initial follow-up is performed at 3 years, the interval increasing to 5 years after a normal examination.

Inflammatory bowel disease

The significantly increased risk of developing colorectal cancer in patients with long-standing ulcerative colitis is now accepted (Kvist et al 1989), the risk increasing with the duration of the disease and its extent (Collins et al 1987,

Table 2.3 Nottingham family history screening protocol

Risk*	Preliminary screen	Surveillance
<1:15	FOB test + flexible sigmoidoscopy	Normal investigation → repeat endoscopy 5-yearly & FOB test biennially Abnormal investigation → full colonoscopy, treat neoplasia & repeat endoscopy & FOBT in 1 year
>1:15	FOB test + colonoscopy	Normal investigation → repeat endoscopy 5-yearly & FOB test biennially. Abnormal investigation → treat neoplasia & repeat endoscopy & FOB test in 1 year

*Population risk – 1:50 risk
One first degree relative > 45 years – 1:17 risk
Two first degree & second degree relatives > 45 years – 1:12 risk
One first degree relative < 45 years – 1:10 risk
Two first degree relatives, one < 45 years – 1:6 risk
Three first degree relatives – 1:2 risk

Lennard-Jones et al 1990). Recent evidence suggests that Crohn's colitis also bears a cancer risk and has a pathological profile comparable with ulcerative colitis (Choi & Zelig 1994). Surveillance programmes were instituted following the development of colonoscopy and the description of the association between colorectal dysplasia and cancer (Morson & Pang 1967). At-risk patients are examined at annual or biennial intervals, by colonoscopy and biopsy, to detect premalignant dysplasia or early cancer.

However, the rationale for these surveillance programmes has been challenged. Lynch et al (1993b) concluded that only one of nine cancers that arose in association with ulcerative colitis during a 12 year surveillance period was detected by the surveillance programme. Their literature review suggested only 13% of the colonic cancers which arose during colonoscopic surveillance programmes represented successes for those programmes (Dukes' A or B tumours). The efficacy of colonoscopic surveillance programmes is therefore questionable; Sachar (1993) concluded 'The desired goal of surveillance programmes is not cancer detection but cancer prevention ... saving colons must always be subordinate to saving lives'.

Screening tests

Faecal occult blood tests

Several classes of faecal occult blood tests have been developed based on (a) the pseudoperoxidase activity of haemoglobin, (b) immunological reactivity to globin and (c) haem–porphyrin assays. All these tests are based on the premise that colonic cancers and adenomas often cause bleeding in excess of the normal range (Macrae & St John 1982). However, between one-quarter and one-third of patients with cancers have average daily blood loss within the normal range of less than 1.5 ml per day (Macrae & St John 1982). There is also a variable quantity of bleeding from day to day in patients with large bowel neoplasia (Farrands & Hardcastle 1983, St John et al 1992) and the blood products present in the stool are often unequally distributed (Rosenfield et al 1979). These factors must be considered when comparing these tests.

Guaiac tests

The most commonly employed test has been Haemoccult. The test consists of a filter paper slide impregnated with guaiac which undergoes phenolic oxidation in the presence of haemoglobin in the stool when hydrogen peroxide is added. A colour change from clear to blue indicates a positive test. The sensitivity of the test is however, reduced by the fact that anything with peroxidase activity – for example, fresh fruit such as bananas and vegetables such as broccoli and radish – can produce a positive reaction (Young et al 1990). Conversely, agents (such as ascorbic acid) that interfere with the oxidation reaction may produce a false-negative result in the presence of haemoglobin.

Screening studies have attempted to reduce these problems by testing or retesting subjects after imposing dietary restrictions. For example, Robinson et al (1993) showed that only 36% of subjects whose initial test was <5 squares positive remained positive following retesting with dietary restriction. In contrast, 88% of subjects whose initial test was ≥5 squares positive remained positive after retesting. Dietary interference is therefore more significant in weakly positive cases and limiting retesting with dietary restriction to this group is likely to both improve test sensitivity and enable rapid investigation of those with strongly positive tests.

Haemoccult will detect losses of 10 ml/day in 67% of cases (Stroehlein et al 1976) and >20 ml/day in 80–90% cases (Doran & Hardcastle 1982), allowing reasonable test sensitivity without resulting in large numbers of false-positives.

Immunological tests

These tests are based on antihuman haemoglobin antibodies detecting stool haemoglobin using a variety of methodologies, including radial immunodiffusion (Frommer et al 1988), ELISA (Turunen et al 1984), haemagglutination-inhibition (St John 1990) and latex agglutination (Vaananen & Tenhunen 1988). They are specific to human haemoglobin and therefore avoid the problems of dietary interference. The likelihood of false-positives from upper gastrointestinal blood loss is also reduced as the immunoreactive haemoglobin is rapidly degraded before it reaches the large bowel. The sensitivity of the various immunological tests ranges from 200 µg to 700 µg haemoglobin per gram faeces (Saito 1992), about 0.2–0.7 ml blood loss per day.

Haem–porphyrin assays

These tests detect the broadest range of blood derivatives, namely deironed haems (haem-derived porphyrins) as well as any intact haem in any form (free or as haemoprotein) (Schwartz et al 1983). It is a quantitative measure, based on the fluorescence of haem-derived porphyrins, of total blood loss into the gastrointestinal tract. While pseudoperoxidase activity does not affect the assay, a strict dietary protocol excluding non-human haem is essential and blood loss from the proximal and distal gastrointestinal tract cannot be distinguished.

Studies comparing FOB tests

Haemoccult has been compared to several immunological tests and the results are summarized in Table 2.4. The guaiac test has consistently failed to detect as many cancers as the immunochemical test but the latter has tended to have a higher positivity rate. The marked exception is Fujita's 1992 study using a guaiac test with approximately twice the sensitivity of Haemoccult. A test with a high positivity rate and low predictive value, even if highly sensitive, is unsuitable for a population screening study because of the increased cost and potential morbidity of investigating large numbers of people with false-positive tests. Even so, the immunological tests appear to outperform standard Haemoccult as far as sensitivity is concerned while retaining an acceptable specificity.

In a recent study, an example of each type of FOBT was compared, including a newer guaiac test, HaemoccultSENSA (St John et al 1993b). The sensitivities of these tests in patients with known colorectal malignancies were: Haemoccult-SENSA 94%, HemeSelect 97%, HaemoQuant 71% and Haemoccult 89%. These results confirm the findings of Ahlquist et al (1993) that Haemoquant is not suitable for colorectal cancer screening. The positivity rates for Haemoccult-SENSA and HemeSelect are shown in Table 2.4

Table 2.4 Comparison of Haemoccult with various immunochemical tests (adapted from Young & St John 1991)

Reference	Test	Immunochemical	Guaiac
Frommer 1992	Radial immunodiffusion		Haemoccult
	n =	13 675	6903
	Positivity rate	7.5%	2.0%
	PPV: cancer (%)	7.5	8.1
Thomas 1992	Detectacol		Not performed
	n =	6323	
	Positivity rate	5.2%	
	PPV: cancer (%)	10	
Fujita 1992	Immudia-Hem Sp		Shionogi B
	n =	15 488	12 520
	Positivity rate	3.2%	20.8%
	PPV: cancer (%)	5.6	0.7
Iwase 1992	Immudia-Hem Sp		Haemoccult
	n =	5715	5715
	Positivity rate	6.8%	1.7%
	PPV: cancer (%)	4.1	5.2[1]
Kawaguchi 1992	Immudia-Hem Sp[2]		Not performed
	n =	29 770	
	Positivity rate	3.0%	
	PPV: cancer (%)	3.2	
St John et al 1993b	HemeSelect		Haemoccult-SENSA
	n =	1355	1355
	Positivity rate	3.0%	5.0%
	PPV: cancer (%)	2.4	1.5
Robinson 1994	HemeSelect		Haemoccult
	n =	1489	1489
	Positivity rate	9.7%	1.1%
	PPV: cancer (%)	6.2	5.9
Armitage 1985	FECA EIA (ELISA)		Haemoccult
	n =	1304	1304
	Positivity rate	8.1%	3.1%
	PPV: cancer (%)	4.5	6.9

PPV = positive predictive value
[1] Only 64% of those with positive Haemoccult tests had complete large bowel examinations
[2] Two day test only

when employed in screening individuals and, although the sensitivity of these two tests has not been published, the estimated specificity is 96.1% for HaemoccultSENSA and 97.8% for HemeSelect. The results are encouraging and, if population screening by FOBT is introduced, an immunological test may provide the best combination of sensitivity and specificity.

Population screening trials

Haemoccult has been used in population screening trials since 1975. The first trial to report mortality figures was the Memorial Sloan–Kettering Cancer Centre–Strang Clinic Trial, New York (Winawer et al 1993a). Patients had been allocated to a study or control group depending on their date of enrolment and, although two trials were commenced, the control and study groups were only sufficiently matched in Trial II for a comparison of colorectal mortality to be performed. The only difference between the two groups was that the study group was offered a FOBT whereas the control group was not. After 9 years follow-up, there was a significant ($p<0.001$) difference in long-term survival between the study and control groups and, although there was a 43% reduction in mortality in the study group from colorectal cancer, this just failed to reach statistical significance ($p<0.053$).

In 1977, a FOBT was added to the annual cancer screening programme in Germany for persons over the age of 45 years. Wahrendorf et al (1993) identified 163 male and 209 female patients (age range 55 to 75 years) who had died of colorectal cancer between 1983 and 1986 and compared their screening histories with a case-matched control group. Twenty nine percent of women in the control group had completed a FOBT compared to only 16% of the study group for the time period 6–36 months prior to diagnosis, a statistically significant result with an odds ratio of 0.43 (95% CI: 0.27, 0.68) implying a protective effect for those completing FOBTs. The data for men were 13% and 14% respectively, suggesting that FOBT screening in men has no effect. The authors explain this discrepancy by the difference in compliance with screening – only 8% men participating in screening compared to 20% women.

Gnauck (1994) has reported the results of screening in Germany for the later period, 1985–90. Compliance with Haemoccult testing has been very low (10% men, 22% women) with positivity rates of 0.9% for women and 1.9% for men. Approximately 1500 colorectal cancers have been found annually, 0.1:1000 female and 0.8:1000 male screenees. This equates to a positive predictive value for cancer of 1.4% in women and 4.2% in men. Unfortunately, polyps are not registered and, due to the absence of a national cancer registry, the effect of this screening on mortality is unknown.

A similar case-control study was performed using data from the Kaiser Permanente Medical Care Program in Northern California (Selby et al 1993). A history of FOBT screening was compared between a total of 485 persons who developed fatal colorectal cancer after 50 years of age and 727 age- and sex-matched controls. The risk for fatal colorectal cancer was reduced by 10–30% among those who had had an FOBT, depending on the time interval since their last FOBT. It was concluded that a 25% reduction in mortality was possible for persons who have a screening FOBT every 1–2 years. However, the confidence intervals were wide and included 1, the observed association therefore conceivably being due to chance.

While case-control studies are unaffected by non-compliance, they introduce confounding variables which may lead persons with a lower risk for colorectal cancer to have screening FOBTs more frequently. This concern is eliminated by randomized controlled trials, five of which have been instigated since 1975. Three of the European studies have reported interim results while the Minnesota trial has published mortality data.

The Danish study (Kronborg et al 1989) randomized 30 970 persons aged 45–74 years to a screening group (Haemoccult) and 30 968 to a control group. The screening interval was 2-yearly, two rescreens were performed and the Haemoccult test was not rehydrated. The results are summarized in Table 2.5. Screen-detected cancers were smaller and at an earlier Dukes'

Table 2.5 Results of the European population screening studies

Centre	Screening round	Number offered screen	Acceptors	Number with positive tests	Neoplastic disease detected Cancers	Polyps
Fuhnen, Denmark	First screen	30 970	20 672 (67%)	215 (1.0%)	37	86
	First rescreen	20 112	18 779 (93%)	159 (0.8%)	13	76
	Second rescreen		17 284	155 (0.9%)	24	n/a
Nottingham, England	First screen	77 226	41 114 (55%)	843 (2.0%)	89	461
	First rescreen	46 371	32 191 (69%)	415 (1.3%)	55	199
	Second rescreen	43 727	26 425 (60%)	217 (1.0%)	32	125
	Third rescreen	36 570	18 589 (51%)	256 (1.4%)	38	93
	Fourth rescreen	10 113	5 169 (51%)	80 (1.5%)	9	61
Goteborg, Sweden	First screen	13 759	9081 (66%)	84 (1.9%) 256[+] (5.8%)	16	58
	First rescreen	13 357	7770 (58%)	497 (6.4%)	19	91

[+]Rehydrated Haemoccult tests

stage than cancers in the control group population (52% vs 8% stage A respectively). Five-year follow-up data from this study (Moller Jensen et al 1992) have detected 81 interval cancers, amounting to 52% of all cancers observed in persons having at least one Haemoccult test. The interval cancers occurred with equal frequency during the 2-year screenings but were no worse than among controls for Dukes' stage and tumour size. Interim mortality data has been published (Kronborg et al 1992) but no definitive results will be available until 1996.

A study in Goteborg, Sweden, was commenced in 1982 in which all the inhabitants between 60 and 64 years of age were randomly divided into a test and control group (Kewenter et al 1988). As part of the study, the test group was further randomized to either rehydrated or non-rehydrated Haemoccult tests. The effect of rehydration on the positivity rate is indicated in Table 2.5. Although significantly more subjects required investigation, the pick-up rate was also significantly higher (50 vs 24 neoplasms). Rehydrating Haemoccult produced a 33% improvement in sensitivity at the cost of a 2% fall in specificity, the overall effect being a decline in positive predictive value from 32% for non-rehydrated tests to 23% for rehydrated tests.

Follow-up of the original cohort has continued and the results of the first 7 years have been published (Kewenter et al 1994). The lead time effect is clearly illustrated by the fact that 61 cancers were detected in the screened group compared to only 20 in the control group. However, during the first 2 years of follow-up, the number of cancers in the test group was only half that in the control group. From the third year of follow-up onwards, the number of cancers diagnosed in the test and control groups were the same. Therefore, in order to take advantage of the lead time effect (diagnosing cancers at a less advanced stage), the maximum time interval between FOBT screening rounds should be 2 years.

The largest of the randomized studies is taking place in Nottingham (Hardcastle et al 1989) (Table 2.5). Over 154 000 persons aged 50–74 years have been randomized to either screening 2-yearly by Haemoccult or a control group. The fall in compliance from the second rescreen onwards reflects a change in protocol at this time, following which previous non-responders were reinvited to complete Haemoccult tests. If compliance for previous responders only is considered, it becomes 88% for the second rescreen, in line with the Danish study.

Similarly, if size of tumour or Dukes' stage are considered, significantly more screen-detected tumours are at a less advanced stage than the control group tumours. For example, 56% screen-detected cancers were stage A or B compared to only 46% of controls at the prevalence screen and this difference has been maintained on rescreens (62% Dukes' A or B compared to 47% in the control group). The effect of rescreening halved the positivity rate initially, which has then remained constant, suggesting that the initial screen detected the cohort of cancers present and subsequent screens are tending only to detect new tumours or tumours which are beginning to bleed. This hypothesis is supported by the fact that the positive predictive value for cancer has gradually increased from 10% to 15% during subsequent screening rounds and also by the fact that the yield of neoplasia has fallen from 10.3 per 1000 at first screening to 1.6 per 1000 at the third.

As was the case in the Danish study, completing a Haemoccult test does not seem to delay symptomatic presentation in the interval between tests. There was no difference between the interval cancers and the control group cancers in terms of Dukes' stage, degree of differentiation or resectability.

The only randomized study to report a statistically significant reduction in mortality from colorectal cancer by FOBT screening is the Minnesota Colon Cancer Control Study (Mandel et al 1993). The trial targeted 50–80 years olds and recruited 46 551 volunteers who were then randomized to receive screening yearly or 2-yearly or to a control group. Compliance was high with 90% completing at least one screening round and 46% completing every screening round in the annual group, the respective figures being 89% and 59% in the 2-yearly group.

Over 13 years of follow-up, 1002 cases of colorectal cancer and 320 deaths from colorectal cancer were observed. Although the cumulative incidence of colorectal cancer was similar in the three groups, the cumulative annual mortality from colorectal cancer was lower in the annually screened group (5.88 per 1000) than in the group screened 2-yearly (8.33 per 1000) and the control group (8.83 per 1000). This translates into a 33% reduction in mortality from colorectal cancer in the annually screened group when compared to the control group. However, in contrast to the European studies, the number of Dukes' stage A and B tumours were identical in the annually screened and control groups (208 cancers). This is surprising when one considers that the aim of screening is to identify colorectal neoplasia before it reaches an advanced stage. In fact, the difference in mortality is attributable to the difference in stage D tumours, twice as many being observed in the control group as were detected in the annually screened group.

Also, in contrast to the Danish and English studies, over 80% of the Haemoccult slides were rehydrated, resulting in a positivity rate of 9.8% overall (compared to 2.4% in the earlier part of the study when the slides were not rehydrated). This increased the sensitivity to 92% (from 81%) but decreased the specificity from 97% to 90%, resulting in a decrease in the positive predictive value for cancer from 5.6% to 2.2%. The consequence of this large number of false positives was a significant increase in the number of patients requiring investigation, 38% of those screened annually and 28% of those screened 2-yearly having at least one colonoscopy. Not only does this affect the cost-benefit analysis for FOBT screening but it raises doubt concerning the mechanism of mortality reduction observed.

Lang and Ransohoff (1994) used a mathematical model to simulate a screening study based on the published data from the Minnesota trial. They concluded that at least one-third to one-half of the benefit was attributable to false-positive FOBT results or chance. The mathematical model suggests that chance only contributes importantly to benefit from FOBT screening when the positivity rate is higher than 5% and this should be borne in mind when interpreting the data from the European studies.

Alternative stool tests

Other markers of colorectal neoplasia have been evaluated in stool. In 1987, Nakayama et al reported the use of albumin as a screening test. Using filter paper smears of stool, a significant difference in the faecal albumin concentrations in 45 normal subjects and 10 patients known to have colorectal cancer was reported.

Further, Thomas (1991) measured faecal albumin concentrations in 144 asymptomatic individuals prior to colonoscopic evaluation of positive FOBTs. Using a predetermined upper limit of normal (95th percentile), a significantly greater proportion of subjects with cancer or an adenoma were positive for faecal albumin than were normal subjects. The amount of faecal albumin detected was independent of cancer stage and tumour site. These results should be interpreted with caution as a specificity of 95% (implied by defining the upper limit of normal as the 95th percentile) is borderline when considering the false-positive rate. Similarly, the results need to be duplicated in a FOBT negative population to exclude selection bias.

Carcinoembryonic antigen (CEA) has also been investigated as a possible faecal marker for colorectal neoplasia. Faecal CEA has been shown to be elevated in patients with colorectal cancer although the elevated faecal levels do not correlate with either Dukes' stage or serum CEA levels (Elias et al 1973, Fujimoto et al 1979). Measurement of faecal CEA in 149 asymptomatic subjects demonstrated that absolute levels were higher in subjects with colorectal neoplasia (Thomas 1991). However, when a discriminating value (95th percentile) was employed, the proportion of subjects with raised faecal CEA levels was similar in those with cancers, adenomas and those with a normal colonoscopy. It seems likely that the normal colonic expression of CEA is too variable to make its faecal level specific enough for a screening test.

The most exciting developments have been in the field of molecular biology. In 1992, Sidransky et al demonstrated that Kirsten-ras oncogene mutations could be detected in the stool of patients with colorectal cancer. Of 24 tumours selected at random, nine (37%) were shown by sequencing to contain K-ras mutations. The mutations were subsequently also identified in DNA isolated from stool in eight out of the nine cases. Similarly, Tokisue et al (1994) identified k-ras mutations in tumour tissue from six (30%) of 20 adenomas and five (31%) of 16 cancers. K-ras mutations were also identified in the stool of three (50%) and four (80%) of these cases respectively. No false-positives were detected and none of the stool samples collected after tumour resection showed mutations.

These results suggest that detecting genetic alterations in stool may provide a more specific test for screening although more than one gene would have to be analysed to ensure adequate sensitivity. Since cells are constantly exfoliated, this type of test would have an advantage over the FOBTs which rely on detecting intermittent bleeding.

Endoscopic screening

No randomized trials comparing endoscopic screening with a control group have been published to date. There are, however, several descriptive and case-control studies which address the role of sigmoidoscopy for screening asymptomatic individuals.

Rigid sigmoidoscopy

In 1960, Hertz et al published details of 26 126 subjects over the age of 45 years who had been screened annually by sigmoidoscopy. Cancers were diagnosed in 58 of those screened and, of the 50 who were followed for 15 years, the 5-year survival rate was reported as 88%.

A second descriptive study (Gilbertson & Nelms 1978) was commenced in 1948 at the University of Minnesota during which 21140 subjects over 45 years old received a total of 113 800 examinations. On initial examination, 27 cancers were detected, the 5-year survival rate being 64%. Subsequent surveillance found only 13 more cancers although the authors calculated 90 were expected and they concluded that 85% of the expected cancers had been prevented by polypectomy.

Two major criticisms can be levelled at these studies. Firstly, inferences are made from assessments of survival rates rather than mortality. Much better survival of a group of screen-detected cancers could result from any one of several biases – lead time, length bias, selection bias or overdiagnosis bias. Also, the expected number of cancers calculated by Gilbertson has been questioned. Miller (1987) estimated that only 38 cancers would be expected, resulting in a more modest reduction in incidence (60%).

More recently, a study was reported describing the long-term risk of developing cancer in a cohort of patients who had previously had adenomas removed but had not subsequently been followed up (Atkin et al 1992). Over 1600 patients were identified who had undergone adenoma excision by means of a 25 cm rigid sigmoidoscope between 1957 and 1980. After an average follow-up of 13.8 years per patient, 49 adenocarcinomas had been identified, 14 in the rectum and 35 in the colon. Patients with small (<1 cm), tubular adenomas (single or multiple) only developed four cancers, half the number expected, whereas those with large (≥1 cm), tubulovillous or villous adenomas (single or multiple) had developed 31 cancers, around three times the number expected. The authors concluded that complete adenoma removal lessened the risk of developing cancer to below that of the general population for the subgroup with good prognostic factors (see Table 2.6) but that those with poor prognostic factors remained at high risk.

Previous exposure to sigmoidoscopy was also examined in a case-controlled study using data from the Kaiser Permanente Medical Care Program (Selby et al 1992). Patients (261) who had died of cancer of the rectum and distal colon between 1971 and 1988 were identified and their exposure to sigmoidoscopy during the 10 years prior to their diagnosis compared to 868 control subjects. Only 8.8% of the case subjects had undergone sigmoidoscopy as compared with 24.2% of the controls (odds ratio 0.30). Even after adjusting for confounding variables, such as a personal or family history of colorectal neoplasia or the number of periodic health check-ups, the odds ratio was still 0.41, implying a 59% reduction in mortality. The apparent benefit of screening by sigmoidoscopy was confined exclusively to the part of the rectum and sigmoid colon that can be viewed with the rigid sigmoidoscope, the percentage of case and control subjects with cancer beyond the reach of the sigmoidoscope being 22.9% and 25.0% respectively. Quoting published data on the percentage of colorectal cancers and adenomatous polyps arising within reach of the 60 cm flexible sigmoidoscope (>50%), the authors concluded 'A screening program using flexible sigmoidoscopy could lead to a reduction of at least 30% in total mortality from colorectal cancer'.

Another study, which is often quoted as a randomized trial of sigmoidoscopy is the Kaiser Permanente Multiphasic Evaluation Study (Selby et al 1988). This is, in fact, a trial of annual urging to obtain a multiphasic health check-up, an optional addition to which was a 25 cm rigid sigmoidoscopy. Approximately 11 000 existing members of the health care programme were randomized to either a study or control group. Between 1964 and 1980, members of the study group received annual urging by telephone to schedule an appointment for a health check-up whereas control group members received their usual health care. On analysis, the study group had both a lower cumulative incidence (4.3 vs 6.7 cases per 1000) and lower mortality from colorectal cancer (1.4 vs 2.7 deaths per 1000) than the control group for tumours within 20 cm reach of the sigmoidoscope. There was no difference in either the cumulative incidence or mortality for tumours beyond 20 cm. In addition,

Table 2.6 Prognostic factors affecting adenoma progression

	Prognosis	
	Good	Poor
Histology	Tubular	Tubulovillous Villous
Degree of dysplasia	Mild Moderate	Severe
Size	<1 cm	≥1 cm
Number	≤3	>3

there was a much more favourable stage distribution amongst the study group for tumours arising within reach of the sigmoidoscope (86% stage B or better, compared to 54%).

However, two features of this study make it unlikely that sigmoidoscopy alone was responsible for the observed difference in mortality. Firstly, the number of polyps detected or removed was the same between the two groups (103 vs 110) whereas 1154 additional examinations in the study group would have been expected to generate a study group excess of at least 34 polyps. The authors account for this by explaining that a majority of the excess sigmoidoscopies were performed on a small group of persons who had five or more examinations in the 10-year period.

Secondly, there was no substantial difference in the exposure to sigmoidoscopy between the two groups (25% in the control group compared to 30% in the study group). The authors calculated that the observed excess rate of exposure to screening sigmoidoscopy in the study group would have prevented only one death in the 18 years of follow-up. This study therefore does not provide evidence either for or against the efficacy of sigmoidoscopic screening in colorectal cancer but suggests that multiphasic health checks are beneficial in improving survival.

Flexible sigmoidoscopy

The rigid sigmoidoscope is limited in its ability to detect colonic cancers by its length, the average depth of insertion being 20 cm (Nicholls & Dube 1982), enabling, at best, visualization of 40% of all colorectal cancers. Attention has recently been focused on the 65 cm flexible sigmoidoscope as a possible alternative screening technique. Flexible sigmoidoscopy has been shown to have better patient acceptance than rigid sigmoidoscopy (Winawer et al 1987) and, although bowel preparation is required (usually a simple enema), it enables examination of the distal 60 cm of the colon, where up to 70% of cancers and large adenomas are found (Hardcastle et al 1989, Kronborg et al 1989).

In a recent publication, the yield of flexible sigmoidoscopy in an asymptomatic population aged 50–65 years following a screening examination was reported (Wherry & Thomas 1994). Over 4000 subjects underwent flexible sigmoidoscopy and 11 carcinomas were detected. Two further carcinomas were detected during completion examinations for subjects who had distal polyps, the overall detection rate being 3.2 carcinomas per 1000 screened. Over 92% of the carcinomas were either stage A or B. In addition, 239 adenomas were detected in 217 individuals, 70% of which were greater than 1 cm. This study illustrates the greater sensitivity of flexible sigmoidoscopy for both cancers (3.2 per 1000 vs 2.3 per 1000 screened) and adenomas (5.4% vs 0.8%) when compared to Haemoccult screening. Unfortunately, no data are available on the subsequent development of left or right-sided cancers in this cohort and so the false-negative rate is unknown.

In a smaller retrospective case-controlled study, the screening histories of 66 subjects who had died of colorectal cancer were compared to 196 age- and sex-matched controls (Newcomb et al 1992). While both rigid and flexible sigmoidoscopy were employed during the study period, the majority of subjects had undergone flexible sigmoidoscopy. Individuals who had a single examination with a sigmoidoscope were found to have a lower risk when compared with those who had never had a screening sigmoidoscopy (odds ratio 0.21). This result should be interpreted with caution as there was also a reduction in mortality from tumours out of reach of the sigmoidoscope (odds ratio 0.36), although this reduction was not statistically significant. It does, however, raise the possibility that the reductions in mortality observed were due to confounding variables, such as self-selection for screening, which is known to occur in individuals at lower risk of disease or mortality (Connor et al 1991).

Utilizing the data described above, the Imperial Cancer Research Fund has suggested that a trial of screening for colorectal cancer by once-only sigmoidoscopy at age 55–60 years should be performed (Atkin et al 1993). Assuming a compliance rate of 70%, the authors calculate that a single flexible sigmoidoscopy would detect 70% of distal colorectal cancers occurring up to age 75 and 50% of cancers occurring between 75 and 79 years. This equates to the prevention of about 5500 colorectal cancer cases and 3500 colorectal cancer deaths per year. Such a trial is likely to be commenced shortly, involving 120 000 participants, with mortality data anticipated in 15 years time.

The shortcoming of screening by flexible sigmoidoscopy is that only the distal segment of the bowel is examined. While approximately 30% of subjects with proximal tumours have 'marker' distal adenomas which would result in a completion examination of the bowel, around 25% of all colorectal cancers would be missed by this technique. In addition, up to 60% of proximal adenomas may also escape detection (Lieberman & Smith 1991). It has therefore been suggested that the sensitivity of flexible sigmoidoscopic screening could be increased by combining it with a FOBT. Applying such a combined approach to the Nottingham screening data, flexible sigmoidoscopy would have been likely to detect 15 of the 22 interval cancers, increasing the sensitivity of cancer detection to 93% – an improvement of 18% over the sensitivity of Haemoccult alone (Hardcastle et al 1989).

A prospective randomized multicentre trial is currently in progress to define the benefit of adding flexible siigmoidoscopy to screening by Haemoccult alone. Interim data are shown in Table 2.7. While the number of cancers detected is too small to comment on, the significantly greater sensitivity of flexible sigmoidoscopy for adenomas is already apparent. However, the improved detection rate is at the cost of compliance and alternative methods of recruitment are currently being investigated to improve compliance.

Colonoscopy

The most sensitive evaluation of the whole colon is by colonoscopy. This is, however, labour-intensive, expensive and associated with potentially lethal complications (perforation and haemorrhage), which have precluded its use as a screening test. It is still the surveillance technique of choice in high-risk individuals (FAP, HNPCC and ulcerative colitis) but, due to its superior sensitivity, its role in screening asymptomatic individuals is being questioned. Lieberman (1991) calculated that the cost of detecting one patient with an adenoma ≥1 cm would be $23 793 by flexible sigmoidoscopy and FOBT compared with $20 254 by colonoscopy, because of the latter's higher detection rate. This extrapolates to a cost of $444 133 per death prevented by flexible sigmoidoscopy/FOBT compared to $347 214 per death prevented by colonoscopy (c.f. breast cancer screening $343 406 per death prevented). The author concludes that colonoscopic screening should be reevaluated as more data on the incidence and prevalence of proximal colonic neoplasia become available.

Table 2.7 Interim results of European flexible sigmoidoscopy

		Goteborg	Greece	Newport	Nuneaton	Odense
Invited	Group 1	738	5000	1738	1098	3000
	Group 2	750	5000	1784	1247	3000
Screened	Grp 1 – S + H	268	1040	385	292	924
	– H only	154	3160	852	208	66
	Grp 2	454	4280	942	654	1265
No. of adenomas >1 cm						
	Grp 1 S+ve, H–ve	4	28	14	2	26
	H+ve, S–ve	1	6	0	0	0
	S & H +ve	3	6	9	2	5
	Grp 2	3	9	7	1	7
No. of cancers						
	Grp 1 S+ve, H–ve	0	1	0	1	2
	H+ve, S–ve	0	1	1	0	0
	S & H +ve	0	1	0	1	2
	Grp 2	0	1	1	1	2

Surveillance

Screening also introduces the problem of following up those individuals who have had adenomas removed. Until recently, surveillance intervals have been based on estimates of rates of progression from adenoma to carcinoma; for example, Stryker et al (1987) suggested a cumulative risk of polyp progression of 2.5%, 8% and 24% at 5, 10 and 20 years respectively. However, a randomized trial of surveillance intervals has suggested that the overall risk may be considerably less than this for the majority of polyps.

In 1978, a prospective randomized trial was initiated to compare follow-up colonoscopy at 3 years only with colonoscopy at 1 and 3 years – the National Polyp Study (Winawer et al 1993b). Over 1400 subjects were randomized following colonoscopic excision of newly diagnosed adenomas. Exclusion criteria included the presence of colorectal cancer, non-adenomatous polyps, malignant polyps, a sessile adenoma with a base longer than 3 cm and the absence of polyps. Although those subjects who underwent two examinations had more polyps overall (41.7% vs 32%), the number of subjects in each group who had adenomas with advanced pathological features (>1 cm, severe dysplasia or invasive cancer) was the same (3.3%). In addition, adenoma size and the extent of the villous component were confirmed to be independent risk factors associated with severe dysplasia.

During the period of follow-up, five asymptomatic colorectal cancers were detected in five patients (Winawer et al 1993c). This observed incidence of 0.6 colorectal cancers per 1000 person-years was compared to calculated incidences using previously published data: the expected incidence was calculated to be 5.8 according to the Mayo Clinic data (Stryker et al 1987), 5.2 according to the St Mark's data (Atkin et al 1992) and 2.5 according to the SEER data (Gloeckler-Ries et al 1990). The authors conclude that colorectal cancer can be prevented by colonoscopic removal of all identified polyps.

However, the populations being compared are different. The Mayo Clinic and St Mark's data are both derived from retrospective cohorts of patients and, in the case of the Mayo Clinic data, were derived from subjects investigated only by barium enema, a technique known to be less sensitive than colonoscopy. Similarly, the National Polyp cohort is highly selected when compared to the SEER database as any patients with colorectal cancer, a malignant polyp, a personal history of colorectal cancer or adenomatous polyps, inflammatory bowel disease or familial polyposis were excluded. For example, if this group of patients were included in the database, the number of cancers observed would have been seven as opposed to the 8.1 expected in the subgroup with small or medium-sized adenomas at enrolment (Atkin 1994, personal communication).

While this study illustrates the difficulty of comparing results with previously published data, the differences in observed and expected rates are so large that it is likely colonoscopic polypectomy has an effect in reducing the incidence of colorectal cancer although it is still too early to predict how large this reduction is. The trial does, however, strongly support 3-yearly surveillance intervals for patients with 'clean colons' following the removal of sporadic adenomas.

Cost-benefit analysis

As has already been discussed, screening by colonoscopy has been calculated to be as cost-effective as breast screening (Liberman & Smith 1991). Walker et al (1991), using the Nottingham data, calculated a cost per cancer detected of £2705 employing Haemoccult screening only. If subsequent screening rounds are incorporated, the cost per cancer detected remains relatively constant at £3128 for round two and £2481 for round three, but the cost per person screened decreases (£5.33 for round one compared to £4.09 for round three). These costs are significantly less than those calculated by Lieberman reflecting the increased cost of screening by colonoscopy.

However, while more expensive, the potential for reducing mortality is greater with endoscopic screening. There are no data available directly comparing endoscopic screening with FOBT tests but two mathematical models have been employed to estimate the potential cost differences (Eddy 190, OTA 1990). Beginning at 50 years of age, FOBT screening alone was calculated to reduce mortality by 23% at a cost of $26 per day of extra life; FOBT plus sigmoidoscopy every 3 years would reduce mortality by 42% at a cost of $75 per day of extra life; and FOBT plus colonoscopy every 3 years would reduce mortality by 69% at a cost of $116 per day of extra life. The ethical dilemma is to select the least costly screening protocol that provides an acceptable effect on incidence and mortality.

Summary

The efficacy of colorectal cancer screening is measured by its ability to reduce colorectal cancer mortality. The application of a screening test is a complex process – the screening test must be applied at the right time to the appropriate population. Moreover, the screening test itself may only be designed to detect a subgroup who subsequently require further evaluation. The effectiveness and cost of screening are directly related to the strategies used to deal with positive tests.

The use of FOBTs has been widely investigated and evidence is accumulating that they are effective in reducing mortality from colorectal cancer although poor sensitivity limits their application at the present time. Screening with flexible sigmoidoscopy is costly but may have a greater impact on mortality, reducing it by around 45%. Screening with colonoscopy may be even more effective, reducing mortality by up to 70%, and could be cost-effective if screening intervals could be extended to 10 years or more.

The way forward continues to rest with research into more sensitive FOBTs, more cost-effective endoscopic protocols and greater knowledge of the biological factors triggering dysplastic changes in large bowel mucosa. Comprehension of the time-scales involved in the adenoma–carcinoma sequence should enable effective screening and surveillance protocols to be developed.

References

Ahlquist DA, Wieand HS, Moertel CG et al 1993 Accuracy of faecal occult blood screening for colorectal neoplasia. Journal of the American Medical Association 269: 1262–1267

Alma T, Lieznerski G 1973 The intestinal polyposes. Clinics in Gastroenterology 2: 577–601

Armitage N, Hardcastle JD, Amar SS, Balfour TW, Haynes J, James PD 1985 A comparison of an immunological faecal occult blood test Fecatwin sensitive/FECA EIA with Haemoccult in population screening for colorectal cancer. British Journal of Surgery 51: 799–804

Atkin WS, Morson BC, Cuzick K 1992 Long-term risk of colorectal cancer after excision of rectosigmoid adenomas. New England Journal of Medicine 326: 658–662

Atkin WS, Cuzick J, Northover J M A, Whynes D K 1993 Prevention of colorectal cancer by once-only sigmoidoscopy. Lancet 341: 736–740

Bond J H 1993 Polyp guideline: diagnosis, treatment and surveillance for patients with non-familial colorectal polyps. Annals of Internal Medicine 119: 836–843

Burt R W, Samowitz W S 1988 The adenomatous polyp and the hereditary polyposis syndromes. Gastroenterological Clinics of North America 17: 657–678

Cancer research campaign handbook 1993 Relative 5-year survival rates for the commonest 10 malignancies, p 1, George Over, London

Cannon-Albright L A, Skolnick M H, Bishop D T et al 1988 Common inheritance of susceptibility to colonic adenomatous polyps and associated colorectal cancers. New England Journal of Medicine 319: 533–537

Choi P M, Zelig M P 1994 Similarity of colorectal cancer in Crohn's disease and ulcerative colitis: implications for carcinogenesis and prevention. Gut 35: 950–954

Collins R H, Feldman M, Fordtran J S 1987 Colon cancer, dysplasia and surveillance in patients with ulcerative colitis: a critical review. New England Journal of Medicine 316: 1654–1658

Connor R L, Prorok P A, Weed P L 1991 The case-control design and the assessment of the efficacy of cancer screening. Journal of Clinical Epidemiology 44: 1215–1221

Deans G T, Patterson C C, Parks T G, Spence R A J 1994 Colorectal carcinoma: importance of clinical and pathological factors in survival. Annals of the Royal College of Surgeons of England 76: 59–64

Doran J, Hardcastle J D 1982 Bleeding patterns in colorectal cancer: the effect of adpirin and implications for faecal occult blood testing. British Journal of Surgery 69: 711–713

Duncan J L, Kyle J 1982 Family incidence of carcinoma of the colon and rectum in north-east Scotland. Gut 23: 169–171

Eddy DM 1990 Screening for colorectal cancer. Annals of Internal Medicine 113: 373–384

Elias EG, Holyoke ED, Ming Chu T 1973 Carcinoembryonic antigen in faeces and plasma of normal subjects and patients with colorectal cancer. Diseases of the Colon and Rectum 17: 38–41

Eng C, Ponder BAJ 1993 The role of gene mutations in the genesis of familial cancers. FASEB Journal 7: 910–919

Farrands P A, Hardcastle J D 1983 Accuracy of occult blood tests over a six-day period. Clinical Oncology 9: 217–225

Feldman W 1990 How serious are the adverse effects of screening? Journal of General Internal Medicine 5 (suppl): S50–S53

Frommer D J, Kapparis A, Brown M K 1983 Improved

screening for colorectal cancer by immunological detection of occult blood. British Medical Journal 296: 1092–1094

Fujimoto S, Kitsukara Y, Itoh K 1979 Carcinoembryonic antigen in gastric juice or faeces as an aid in the diagnosis of gastrointestinal cancer. Annals of Surgery 189: 34–38

Fujita M 1992 Feasibility of 3-day faecal occult blood testing using immunochemical haemagglutination method in mass screening for colorectal cancer. In: Young GP, Saito H (eds) Faecal occult blood tests: current issues and new tests. SmithKline Diagnostics, San José, p 82–89

Gilbertson V A, Nelms J M 1978 The prevention of invasive cancer of the rectum. Cancer 41: 1137–1139

Gloeckler-Ries LA, Hankey B F, Edwards B K 1990 Cancer Statistics Review 1973–1987. Department of Health and Human Services, Bethesda, Md (DHHS publication No. (NIH) 90–2789)

Gnauck R 1994 Colon cancer screening in Germany – six year review (abstr). Gut 35 (suppl 4): A63

Groden J, Thliveris A, Samowitz W S et al 1991 Identification and characterisation of the adenomatous polyposis coli gene. Cell 66: 589–600

Hardcastle JD, Thomas WM, Chamberlain J et al 1989 Randomised controlled trial of faecal occult blood screening for colorectal cancer. Lancet i: 1160–1164

Hertz RE, Deddish MR, Day E 1960 Value of periodic examinations in detecting cancer of the rectum and colon. Postgraduate Medicine 27: 290–294

Iwase T 1992 The evaluation of an immunochemical faecal occut blood test by reversed passive haemagglutination compared with Haemoccult II in screening for colorectal cancer. In: Young GP, Saito H (eds) Faecal occult blood tests: current issues and new tests. SmithKline Diagnostics, San José, p 90–94

Jarvinen HJ 1992 Epidemiology of familial adenomatous polyposis in Finland: impact of family screening on the colorectal cancer rate and survival. Gut 33: 357–360

Kawaguchi H 1992 Mass screening for colorectal cancer by immunochemical occult blood test employing reversed passive haemagglutination. In: Young GP, Saito H (eds) Faecal occult blood tests: current issues and new tests. SmithKline Diagnostics, San José, p 96–100

Kewenter J, Bjork S, Haglind E, Smith L, Svanvik J, Ahren C 1988 Screening and rescreening for colorectal cancer. Cancer 62: 645–651

Kewenter J, Brevinge H, Engaras B, Haglind E, Ahren C 1994 Follow-up after screening for colorectal neoplasms with faecal occult blood testing in a controlled trial. Diseases of the Colon and Rectum 37: 115–119

Kronborg O, Fenger C, Olsen J et al 1989 Repeated screening for colorectal cancer with faecal occult blood test. Scandinavian Journal of Gastroenterology 24: 599–606

Kronborg O, Fenger C, Worm J et al 1992 Causes of death during the first five years of a randomized trial of mass screening for colorectal cancer with faecal occult blood test. Scandanavian Journal of Gastroenterology 27: 47–52

Kvist N, Jacobsen O, Kvist HK et al 1989 Malignancy in ulcerative colitus. Scandinavian Journal of Gastroenterology 24: 497–506

Lang CA, Ransohoff DF 1994 Faecal occult blood screening for colorectal cancer: is mortality reduced by chance selection for screening colonoscopy? Journal of the American Medical Association 271: 1011–1013

Leach FS, Nicolaides NC, Papadopoulos N et al 1993 Mutations of a mutS homolog in hereditary nonpolyposis colorectal cancer. Cell 75: 1215–1225

Lennard-Jones JE, Nelville DM, Morson BC et al 1990 Precancer and cancer in extensive ulcerative colitis: findings among 401 patients over 22 years. Gut 31: 800–806

Lieberman DA, Smith FW 1991 Screening for colon malignancy with colonoscopy. American Journal of Gastroenterology 86: 946–951

Lindblom A, Tannergård P, Werelius B, Nordenskjöld M 1993 Genetic mapping of a second locus predisposing to hereditary nonpolyposis colon cancer. Nature Genetics 5: 279–282

Lynch HT, Kimberling WI, Albano WA et al 1985 Hereditary nonpolyposis colorectal cancer (Lynch syndromes I and II): clinical description of resource. Cancer 56: 934–938

Lynch HT, Smyrk TC, Lanspa SJ et al 1990 Phenotypic variation in colorectal adenoma/cancer expression in two families. Hereditary flat adenoma syndrome. Cancer 66: 909–915

Lynch HT, Smyrk TC, Watson P et al 1993a Genetics, natural history, tumour spectrum and pathology of hereditary nonpolyposis colorectal cancer: an updated review. Gastroenterology 104: 1535–1549

Lynch DAF, Lobo AJ, Sobala GM et al 1993b Failure of colonoscopic surveillance in ulcerative colitis. Gut 34: 1075–1080

Macrae FA, St John DJB 1982 Relationship between patterns of bleeding and Haemoccult sensitivity in patients with colorectal cancers and adenomas. Gastroenterology 82: 891–898

Mandel JS, Bond JH, Church TR et al 1993 Reducing mortality from colorectal cancer by screening for faecal occult blood. New England Journal of Medicine 328: 1365–1371

Miller AB 1987 Review of sigmoidoscopic screening for colorectal cancer. In: Chamberlain J, Miller A B (eds) Screening for gastrointestinal cancer. Hans Huber, Toronto.

Moller Jensen B, Kronborg O, Fenger C 1992 Interval cancers in screening with faecal occult blood test for colorectal cancer. Scandinavian Journal of Gastroenterology 27: 779–782

Morson BC, Pang LSC 1967 Rectal biopsy as an aid to cancer control in ulcerative colitis. Gut 8: 423–434

Nagase H, Miyoshi Y, Horii A et al 1992 Correlation between the location of germ-line mutations in the APC gene and the number of polyps in familial adenomatous polyposis patients. Cancer Research 52: 4055–4057

Nakayama T, Yasuoka H, Kishino T 1987 Enzyme linked immunosorbent assay of human faecal occult albumin. Lancet i: 1368–1369

Newcomb PA, Norfleet RG, Storer BE, Surawicz TS, Marcus PM 1992 Screening sigmoidoscopy and colorectal mortality. Journal of the National Cancer Institute 84: 1572–1575

Nicholls RJ, Dube S 1982 The extent of the examination by rigid sigmoidoscopy. British Journal of Surgery 69: 438

Office of Population Censuses and Surveys 1980 Cancer survival 1953–1973 registrations. OPCS Monitor MB1. OPCS, London

Office of Population Censuses and Surveys 1993 Mortality statistics 1992. Series DH2, 16. OPCS, London

Office of Population Censuses and Surveys 1993 Cancer statistics: registrations 1988. Series MB1, 21. OPCS, London

Office of Technology Assessment 1990. Costs and effectiveness of colorectal cancer screening in the elderly: background paper. US Government Printing Office, Washington DC. Publication no. (OTA) BP-H-74: 7–56

Papadopoulos N, Nicolaides NC, Wei Y-F et al 1994 Mutation of a mutL homolog in hereditary colon cancer. Science 263: 1625–1629

Powell SM, Petersen GM, Krush AJ et al 1993 Molecular diagnosis of familial adenomatous polyposis. New England Journal of Medicine 329: 1982–1987

Robinson MHE, Thomas WM, Pye G et al 1993 Is dietary restriction always necessary in Haemoccult screening for colorectal neoplasia? European Journal of Surgical Oncology 19: 539–542

Robinson MHE, Marks CG, Farrands PA et al 1994 Population screening for colorectal cancer: comparison between guaiac and immunological faecal occult blood tests. British Journal of Surgery 82: 448–451

Rosenfield RE, Kochwa S, Kaczera Z et al 1979 Nonuniform distribution of occult blood in faeces. American Journal of Clinical Pathology 71: 204–209

Sachar DB 1993 Clinical and colonoscopic surveillance in ulcerative colitis: are we saving colons or saving lives? Gastroenterology 105: 588–589

St John DJB 1990 Faecal occult blood tests: a critical review. In: Hardcastle JD (ed) Screening for colorectal cancer. Proceedings of International Meeting. Normed Verlag, Bad Homburg, p 55–68

St John DJB, Young GP, McHutchison JG et al 1992 Comparison of the sensitivity and specificity of Haemoccult and HemoQuant: studies in healthy volunteers and patients with colorectal neoplasia. Annals of Internal Medicine 117: 376–382

St John DJB, McDermott FI, Hopper JL et al 1993a Cancer risk in relatives of patients with common colorectal cancer. Annals of Internal Medicine 118: 785–790

St John DJB, Young GP, Alexeyeff MA et al 1993b Evaluation of new occult blood tests for detection of colorectal neoplasia. Gastroenterology 104: 1661–1668

Saito H 1992 Essentials of immunochemical occult blood tests. In: Young GP, Saito H (eds) Faecal occult blood tests: current issues and new tests. SmithKline Diagnostics, San José, p 60–69

Schwartz S, Dahl J, Ellefson M et al 1983 The HemoQuant test: a specific and quantitative determination of heme (haemoglobin) in faeces and other materials. Clinical Chemistry 35: 2290–2296

Selby JV, Friedman GD, Collen MF 1988 Sigmoidoscopy and mortality from colorectal cancer: the Kaiser Permanente multiphasic evaluation study. Journal of Clinical Epidemiology 41: 427–434

Selby JV, Friedman GD, Quesenberry CP, Weiss NS 1992 A case-control study of screening sigmoidoscopy and mortality from colorectal cancer. New England Journal of Medicine 326: 653–657

Selby JV, Friedman GD, Quesenberry CP, Weiss NS 1993 Effect of faecal occult blood testing on mortality from colorectal cancer. Annals of Internal Medicine 118: 1–6

Sidransky D, Tokino T, Hamilton S R et al 1992 Identification of ras oncogene mutations in the stool of patients with curable colorectal tumours. Science 256: 102–105

Stephenson BM, Finan PJ, Gascoyne J et al 1991 Frequency of familial colorectal cancer. British Journal of Surgery 78: 1162–1166

Stroehlein JR, Fairbanks VF, McGill BD et al 1976 Haemoccult detection of faecal occult blood quantitated by radioassay. American Journal of Digestive Diseases 21: 841–844

Stryker SJ, Wolff BG, Culp CE et al 1987 Natural history of untreated colonic polyps. Gastroenterology 93: 1009–1013

Thomas D 1992 Colon cancer screening based on the radial immunodiffusion test 'Detectacol'. In: Young GP, Saito H (eds) Faecal occult blood tests: current issues and new tests. SmithKline Diagnostics, San José, p 76–81

Thomas WM 1991 Faecal screening tests for colorectal cancer. DM thesis, University of Nottingham

Tokisue M, Yasutake K, Oya M et al 1994 Detection of K-ras gene mutations in the stool sample of patients with colorectal tumours (abstr). Gut 35 (suppl 4): A70

Turunen MJ, Liewendahl K, Partanen P, Adlercreutz H 1984 Immunological detecting of faecal occult blood in colorectal cancer. British Journal of Cancer 49: 141–148

Vaananen P, Tenhunen R 1988 Rapid immunochemical detection of faecal occult blood by use of a latex-agglutination test. Clinical Chemistry 34: 1763–1766

Wahrendorf J, Robra B-P, Wiebelt H et al 1993 Effectiveness of colorectal cancer screening: results from a population-based case-control evaluation in Saarland, Germany. European Journal of Cancer Prevention 2: 221–227

Walker A, Whynes D K, Chamberlain J O, Hardcastle J D 1991 The cost of screening for colorectal cancer. Journal of Epidemiology and Community Health 45: 220–224

Wherry DC, Thomas WM 1994 The yield of flexible fibreoptic sigmoidoscopy in the detection of asymptomatic colorectal neoplasia. Surgical Endoscopy 8: 279–281

Winawer SJ, Miller C, Lightdale C et al 1987 Patient response to sigmoidoscopy: a randomized trial of rigid and flexible sigmoidoscopy. Cancer 60: 1905–1908

Winawer SJ, Zauber AG, Stewart M, O'Brian MJ 1991 The natural history of colorectal cancer: opportunities for intervention. Cancer 67: 1143–1149

Winawer SJ, Flehinger BJ, Schottenfeld D, Miller D G 1993a Screening for colorectal cancer with faecal occult blood testing and sigmoidoscopy. Journal of the National Cancer Institute 85: 1311–1318

Winawer SJ, Zauber AG, O'Brien MJ et al 1993b Randomized comparison of surveillance intervals after colonoscopic removal of newly diagnosed adenomatous polyps. New England Journal of Medicine 328: 901–906

Winawer SJ, Zauber AG, Ho MN et al 1993c Prevention of colorectal cancer by colonoscopic polypectomy. New England Journal of Medicine 329: 1977–1981

Young GP, St John DJB, Rose IS, Blake D 1990 Haem in the gut. II. Faecal excretion of haem and haem-derived porphyrins and their detection. Journal of Gastroenterology and Hepatology 5: 194–203

Young GP, St John JB 1991 Selecting an occult blood test for use as a screening tool for large bowel cancer. Frontiers in Gastrointestinal Research 18: 135–156

3 Colorectal polyps and their management

S. NIVATVONGS   S. DORUDI

Introduction

The word 'polyp' is a non-specific clinical term that describes any projection from the surface of the intestinal mucosa regardless of its histologic nature. There are several types of polyps, classified by their histologic appearance:

1. Neoplastic – tubular adenoma, villous adenoma, tubulovillous adenoma. These may occur as (a) sporadic or (b) part of familial adenomatous polyposis (FAP).
2. Hyperplastic.
3. Hamartomatous – juvenile polyp, Peutz–Jeghers syndrome, Cronkhite–Canada syndrome, Cowden's disease.
4. Inflammatory – inflammatory polyp or pseudopolyp, benign lymphoid polyp.

A neoplastic polyp is the most important kind since it can evolve into an invasive carcinoma. Although the polyps in familial adenomatous polyposis are also neoplastic, the management of this condition is discussed separately. Hyperplastic, hamartomatous and inflammatory polyps are non-neoplastic and have no malignant potential (except Peutz–Jeghers polyp).

Neoplastic polyps – (a) sporadic

A neoplastic polyp is an epithelial tumour composed of abnormal glands of the large bowel. A neoplastic polyp has been termed an adenoma which is classified into three types by the World Health Organization (Jass & Sobin 1989), according to its histology.

A *tubular adenoma* is composed of branching neoplastic tubules embedded in lamina propria and occupying at least 80% of the tumour (Fig. 3.1).

A *villous adenoma* is composed of at least 80% of fingerlike long tubules (Fig. 3.2), while a *tubulovillous adenoma* is composed of tubules as well as villous structures, each contributing more than 20% of the tumour mass (Fig. 3.3). Tubular adenoma accounts for 75% of all neoplastic polyps, villous adenoma 10% and tubulovillous adenoma 15% (Morson 1974).

Dysplasia is the term describing the histologic abnormality of an adenoma according to the degree of atypical cells, categorized as mild, moderate and severe. Thus, severe dysplasia designates the condition one step away from an invasive carcinoma.

Neoplastic polyps are common. In autopsy series, the adenomas are present in 34–52% of males and 29–45% of females over 50 years of

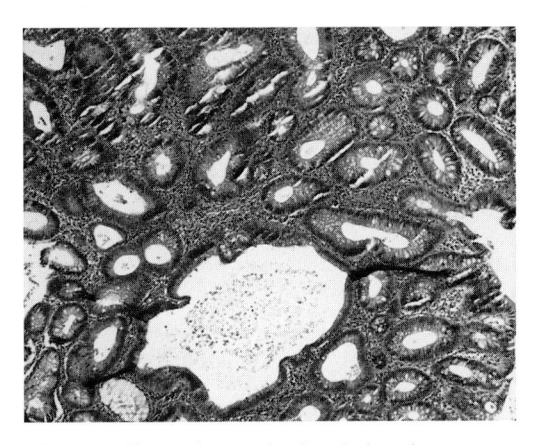

Fig. 3.1 Photomicrograph of a tubular adenoma.

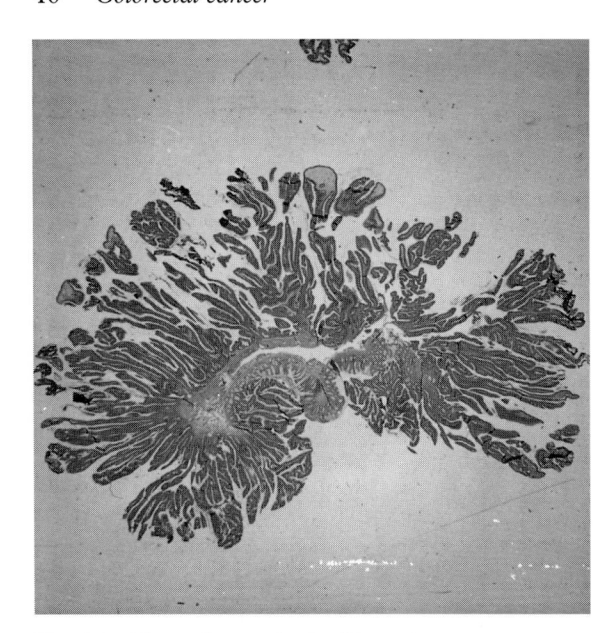

Fig. 3.2 Photomicrograph of a villous adenoma.

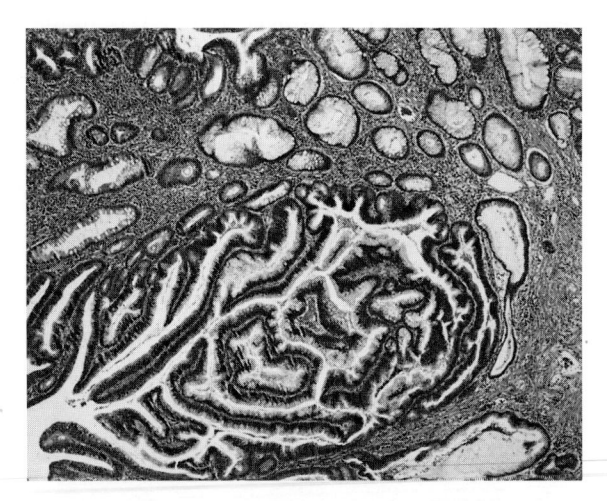

Fig. 3.3 Photomicrograph of a tubulovillous adenoma.

colonoscopy (O'Brien et al 1990). This study gives valuable information regarding the natural history and characteristics of polyps: 66.5% of the polyps are adenomas, 11.2% hyperplastic and 22.3% are classified as 'other' (normal mucosa, inflammatory and juvenile polyps, lymphoid hamartoma, submucosal lipoma, carcinoid and leiomyoma). The majority (65%) of the polyps are in the left colon (Table 3.1) and the size of the adenomas is shown in Table 3.2. It is important to note that size, extent of villous component and increasing age are independent risk factors for high-grade dysplasia. The increased frequency of high-grade dysplasia in adenomas located distal to the splenic flexure is attributable mainly to increased size and villous component rather than to location per se (O'Brien et al 1990). Multiplicity of adenomas affects the risk of high-grade dysplasia but is dependent on adenoma size and villous component and is not an independent factor. Increasing age is associated with risk for high-grade dysplasia and this effect is independent of the size and histologic type (O'Brien et al 1990). Invasive carcinomas are uncommon in adenomas <1 cm and the incidence increases with increased size of the polyps (Grinnell & Lane 1958, Muto et al 1975) (Table 3.3).

age (Rickert et al 1979, Williams et al 1982). Most adenomas (87–89%) are <1 cm in size (Rickert et al 1979, Williams et al 1982). The number, but not the size, of polyps increases with age (Rickert et al 1979). Carcinomas are found in 0–4% (Eide & Stalsberg 1978, Rickert et al 1979, Vatn & Stalsberg 1982, Williams et al 1982).

The National Polyp Study, a multicentre randomized clinical trial in the United States, includes 3371 adenomas from 1867 patients detected by

Table 3.1 Distribution of colorectal adenomas by colonoscopy (O'Brien et al 1990)

	%
Caecum	8
Ascending colon	9
Hepatic flexure	4
Transverse colon	10
Splenic flexure	4
Descending colon	14
Sigmoid colon	43
Rectum	8
TOTAL	100

Table 3.2 Size of adenoma by colonoscopy (O'Brien et al 1990)

	%
≤0.5 cm	38
0.6–1.0 cm	37
≥1 cm	25
TOTAL	100

Table 3.3 Relationship between size of adenoma and carcinoma (Muto et al 1975)

Size (cm)	Adenoma (no.)	Invasive carcinoma (%)
<1	1479	1.3
1–2	580	9.5
≥2	430	46

Aetiology

Although the aetiological mechanisms of adenoma formation remain incompletely understood, the last 5 years have witnessed significant advances in elucidating the molecular basis of colorectal tumourigenesis (see Ch. 1). Indeed, colorectal cancer has proved to be a paradigm amongst malignancies for the molecular description of tumour progression. This has largely evolved because of the epidemiological importance of this tumour and also because of three important factors regarding its natural history. Firstly, the progression of this cancer in terms of the adenoma–carcinoma sequence is well delineated. Secondly, well-characterized inherited syndromes exist that predispose to colorectal cancer indicating a genetic basis in their aetiology. Finally, and perhaps most importantly, the tumours themselves and their precursors (i.e. adenomas) are very amenable to colonoscopic sampling, thus providing material for analysis.

The known molecular events in the progression of this disease from normal epithelium to invasive cancer have already been authoritatively reviewed in Chapter 1 but are illustrated in Figure 3.4 to allow further discussion of molecular mechanisms of adenoma formation. It is now accepted that tumours derive from single clones and such clonal dominance has been elegantly demonstrated in human tumours growing in nude mice by 'tagging' tumour cells with unique genetic markers using retroviral gene transfer (Waghorne et al 1988). Analysis of the clonal composition of colorectal cancers has similarly demonstrated that tumours, including small adenomas, have a monoclonal composition (Fearon et al 1987). In contrast, normal epithelium has a polyclonal nature as it has originated from numerous stem cells. Thus, adenomas arise from the clonal expansion of a small number of cells from a single intestinal crypt through selection by a microevolutionary process

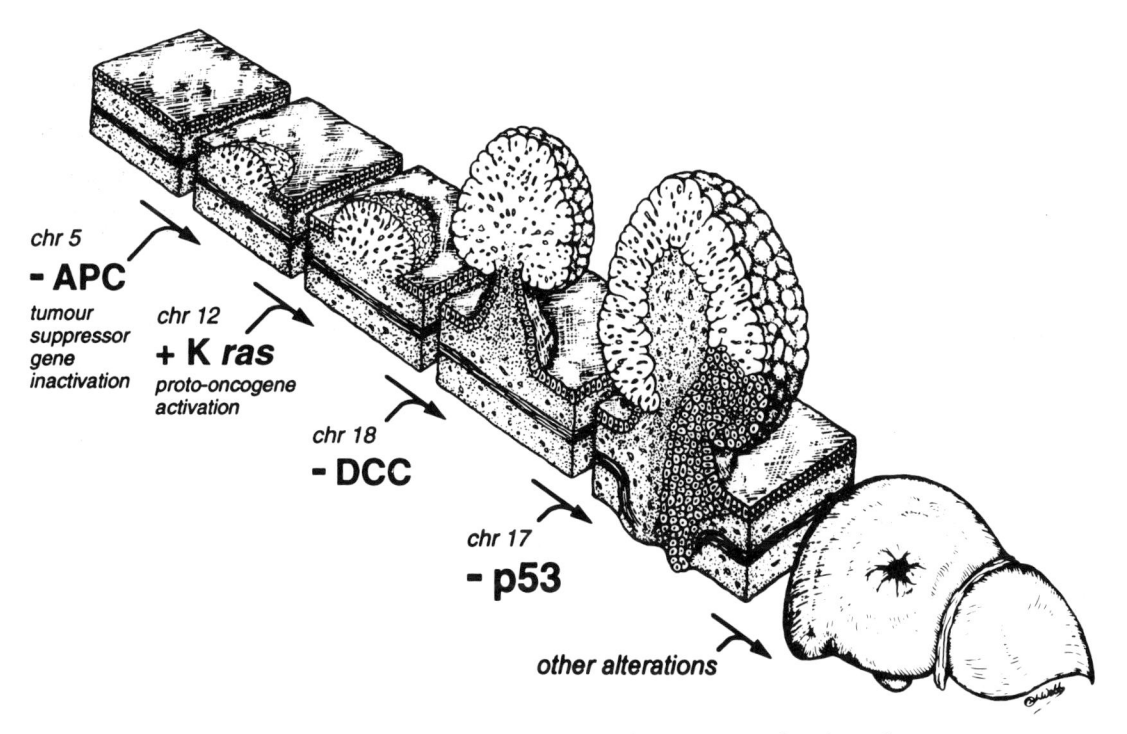

Fig. 3.4 Molecular events in the progression of the adenoma–carcinoma sequence in colorectal cancer.

that may be initiated by environmental (luminal) factors and sustained by the effects of subsequent molecular alterations. The molecular basis of this clonal expansion remains unclear but there has been intense interest in the identification of somatic alterations in colorectal tumour cells at various stages of tumour progression.

Amongst the earliest detectable molecular abnormalities that may initiate adenoma formation, inasmuch as they are present in very small adenomas (0.5 cm or less), are alterations in DNA methylation and in the adenomatous polyposis coli (APC) gene which has been cloned and sequenced. The frequency of APC mutations does not alter between adenomas and carcinomas (Powell et al 1992), an observation that is supportive of the early role of APC abnormalities in adenoma formation. Significant loss of DNA methylation occurs early on in colorectal tumourigenesis. Indeed, even very small adenomas have been demonstrated to have significant loss of methyl groups as compared to normal mucosa (Feinberg et al 1988). It has been suggested that hypomethylated DNA in premalignant cells is more susceptible to mutagenesis, perhaps because of less tight chromatin packing and therefore enhanced carcinogen access (Jones & Buckley 1990). However, even non-malignant (normal) mucosa of patients with colon cancer exhibits abnormalities of DNA methyltransferase, the enzyme responsible for cytosine methylation in DNA (El-Deiry et al 1991). This finding would suggest that alterations in DNA methylation may play an important role in early tumourigenic events.

Germline mutations in the APC gene are responsible for the hereditary condition familial adenomatous polyposis (FAP) which confers susceptibility to colorectal cancer (see Ch. 1). Although FAP accounts for less than 1% of all colorectal cancers, the importance of this gene product is underscored by the finding that APC mutations are common in *sporadic* adenomas and carcinomas (Miyoshi et al 1992). Over 90% of such mutations result in truncation of the APC gene product with loss of the carboxy-terminal region (Nagese & Nakamura 1993). Recently, two important findings have shed light on the function of the APC gene product and the mechanisms by which dysfunction of mutant APC may enhance early tumourigenesis. Firstly, APC protein has been shown to be associated with cytoplasmic proteins (α- and β-catenins) that link the cell adhesion molecule, and putative tumour suppressor gene, E-cadherin to the cell cytoskeleton (Rubinfeld et al 1993, Su et al 1993). Secondly, wild-type APC protein, but not mutant protein lacking the carboxy-terminal region, appears to be associated with the microtubule cytoskeleton (Munemitsu et al 1994, Smith et al 1994).

An intriguing possibility regarding the functional implications of these recent data is that APC may modulate intercellular signals passing along the cadherin–catenin–cytoskeleton axis that are responsible for cell growth and differentiation. Thus, mutant APC proteins that have reduced or no affinity for α- and β-catenins may contribute to formation of adenomatous polyps by loss of intercellular contact or communication, processes that may be dependent on association of the intact APC gene product with these catenins. Alternatively, adenoma formation, which is associated with a defective APC gene, may be partly attributable to the inability of mutant APC protein to interact with the cytoplasmic microtubule network. In this context, it is of interest that the assembly and reorganization of microtubules are closely coordinated with cell divisions and it has been suggested that disassembly of the microtubule network may activate initiation of DNA synthesis and thus increase cell proliferation (Munemitsu et al 1994). Moreover, the major effect of APC gene inactivation in colonic epithelium may not necessarily result in the induction of a malignant phenotype per se; rather, it may cause an increased proliferation rate in affected cells which provides an expanded cell population at risk of subsequent transformation events.

It can be seen that our understanding of the precise mechanisms by which luminal factors induce DNA damage or modify epithelial gene expression and how these ensuing molecular alterations themselves affect mucosal biology is still far from complete. However, the near future will undoubtedly yield further information on the function of the APC gene product which promises to play a central role in early tumourigenic events. Additionally, the inevitable discovery of other, as yet unidentified genetic lesions will not only help to complete the picture but may also provide some targets for the design of rational drug treatment or even gene therapy.

Diagnosis of colorectal adenomas

Adenomas of the large bowel are usually asymptomatic and are frequently discovered during routine endoscopic examination or barium enema studies. Bleeding per rectum is most common finding if the polyp is situated in the rectum or sigmoid colon. A large pedunculated polyp in the lower part of the rectum may prolapse through the anus. A large villous adenoma may manifest as watery diarrhoea; in rare instances, it causes fluid and electrolyte imbalance. Intermittent abdominal pain from recurrent intussusception or spasm may occur with a large colonic polyp but is unusual. Mild anaemia may follow chronic bleeding from an ulcerated polyp. With a small polyp up to 8 mm, biopsy and electrocoagulation can be performed, preferably using a 'hot' biopsy forceps for histopathologic examination. A large polyp should be completely snared or excised. Biopsies of a large polyp do not represent the entire lesion and may present difficulty in interpretation of an invasive carcinoma. Occasionally, biopsy may cause displacement of the gland into the submucosa and can be misinterpreted as an invasive carcinoma. An alternative diagnostic method is a barium enema, preferably air contrast barium enema. This should be preceded by a rigid proctosigmoidoscopy or a flexible sigmoidoscopy since the anorectum and the sigmoid colon are difficult to examine by barium enema study.

Why remove a polyp?

It has generally been accepted that most, if not all, colorectal carcinomas are derived from benign adenomas through the adenoma–carcinoma sequence. It takes 5 years from a clean colon to the development of an adenoma and 10 years from clean colon to the development of invasive carcinoma (O'Brien et al 1990). Thus, removal of an adenoma is prophylactic against the development of colorectal carcinoma. Gilbertson (1974), in a retrospective study, shows that removal of rectal polyps in patients under surveillance with yearly rigid proctosigmoidoscopy results in a lower than expected incidence of rectal carcinoma. This result is confirmed by Selby et al (1992): in a case-controlled study using rigid proctosigmoidoscopy, screening examination produces a 70% reduction in the risk of death from rectal and distal sigmoid cancer. The National Polyp Study also shows that colonoscopic polypectomy results in a lower than expected incidence of colorectal carcinoma (Winawer et al 1993).

Most adenomatous polyps found on routine examination with rigid proctosigmoidoscopy or flexible sigmoidoscopy are small and in themselves have minimal risk of harbouring a carcinoma. Because we do not know whether these small adenomas will continue to grow with eventual degeneration into an invasive carcinoma, their removal is logical provided it can be performed with minimal or no risk of complications.

Another question is whether the patient has a synchronous polyp or polyps more proximally and if so, whether it is important to have it removed. The incidence of synchronous polyps beyond the reach of the rigid proctoscope and flexible sigmoidoscope is about 50% (O'Brien et al 1990). However, most of these polyps are small and have little clinical significance. Using death from cancer as the endpoint. Atkin et al (1992) showed that the risk of development of carcinoma in the more proximal colon is significant if the polyp found in the rectum or sigmoid colon is larger than 1 cm, if the polyp has a villous component and if there are multiple adenomas. They also found that the risk is insignificant if a tubular adenoma in the rectum and sigmoid colon is smaller than 1 cm.

There has been no randomized controlled study to discover whether a total colonoscopy should be performed if a polyp is found in the rectum or sigmoid colon, but it is reasonable to individualize and tailor the practice to each patient. If the patient is young (e.g. <40 years old) or if the patient has a high risk of developing a carcinoma more proximally as discussed by Atkin et al (1992), a total colonoscopy along with removal of polyp should be the method of choice.

44 Colorectal cancer

Management of benign colorectal adenomas

Fibreoptic colonoscopy has revolutionized the management of large bowel polyps. Most polyps throughout the entire colon and rectum can be snared through the colonoscope with minimal morbidity. At the present time, colonic resection or colotomy and polypectomy are reserved for cases in which colonoscopic polypectomy cannot be done, such as lesions that are too large or too flat or when the colonoscope cannot be passed to the site of the polyp.

Clinically, there are two morphologic types of polyps, pedunculated and sessile. The pedunculated polyp has a stem lined with normal mucosa, called a stalk or a pedicle, and has the appearance of a mushroom (Fig. 3.5). A sessile polyp grows flat on the mucosa (Fig. 3.6). A pedunculated polyp is rarely >4 cm in diameter, whereas a sessile polyp can be huge, encompassing the entire circumference of the large bowel. Most pedunculated polyps can be snared in one piece since the pedicles are rarely >2 cm in diameter (Fig. 3.7). Sessile polyps <2 cm usually can be snared in one piece. Large sessile polyps should be snared piecemeal and in more than one session as appropriate (Fig. 3.8). The excised polyps must be prepared properly and sectioned so that all of the

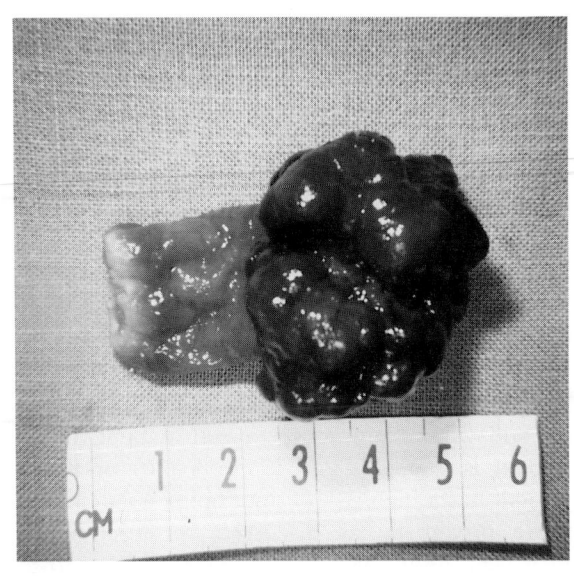

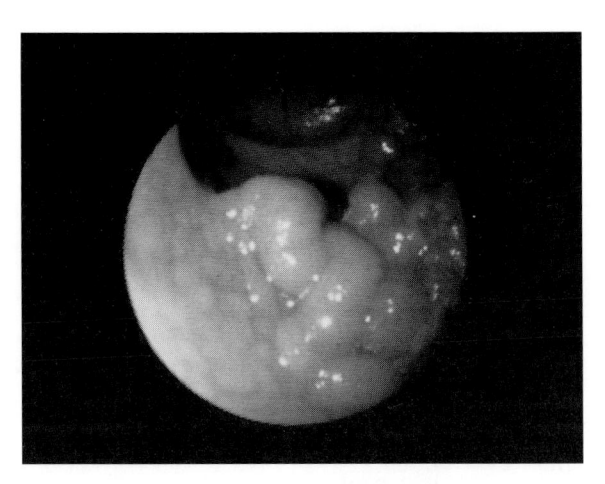

Fig. 3.6 Gross appearance of a sessile polyp in situ.

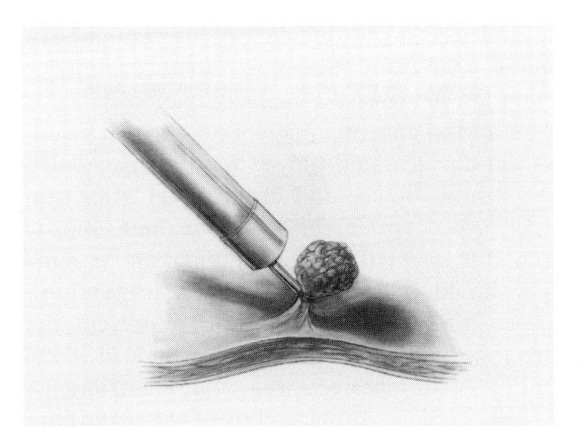

Fig. 3.7 Snare wire around the pedicle of a polyp. (From Nivatvongs S 1992 In: Gordon PH, Nivatvongs S (eds) Principles and practice of surgery for the colon, rectum and anus. Quality Medical Publishing, St Louis, with permission.)

Fig. 3.5 Gross appearance of an excised pedunculated polyp.

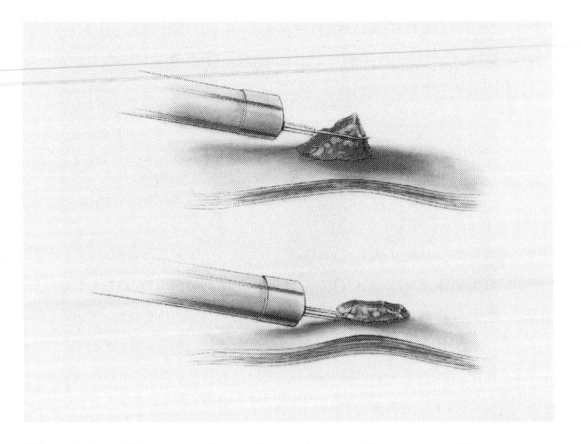

Fig. 3.8 Piecemeal snaring of a sessile polyp. (From Nivatvongs S 1992 In: Gordon PH, Nivatvongs S (eds) Principles and practice of surgery for the colon, rectum and anus. Quality Medical Publishing, St Louis, with permission.)

layers can be examined microscopically and the evidence of invasive carcinoma detected.

In 1985, Muto et al called attention to a separate polyp called a 'flat' adenoma. This type of polyp is unique in that it is usually small and flat, often with a central depression, and is difficult to detect with colonoscopy or even in the resected colon and rectal specimens. Ninety percent of flat adenomas are smaller than 1 cm and more than half are less than 5 mm (Muto & Watanabe 1993). The significance of flat adenomas is the high incidence of carcinomas, which occur at 5.8% even when the lesions are as small as 2–4 mm and rapidly rise to 36.4% when the lesions are 9–10 mm (Table 3.4). About 10% of adenomas in the Muto series are flat adenomas. They are most frequently located in the left colon and the rectum (Muto & Watanabe 1993). Lynch et al (1988) found similar flat adenomas in patients from a kindred under study for hereditary nonpolyposis colon and rectal cancer. Most of their lesions are in the right colon. The flat adenomas, originally thought to occur mostly among Japanese, have been found in studies from Australia, Canada and the United Kingdom (Muto & Watanabe 1993). The so-called de novo carcinomas may well arise from preexisting flat adenomas through the adenoma–carcinoma sequence. The management of flat adenomas is the same as for sessile adenomas. Interestingly, recent molecular analysis of such flat adenomas suggests that these superficial-type colorectal tumours are aetiologically distinct from other polypoid tumours (Minamoto et al 1994), as the mutation rate in the k-ras gene was both significantly reduced (16% in flat adenomas compared to 50% in ordinary colorectal adenomas) and did not occur in the same codons.

Adenomas of the rectum present a unique situation. Many of these lesions can be palpated with finger, suction tube or endoscope. If the lesion is soft, regardless of size, it has a 90% chance of being benign (Galandiuk et al 1987, Nivatvongs et al 1980). There are a number of ways to remove a large ademona in the rectum, including snaring through a rigid proctosigmoidoscope or a colonoscope. A low rectal lesion (up to 7 cm from the anal verge) can be excised per anally (Fig. 3.9). A lesion in the midrectum (7–10 cm from the anal verge) can be excised via a posterior

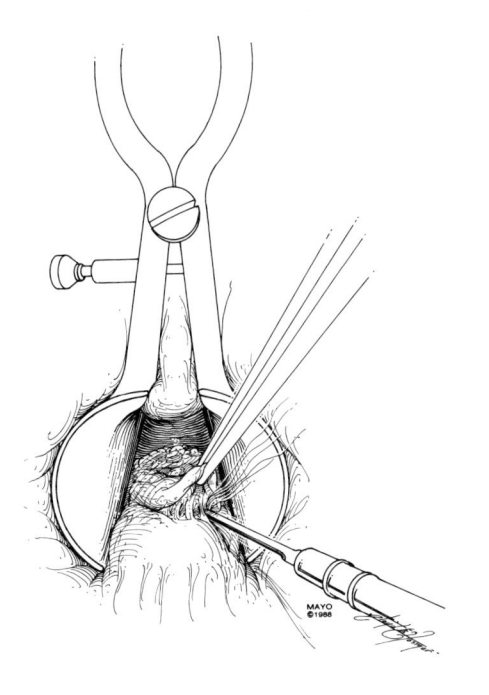

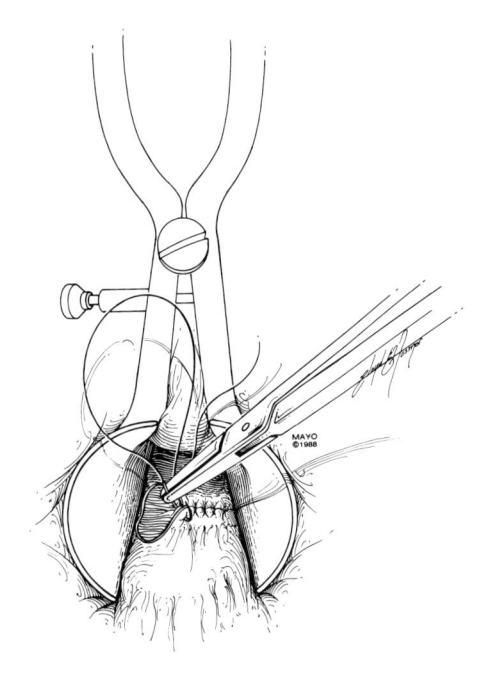

Fig. 3.9 (A) Per anal excision of a sessile polyp in low rectum, using electrocautery in the submucosal plane. (B) The wound is closed transversely with a 3–0 synthetic absorbable suture.

Table 3.4 Size and grade of atypia in flat adenoma (Muto & Watanabe 1993)

Size (mm)	Mild	Moderate	Severe	Total	Malignancy rate (%)
2–4	43	6	3	52	5.8
5–6	31	6	4	41	9.8
7–8	12	6	6	24	25.0
9–10	5	2	4	11	36.4
	91	20	17	128	13.3

proctotomy (Fig. 3.10). A large polyp in the upper rectum that cannot be snared via an endoscope should have an anterior rectosigmoidectomy.

Patients with a neoplastic polyp have a higher risk of developing another polyp, so follow-up colonoscopy is advised. After the colon or rectum is cleared of polyps, follow-up colonoscopy every 3–5 years is adequate. A large sessile polyp, particularly the villous type, is prone to recur and a follow-up check of the polypectomy site should be done every 3–6 months for the first year, every 6–12 months for the second year and every year thereafter to the fifth year, when colonoscopic examination every 3–5 years is appropriate.

Management of polyps with invasive carcinoma

The term 'invasive' carcinoma is applied only when the malignant cells have invaded a polyp, either sessile or pedunculated, partially or totally, through the muscularis mucosa (Fig. 3.11). Carcinoma above the muscularis mucosa does not metastasize and should be classified as dysplasia rather than carcinoma in situ or superficial carcinoma (Morson 1974). For this type of lesion, complete excision is all that is necessary. Follow-up of these polyps is the same as for benign polyps.

A sessile polyp with invasive carcinoma has an overall 10% risk of lymph node metastasis. Bowel

Fig. 3.10 Transsphincteric posterior proctotomy. (a) Line of skin incision, with patient in prone position. (b) The external sphincter muscles and the levator ani muscles are divided and marked with stay sutures. (c) The posterior rectal wall is opened, exposing the anorectal lumen. (d) The lesion in mid rectum is excised in the submucosal plane. (e) The wound is closed in layers with 3–0 synthetic absorbable sutures.

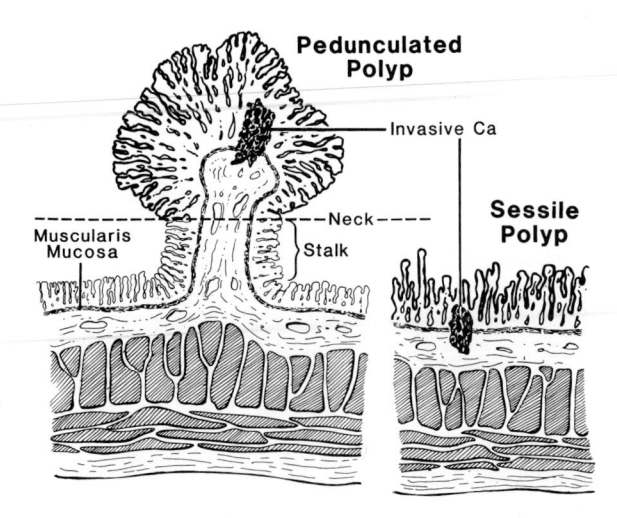

Fig. 3.11 Schematic picture of adenomas with invasive carcinomas.

resection should be considered in most of these patients (Nivatvongs et al 1991). A pedunculated polyp with invasion limited to the head or stalk has a low risk of lymph node metastasis so a complete polypectomy is adequate if there are no other adverse factors. A close follow-up examination with colonoscopy to detect a local recurrence should be done every 3–6 months for the first year. This period can be extended to every 6–12 months in the second and third years and two every year for the next 2 years. Thereafter, colonoscopy every 3 years is adequate.

There have been reports in the literature that undifferentiated carcinoma and invasion of the malignancy into the lymphatic or vascular channels have a high risk of lymph node metastasis (Coverlizza et al 1989, Muto et al 1991, Morson et al 1984, Richards et al 1987). In such situations, bowel resection should be considered even if the invasion is limited to the head of the polyp. A recent study from the Mayo Clinic showed that the risk of lymph node metastasis in a pedunculated polyp is not significant until the invasion reaches down to the submucosa at the base of the stalk (Nivatvongs et al 1991). Bowel resection should be considered in good operative risk patients.

Natural history of untreated colorectal adenomas

A retrospective review of patients from the pre-colonoscopic era by Stryker et al (1987) analysed 226 patients who had colorectal polyps ≥10 mm in diameter in whom periodic radiographic examination of the colon was elected over excision. During a follow-up that ranged from 12 to 229 months (mean 68 months), 37% of the polyps enlarged. Twenty one invasive carcinomas were identified at the site of the index polyp at a mean follow-up of 108 months (range 24–225 months). Actuarial analysis revealed that the cumulative risks of diagnosis of carcinoma at the polyp site at 5, 10 and 20 years are 2.5%, 8% and 24% respectively. In addition, 11 invasive carcinomas were found at a site remote from the index polyp during the same follow-up period. These data further support the recommendation of excision of all colorectal polyps ≥1 cm in diameter and a periodic examination of the entire colon. Although this study has limitations inherent in any retrospective analysis, comparable prospective data are unlikely to be available in the future because of the widespread availability of colonoscopy and the compelling evidence to recommend the removal of neoplastic polyps.

Neoplastic polyps – (b) familial adenomatous polyposis (FAP)

Introduction

FAP is an autosomal dominantly inherited disease that predisposes the carrier to a high probability of colorectal cancer. As already discussed, germline mutations in the APC gene are responsible for this condition which predominantly cause premature truncation of the APC protein, either by a small insertion or deletion resulting in a frame shift or by a point mutation that creates a premature stop codon. Further studies will be necessary to determine whether specific mutations are associated with different phenotypes (e.g. early age of onset, high frequency of extracolonic lesions).

FAP should be regarded as a multisystem disorder as affected individuals exhibit numerous benign and malignant manifestations, although other unknown genetic lesions may well contribute to the final FAP phenotype. Osteomas, epidermoid cysts, congenital hypertrophy of the retinal pigment epithelium (CHRPE), gastric and duodenal polyps and extraintestinal malignancies can all occur. Indeed, in this context, FAP has been aptly described by Jagelman (1987) as a generalized growth disorder. The recognition of numerous other extracolonic lesions associated with multiple adenomas and colorectal cancer has led to the description of a number of eponymous FAP phenotypes: Gardner's syndrome – multiple osteomas and epidermoid cysts; Turcot's syndrome – brain tumours; Zanca's syndrome – cartilaginous exostoses; and Oldfield's syndrome – sebaceous cysts.

Diagnosis

As the most common manifestation, individuals with this condition develop multiple adenomas in the large bowel. Bussey originally defined 'multiple' as greater than 100 because all the patients in the St Mark's Hospital Polyposis Registry had more than 100 adenomas (Bussey 1975). However, Bussey's data were based on careful counting of resected specimens whereas in present practice polyp counts are performed endoscopically. This has important implications in the diagnosis of this condition as most adenomas in FAP are less than 1 cm and many smaller than 0.5 cm. Thus, colonoscopy is likely to underestimate the number of adenomas and even if the endoscopist counts 50 polyps, the patient may still have FAP.

The adenomas of FAP occur in all parts of the colon with a tubular architecture as the predominant histological appearance, while purely villous adenomas are rare in FAP (Boman & Levin 1986). Importantly, even macroscopically flat or 'normal' mucosa may exhibit adenomatous change if biopsied. Colorectal carcinoma invariably develops in untreated patients. Adenomas can also occur in the small bowel, particularly the duodenum, and the stomach. Indeed, periampullary carcinoma is the second most common malignancy in FAP although the incidence of gastric cancer does not appear to be significantly increased (Lynch et al 1991).

Management of FAP

Arguably, the most important aspect in the management of patients with FAP is detailed genetic counselling and education. Once the pedigree is compiled, high-risk patients can be readily identified. Such individuals will be those who have a parent, sibling or progeny who manifest the florid polyposis phenotype. Ideally, these initial interviews are best conducted under the auspices of a family cancer clinic where dedicated personnel can document and centralize the data, contact appropriate relatives and coordinate all subsequent screening investigations and treatment.

Following genetic counselling, a screening sigmoidoscopy (preferably flexible) programme can be initiated at 12–14 years of age and continued on an annual basis until the age of 35. The majority of patients with germline APC dysfunction will manifest colonic polyps by 30 with adenomas initially appearing most frequently in the rectosigmoid region (Lynch et al 1991). Unfortunately, there does not appear to be an unequivocal upper age limit at which it can be safely assumed that the absence of colorectal polyps also indicates an intact and fully functional APC gene.

Genetic screening

Genetic screening with the use of microsatellite probes within the APC gene may prove to be beneficial in obviating the need for repeated endoscopic examinations, particularly in individuals over the age of 30. However, the APC gene in FAP does not appear to exhibit any particular mutational hotspots; rather, mutations are distributed over large regions of the coding DNA (Miyoshi et al 1992), limiting the present usefulness of genetic screening to a research setting. Current techniques allow APC mutations to be identified in approximately 70% of APC patients (Miyoshi et al 1992), but it is anticipated that the technical problems preventing identification of mutations in 100% of individuals will be solved in the near future, allowing a definitive test to be available within the next few years.

Clearly, accurate presymptomatic genetic screening will provide welcome information for those high-risk individuals from FAP families who test negative for APC mutations. It should be emphasized that treatment for individuals who test positive will not be altered in that prophylactic removal of the colon at the first sign of polyps or very soon thereafter continues to be an absolute necessity (see below). However, presymptomatic diagnosis may, at the very least, allow the use and assessment of other treatment modalities (e.g. sulindac or its derivatives) in the prevention of polyp formation (see below). At present, therefore, positive sigmoidoscopy remains the gold standard for diagnosis in high-risk individuals, although experience with genetic screening is rapidly growing.

Surgery

As already stated, once the polyposis phenotype has been detected, the patient should undergo prophylactic colectomy. If local expertise is available, and particularly if numerous polyps are present in the rectum, then a restorative proctocolectomy with formation of an ileoanal pouch should be strongly considered. Such a restorative procedure precludes the need for lifelong rectal surveillance; however, the theoretical risk of adenoma or even carcinoma formation in the remnant cuff of rectal mucosa at the anorectal junction remains. Alternatively, the operation of choice is colectomy with formation of an ileorectal anastomosis. Clearly, patients undergoing this latter procedure will require careful endoscopic surveillance of their rectal mucosa with sigmoidoscopy at 6-monthly intervals.

Resolution of polyps with sulindac

Waddell and Loughry (1983) first reported that sulindac reduces the size and number of rectal polyps in individuals with FAP who had undergone colectomy and formation of an ileorectal anastomosis (1983). Recently, sulindac administration has been shown to result in a reduction of polyp size and number in both the colon and rectum (Giardiello et al 1993). These data would suggest that sulindac is inhibiting an event early on in colorectal tumourigenesis. Interestingly, the reduced form of sulindac is an inhibitor of the cyclooxygenase, a key enzyme in arachidonic metabolism. The predominant site of sulindac reduction is in the colon by local microflora to sulindac sulphide, which is a potent cyclooxygenase inhibitor. Thus, the effect of sulindac in inducing polyp regression would appear to provide evidence for the hypothesis that cyclooxygenase inhibition is germane to the reported ability of aspirin in reducing colon cancer mortality (reviewed in Marnett 1992).

In support of the protective role of cyclooxygenase inhibition in colorectal tumourigenesis, there are reports of elevated levels of prostaglandins in colorectal cancers as compared to adjacent normal mucosa (Marnett 1992). Additionally, a recent study has demonstrated a significant upregulation in the expression of the cyclooxygenase 2 gene (at the mRNA level) in over 80% of colorectal cancers and 50% of adenomas examined (Eberhart et al 1994). Clearly, none of these data provide a causal role for prostaglandins, or a disturbance in their metabolism, in colorectal tumourigenesis in individuals with FAP (or sporadic colorectal cancer). Indeed, the mechanisms by which abnormalities of prostaglandin metabolism are translated into alterations of cell signalling, cell differentiation, cell proliferation and finally tumour formation remain poorly understood. The long-term risks and benefits have yet to be assessed carefully and certainly at present, this treatment modality is not an alternative to surgery in the prevention of colorectal cancer in the management of individuals with FAP.

Management of upper gastrointestinal tract lesions

As our understanding of the full FAP phenotype has become clear it is now recognized that adenomas also occur in the stomach, duodenum and small bowel in FAP individuals. Cancer of the duodenum does occur and, as already discussed, cancer of the periampullary region is the second most common cancer affecting FAP patients (Lynch et al 1991). Ileal and jejunal cancers are very rare but gastric adenocarcinoma and carcinoids have been reported, though gastric polyps are usually fundic gland polyps rather than adenomas (Lynch et al 1991).

The published figures for the incidence of upper gastrointestinal lesions from different centres range from 44% to 90% (Lynch et al 1991) but further studies are needed to delineate more accurately the risk of upper gastrointestinal cancer in FAP patients. In individuals with colonic polyposis upper gastrointestinal endoscopy is recommended every 3 years with annual endoscopy and biopsy in patients who subsequently develop gastric or duodenal polyps. Lynch has suggested an initial examination with a forward-viewing endoscope immediately followed by side-viewing endoscopy, allowing clearer visualization of the ampulla (Lynch et al 1991).

Hyperplastic polyps

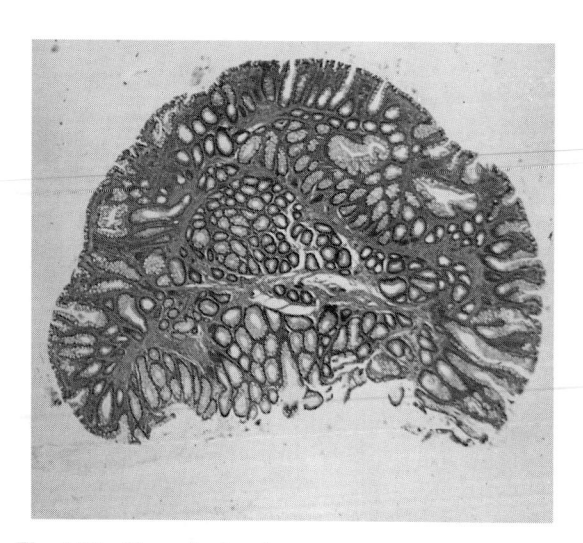

Hyperplastic polyps are non-neoplastic polyps commonly found in the rectum as small, pale and glassy mucosal nodules. Most of them are 3–5 mm in size, although larger ones can be seen in the more proximal part of the colon. Studies (O'Brien et al 1990) using histologic evidence have shown that the majority of small polyps, particularly those in the more proximal colon, are adenomatous polyps in contrast to previous impressions that most small polyps are of the hyperplastic type. Histologic differentiation from neoplastic polyps presents no problem. The characteristic picture is a saw-tooth appearance of the lining of epithelial cells, producing a papillary outline. There is no clear dysplasia and, thus, no potential for malignancy and their removal is unnecessary (Fig. 3.12). However, if their gross appearance is not typical for hyperplastic polyps, a biopsy should be taken to rule out an adenoma.

Hamartomatous polyps

A hamartoma is a malformation or inborn error of tissue development characterized by an abnormal mixture of tissues endogenous to the part, with an excess of one or more of these tissues. It may show itself at birth or by extensive growth in the postnatal period.

Juvenile polyps

Juvenile polyps characteristically occur in children, although they may present in adults at any age. This type of polyp is a hamartoma and is not premalignant. Macroscopically they are pink, smooth, round and usually pedunculated. The cut section shows a cheeselike appearance caused by dilated cystic spaces. Microscopic pictures show dilated glands filled with mucus and an abnormality of the lamina propria which has a mesenchymal appearance (Fig. 3.13). Bleeding from the rectum is a common finding and a moderate amount of bleeding can occur if the polyp is amputated, a phenomenon not seen in other types of polyps. Intussusception of the colon occasionally occurs if the polyp is large. Treatment is by excision or snare through the rigid proctosigmoidoscope or the colonoscope,

Fig. 3.12 Hyperplastic polyp.

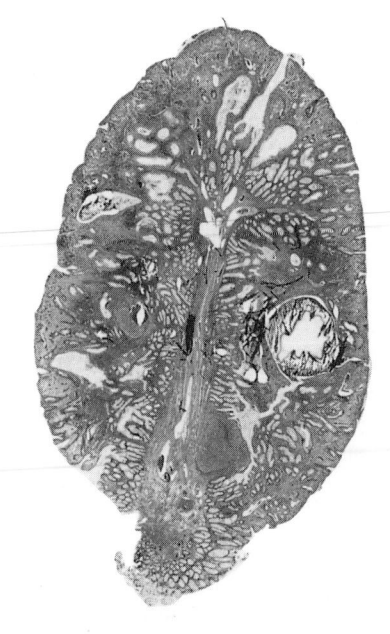

Fig. 3.13 Juvenile polyp.

depending on the location of the polyps.

Familial juvenile polyposis coli is a recognized entity distinct from other polyposes (Gilinsky et al 1986, Grosfeld & West 1986). Hundreds or even thousands of polyps are distributed throughout the entire colon and rectum and the disease may also involve the stomach and small bowel. Inheritance is autosomal dominant. Rectal bleeding is the most common symptom but prolapse or protrusion of a rectal mass, intestinal or colonic intussusception, abdominal pain, diarrhoea and protein loss can also be present. Unlike solitary juvenile polyposis which is not premalignant, diffuse juvenile polyposis can degenerate to adenomas and eventually carcinoma. Sometimes adenomatous polyps coexist in the same patient. The treatment is subtotal colectomy with ileorectal anastomosis. If the rectum is lined with polyps, a proctocolectomy with ileoanal pouch procedure is indicated.

Peutz–Jeghers syndrome

The Peutz–Jeghers syndrome was originally described by Peutz in 1921, but it was not clearly identified until attention was brought to it by Jeghers et al in 1949. The syndrome comprises melanin spots on the buccal mucosa and lips; the face and digits may be involved to a variable extent, but the mouth pigmentation is the sine qua non of this portion of the syndrome. The presence of polyps in the small bowel is a constant finding of this syndrome, but the stomach, colon and rectum may also be involved.

The characteristic Peutz–Jeghers polyp has an abnormal muscularis mucosa branching into the lamina propria, giving the appearance of a Christmas tree (Fig. 3.14). Inheritance is in a Mendelian-dominant manner. The polyp is considered a hamartoma, which generally should not degenerate to malignancy. However, in the past a few cases have been documented of Peutz–Jeghers polyps degenerating into invasive adenocarcinomas (Dozois et al 1969, Giardiello et al 1987). Most polyps are in the small bowel and their removal is not indicated unless an intussusception or severe haemorrhage ensues. Large polyps

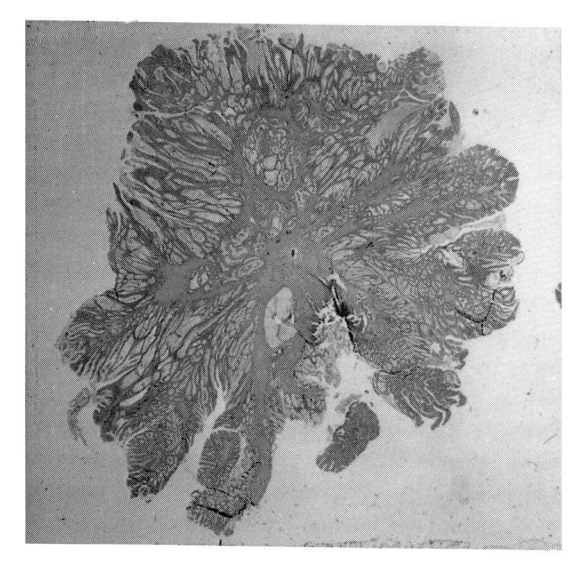

Fig. 3.14 Peutz–Jeghers polyp.

in the colon and rectum should be snared via colonoscopy to prevent bleeding and intussusception, if it can be performed with minimal risk.

Cronkhite–Canada syndrome

The Cronkhite–Canada syndrome is characterized by generalized gastrointestinal polyposis in association with alopecia, cutaneous pigmentation and atrophy of fingernails and toenails (Cronkhite & Canada 1955). It is not inherited and is considered a hamartoma. Diarrhoea is a prominent feature and vomiting, malabsorption and protein-losing enteropathy are the common clinical manifestations. The polyps consist of cystic dilatation of the epithelial tubules similar to that of juvenile polyps, but the lesions are usually smaller and do not show a marked excess of lamina propria. Most patients die within a relatively short time following the diagnosis, but there have been a few reports of spontaneous remission (Russell et al 1983). Colon carcinoma in patients with Cronkhite–Canada syndrome has been reported (Rappaport et al 1986).

The cause of Cronkhite–Canada syndrome is not always clear but may be related to fat, protein and carbohydrate malabsorption. The treatment is symptomatic. Bowel resection is reserved for cases in which complications such as bowel obstruction develop.

Cowden's disease

Cowden's disease is an uncommon familial syndrome of combined ectodermal, endodermal and mesodermal hamartomas. The disease was named after the family name of the propositus by Lloyd and Dennis (1963). Cutaneous and oral verrucous papules are regular and diagnostic findings (Thyresson & Doyle 1981).

Polyps in patients with Cowden's disease are small, typically <5 mm in diameter. Microscopic features are consistent with hamartomas, characterized by disorganization and proliferation of the muscularis mucosa with minimally abnormal overlying mucosa (Carlson et al 1984). The important aspect of this disease is its association with other lesions, particularly carcinoma of the breast, thyroid neoplasms, ovarian cysts and other gastrointestinal polyps (Thyresson & Doyle 1981). Since the risk of carcinoma in these small polyps is negligible, their removal is unnecessary.

Inflammatory and lymphoid polyps

Inflammatory polyps, or pseudopolyps, may look grossly like adenomatous polyps. However, microscopic examination shows islands of normal mucosa or mucosa with slight inflammation. They are caused by previous attacks of any form of severe colitis (ulcerative, Crohn's, amoebic, ischaemic or schistosomal), resulting in partial loss of mucosa and leaving remnants or islands of relatively normal mucosa.

Radiologically, both the acute and chronic forms appear similar. Distinction can be made with the rigid proctosigmoidoscope, but in the chronic stage a biopsy may be necessary to distinguish the condition from familial polyposis. Inflammatory polyps are not premalignant and their presence in no way influences the potential malignant status of the patient with ulcerative colitis, a development that remains related to the extent, age of onset and duration of disease. That these polyps are not premalignant in ulcerative colitis is relative; the potential carcinomatous status of the pseudopolyp in this condition is no more or less than that of the adjacent mucosa (Morson & Bussey 1970).

Benign lymphoid polyps are an enlargement of lymphoid follicles commonly seen in the rectum. They may be solitary or diffuse and their cause is unknown. Lymphoid polyps must not be confused with familial adenomatous polyposis. The histologic criteria set out by Dawson et al (1961) for the diagnosis of benign lymphoid polyps is as follows. Lymphoid tissue must be entirely within the mucosa and submucosa; there must be no invasion of the underlying muscle coat; at least two germinal centres must be present; and if the rectal biopsy fails to include the muscle coat and no germinal centres are seen, the diagnosis is inconclusive. Treatment of lymphoid polyps is not indicated other than their removal to make the diagnosis and differentiate them from other types of polyps.

References

Atkin WS, Morson BC, Cuzick J 1992 Long-term risk of colorectal cancer after excision of rectosigmoid adenomas. New England Journal of Medicine 326: 658–662

Boman BM, Levin B 1986 Familial polyposis. Hospital Practice 21: 155–170

Bussey HJR 1975 Familial polyposis coli. Johns Hopkins University Press, Baltimore, MD

Carlson GJ, Nivatvongs S, Snover DC 1984 Colorectal polyps in Cowden's disease (multiple hemartoma syndrome). American Journal of Surgery and Pathology 8: 763–770

Coverlizza S, Risio M, Ferrari A, Fenoglio-Preiser CM, Rossini FP 1989 Colorectal adenomas containing invasive carcinoma. Pathologic assessment of lymph node metastatic potential. Cancer 64: 1937–1947

Cronkhite LW Jr, Canada WJ 1955 Generalized gastrointestinal polyposis. An unusual syndrome of polyposis, pigmentation, alopecia and onychotrophia. New England Journal of Medicine 252: 1011–1015

Dawson IM, Cornes JS, Morson BC 1961 Primary malignant lymphoid tumours of the intestinal tract. Report of 37 cases with study factors influencing prognosis. British Journal of Surgery 49: 80–89

Dozois RR, Judd ES, Dahlin DC, Bartholomew LG 1969 The Peutz–Jeghers syndrome. Is there a predisposition to the development of intestinal malignancy? Archives of Surgery 98: 509–517

Eberhart CE, Coffey RJ, Radhika A, Giardiello FM, Ferrenbach S, Dubois RN 1994 Up-regulation of cyclooxygenase 2 gene expression in human colorectal adenomas and adenocarcinomas. Gastroenterology 107: 1183–1188

Eide TJ, Stalsberg H 1978 Polyps of the large intestine in Northern Norway. Cancer 42: 2839–2848

El-Deiry WAS, Nelkin BD, Celano P, Yen R-WC, Falco JP, Hamilton SR 1991 High expression of the DNA methyltransferase gene characterizes human neoplastic cells and progression stages of colon cancer. Proceedings of the National Academy of Sciences USA 88: 3470–3474

Fearon ER, Hamilton SR, Vogelstein B 1987 Clonal analysis of human colorectal tumors. Science 238: 193–197

Feinberg AP, Gehrke CW, Kuo KC, Ehrlich M 1988. Reduced genomic 5-methylcytosine content in human colonic neoplasia. Cancer Research 48: 1159–1161

Galandiuk S, Fazio VW, Jagelman DG et al 1987 Villous and tubulovillous adenomas of the colon and rectum. A retrospective review, 1964–1985. American Journal of Surgery 153: 41–46

Giardiello FM, Welsh SB, Hamilton SR, Offerhaus GJA, Gittelsohn AM, Booker SV 1987 Increased risk of cancer in Peutz–Jeghers syndrome. New England Journal of Medicine 316: 1511–1514

Giardiello FM, Hamilton SR, Krush AJ et al 1993 Treatment of colonic and rectal adenomas with sulindac in familial adenomatous polyposis. New England Journal of Medicine 328: 1313–1316

Gilbertson VA 1974 Proctosigmoidoscopy and polypectomy in reducing the incidence of rectal cancer. Cancer 34 (suppl): 936–939

Gilinsky NH, Elliott MS, Price SK, Wright JP 1986 The nutritional consequences and neoplastic potential of juvenile polyposis coli. Diseases of the Colon and Rectum 29: 417–420

Grinnell RS, Lane N 1958 Benign and malignant adenomatous polyps and papillary adenomas of the colon and rectum: an analysis of 1856 tumors in 1335 patients. International Abstracts of Surgery 106: 519–538

Grosfeld JL, West KW 1986 Generalized juvenile polyposis coli. Archives of Surgery 121: 530–534

Jagelman DG 1987 Extracolonic manifestations of familial polyposis coli. Cancer Genetics and Cytogenetics 27: 319–325

Jass JR, Sobin LH 1989 Histological typing of intestinal tumours, 2nd edn. World Health Organization/Springer-Verlag, London, p 29–30

Jeghers H, McKusick VA, Katz KH 1949 Generalized intestinal polyposis and melanin spots of the oral mucosa, lips and digits. A syndrome of diagnostic significance. New England Journal of Medicine 241: 993–1005

Jones PA, Buckley JD 1990 The role of DNA methylation in cancer. Advances in Cancer Research 54: 1–23

Lloyd KM II, Dennis M 1963 Cowden's disease: a possible new symptom complex with multiple system involvement. Annals of Internal Medicine 58: 136–142

Lynch HT, Smyrk T, Lanspa SJ et al 1988 Flat adenomas in a colon cancer-prone kindred. Journal of the National Cancer Institute 80: 278–282

Lynch HT, Smyrk T, Watson P et al 1991 Hereditary colorectal cancer. Seminars in Oncology 18: 337–366

Marnett LJ 1992 Aspirin and the potential role of prostaglandins in colon cancer. Cancer Research 52: 5575–5589

Minamoto T, Sawaguchi K, Mai M, Yamashita N, Sugimura T, Esumi H 1994 Infrequent K-ras activation in superficial-type (flat) colorectal adenomas and adenocarcinomas. Cancer Research 54: 2841–2844

Miyoshi Y, Ando H, Nagase H et al 1992 Germ-line mutations of the APC gene in 53 familial adenomatous polyposis patients. Proceedings of the National Academy of Sciences 89: 4452–4456

Morson BC 1974 The polyp–cancer sequence in the large bowel. Proceedings of the Royal Society of Medicine 67: 451–457

Morson BC, Bussey HJR 1970 Predisposing causes of intestinal cancer. Current Problems in Surgery Feb, p 1–46

Morson BC, Whiteway JE, Jones EA, Macrae FA, Williams CB 1984 Histopathology and prognosis of malignant colorectal polyps treated by endoscopic polypectomy. Gut 25: 437–444

Munemitsu S, Souza B, Muller O, Albert I, Rubinfeld B, Polakis P 1994 The APC gene product associates with microtubules in vivo and promotes their assembly in vitro. Cancer Research 54: 3676–3681

Muto T, Watanabe T 1993 Flat adenomas and minute carcinomas of the colon and rectum. Perspectives in Colon and Rectal Surgery 6: 117–132

Muto T, Bussey HJ, Morson BC 1975 The evolution of cancer of the colon and rectum. Cancer 36: 2251–2270

Muto T, Kamiya J, Sawada T et al 1985 Small flat adenoma of the large bowel with special reference to its clinicopathologic features. Diseases of the Colon and Rectum 28: 847–851

Muto T, Sawada T, Sukihara K 1991 Treatment of carcinoma in adenoma. World Journal of Surgery 15: 35–40

Nagese H, Nakamura Y 1993 Mutations of the APC (adenomatous polyposis coli) gene. Human Mutations 2: 425–434

Nivatvongs S, Nicholson JD, Rothenberger DA et al 1980 Villous adenoma of the rectum: the accuracy of clinical assessment. Surgery 87: 549–551

Nivatvongs S, Rojanasakul A, Reiman HM et al 1991 The risk of lymph node metastasis in colorectal polyps with invasive adenocarcinoma. Diseases of the Colon and Rectum 34: 323–328

O'Brien MJ, Winawer SJ, Zauber AG et al 1990 The national polyp study. Patient and polyp characteristics associated with high-grade dysplasia in colorectal adenomas. Gastroenterology 98: 371–379

Powell SM, Silz N, Beazer-Barclay Y, Bryan TM, Hamilton SR, Thibodeau SN, Kinzler KW 1992 APC mutations occur early during colorectal tumourigenesis. Nature 359: 235–237

Rappaport LB, Sperling HV, Stavrides A 1986 Colon cancer in Cronkhite–Canada syndrome. Journal of Clinical Gastroenterology 8: 199–202

Richards WO, Webb WA, Morris SJ, Davis RC, McDaniel L, Jones L, Littauer S 1987 Patient management after endoscopic removal of the cancerous colon adenoma. Annals of Surgery 205: 665–672

Rickert RR, Averbach O, Garfinkel L, Hammond EC, Frasca JM 1979 Adenomatous lesions of the large bowel: an autopsy survey. Cancer 43: 1847–1857

Rubinfeld B, Souza B, Albert I et al 1993 Association of the APC gene product with β-catenin. Science 262: 1731–1734

Russell DM, Bhathal PS, St John DJB 1983 Complete remission in Cronkhite–Canada syndrome. Gastroenterology 85: 180–185

Selby JV, Friedman GD, Quesenberry CP Jr, Weiss NS 1992 A case-control study of screening sigmoidoscopy and mortality from colorectal cancer. New England Journal of Medicine 326: 653–657

Smith KJ, Levy DB, Maupin P, Pollard TD, Vogelstein B, Kinzler KW 1994 Wild-type but not mutant APC associates with the microtubule cytoskeleton. Cancer Research 54: 3672–3675

Stryker SJ, Wolff BG, Culp CE, Libbe SD, Ilstrup DM, MacCarty RL 1987 Natural history of untreated colonic polyps. Gastroenterology 93: 1009–1013

Su L-K, Vogelstein B, Kinzler KW 1993 Association of the APC tumor suppressor protein with catenins. Science 262: 1734–1737

Thyresson HN, Doyle JA 1981 Cowden's disease (multiple hamartoma syndrome). Mayo Clinic Proceedings 56: 179–184

Vatn MH, Stalsberg H 1982 The prevalence of polyps of the large intestine in Oslo: an autopsy study. Cancer 49: 819–825

Waddell WR, Loughry RW 1983 Sulindac for polyposis of the colon. Journal of Surgical Oncology 24: 83–87

Waghorne C, Thomas M, Legarde A, Kerbel RS, Breitman ML 1988 Genetic evidence for progressive selection and overgrowth of primary tumors by metastatic cell populations. Cancer Research 48: 6109–6114

Williams AR, Balasooriya BAW, Day DW 1982 Polyps and cancer of the large bowel: a necropsy study in Liverpool. Gut 23: 835–842

Winawer SJ, Zauber AG, Ho MN et al 1993 Prevention of colorectal cancer by colonoscopic polypectomy. New England Journal of Medicine 329: 1977–1981

4 Clinicopathological staging

R. C. NEWLAND   P. H. CHAPUIS   O. F. DENT

Introduction

Staging in this context refers to the classification of colorectal cancer following resection according to the anatomical extent of tumour spread in a manner which has a clinically useful correlation with prognosis. Each tumour stage should define a group of patients who are expected to have a similar prognosis. The use of alphabetical or numerical symbols for the various stages of tumour spread provides a shorthand means of conveying this information.

The applications of staging fall into three main categories, namely patient management, quality assurance and research. Tumour stage influences patient management in that it gives the clinician a guide to prognosis and serves as a basis for the selection of patients who may benefit from postoperative adjuvant therapy. Staging is required for monitoring the results of established methods of treatment so it has an important role in quality assurance. Meaningful comparisons of the results of treatment between institutions are only possible when staging methods have been standardized. Research into the effectiveness of new methods of treatment and into the importance of new prognostic variables is dependent on uniformity and precision in staging.

There has been justifiable criticism of those who propose staging systems which have not been rigorously tested (Goligher 1976). The validation of a staging system requires the collection of a large series of patients treated by comparable methods whose tumour pathology has been carefully documented and whose survival has been determined by follow-up over several years. It is highly desirable that the data be collected prospectively in a single institution using standardized methods. This approach largely avoids the problems of incomplete data and the confounding effects of variables which are unrelated to tumour stage but which may influence survival.

Given the time and effort required to accumulate the necessary data it is not surprising that the debate over what constitutes the optimum staging system has been lengthy and to date is unresolved. The application of modern methods of data handling and statistical analysis has added a new level of sophistication in the debate. With the increasing use of adjuvant therapy and the surgical treatment of liver metastases the opportunity to collect data on a large number of patients whose only treatment has been resection of their primary tumour has become greatly restricted. For this reason there is a pressing need now to define and agree on what constitutes the essential elements of a staging system.

In our view the attributes of a useful staging system are that it must be objective and reproducible; easy to apply and recall; meet a variety of needs (e.g. those of the surgeon, oncologist, general practitioner, tumour registry) and it must sharply separate patients into groups where survival declines in a stepwise manner.

Staging should not be confused with attempts at constructing a prognostic index for colorectal cancer. Such an index comprises several variables which, when combined in a mathematical formula, allow a prediction to be made about the likelihood of a patient surviving for a specific time period. A prognostic index does not depend on the identification of pathological or clinical stages.

Early attempts at staging colorectal cancer were based entirely on the extent of tumour spread within the resected bowel. Recently there has been a trend toward the use of clinicopathological (CP) staging in which the clinical extent of spread is also taken into account. The intention here is to review the background to the development of CP staging and to share our experience of this relatively new approach.

A historical perspective on staging

The first recorded attempts to stage large bowel cancer were made at St Mark's Hospital, London. Initially, Lockhart-Mummery (1927) described how rectal cancer could be staged using clinical observation on the extent of tumour spread. A three-stage classification was proposed and the stages were designated A, B and C respectively in order of worsening prognosis. This approach was taken up by Dukes (1932) who defined a system of staging based on the histological extent of tumour spread within the resected specimen. Dukes also used a three-stage classification: stage A, growth limited to the rectum; stage B, extension into the perirectal fat but no lymph node metastases; stage C, lymph node involvement by tumour irrespective of the extent of direct spread. Dukes provided early statistical support for his classification which is based on the two variables, direct spread of tumour and lymph node metastases within the bowel resection specimen.

The method gained widespread acceptance as it correlated well with prognosis and was easy to recall. Dukes' staging, however, has attracted criticism as the issue of cancer confined to the mucosa was not addressed, the rectal wall was not precisely defined and the classification of tumours in which the surgical margins were involved was not considered (Davis & Newland 1983). In this purely pathological staging system the presence of known metastases remaining after bowel resection was ignored. Failure to account for the presence of residual tumour is a major limitation of all purely pathologic staging systems.

Dukes subsequently modified his staging system by recommending the subclassification of stage C tumours into C1 and C2 (Gabriel et al 1935).

The C2 tumours were defined as having nodal metastases at the apex of the vascular pedicle while in C1 tumours the apical node was not involved. The assumption was that patients with C2 tumours had a worse prognosis. The definitive paper by Dukes & Bussey (1958) on the staging of rectal cancer employed data prospectively collected on 2447 patients treated at St Mark's Hospital over a 24-year period. This paper provided further validation for Dukes' staging and is a testimony to the quality of data collection in that institution. In subsequent studies from St Mark's Hospital the results of 'radical' operations have been reported, that is, those operations in which the surgeon decided at the time of operation 'that all known growth had been removed' (Nicholls et al 1979). It should be appreciated that in these circumstances, staging performed on the specimen is a modification of Dukes' staging due to patient selection. This point must be taken into account when comparisons are made between series. Unfortunately Dukes' staging, despite its simplicity, has often been misquoted, resulting in a further source of confusion (Goligher 1976).

The applicability of the principles of Dukes' staging to colonic cancer was demonstrated by Simpson & Mayo (1939) in a retrospective study of 120 patients who underwent 'curative' resections at the Mayo Clinic. These authors also showed that the extent of tumour penetration, the presence of lymph node metastases and the grade of malignancy are correlated but suggested that each variable might nevertheless have an independent effect on prognosis.

In a study aimed primarily at determining the effect of tumour site in relation to the peritoneal reflection as a prognostic determinant, Kirkland et al (1949) introduced a modification of Dukes' staging which has been widely used in the United States. This system recognized tumour confined to the mucosa (stage A), spread into but not beyond the muscularis propria (stage B1), spread beyond the muscularis propria (stage B2) and involvement of lymph nodes (stage C). In this study the authors used retrospective data from 131 patients with cancer of the rectum, rectosigmoid or lower sigmoid colon and who had undergone a 'curative' abdominoperineal resection at the Mayo Clinic between 1916 and 1940. A similar progressive fall in survival with advance in stage was recorded both for tumours above or below the peritoneal reflection. Deficiencies of this staging system are that it creates a stage for an infrequent group of tumours which for practical purposes have no metastatic potential (mucosal cancer) and it makes no provision for tumours which extend into the submucosa only.

Another modification of Dukes' staging was described by Astler & Coller (1954). This classification differed from that of Kirkland et al only in that stage C tumours were substaged into C1 and C2 depending on the extent of direct spread. For C1 tumours, direct spread did not extend beyond the muscularis propria while C2 tumours did involve direct spread beyond the muscularis propria. Astler & Coller illustrated the value of their classification by use of a retrospective series of 352 patients treated by curative or palliative resection at the University of Michigan between 1940 and 1944.

Like Dukes' classification, the Astler–Coller modification is purely pathological. It suffers the same shortcomings as have been attributed to the Kirkland et al classification and has led to some confusion by using the same symbols to subclassify stage C tumours according to the extent of direct spread as had previously been used by Dukes to indicate level of nodal involvement. The main contribution made by Astler–Coller staging was to stress the prognostic importance of the level of direct spread in stage C tumours. This has been confirmed by a number of subsequent studies (Jass & Love 1989, Newland et al 1994, Wolmark et al 1984). Others have further modified the Astler–Coller system specifically to identify those patients at greatest risk of developing pelvic recurrence from rectal cancer (Gunderson & Sosin 1974).

A major conceptual change in staging was introduced by Turnbull et al (1967) in an evaluation of the 'no touch isolation technique' for treating colonic cancer. For this analysis Turnbull created a stage D in which he categorized tumours found at operation to have either distant metastases or irremovable tumour because of parietal invasion or adjacent organ invasion. Modified Dukes' staging was used for less advanced tumours. Although Turnbull's retrospective analysis of 896 patients treated at the Cleveland Clinic was not primarily concerned with staging, his use of clinical findings at the time of operation to classify separately patients with incurable tumours or advanced local spread aroused interest in CP staging. As parietal or adjacent organ invasion by tumour does not necessarily imply incurability (Polk 1972), Turnbull's stage D contains a prognostically diverse group of patients. Turnbull himself stated that some of those patients he classified as having stage D tumour due to adjacent organ invasion were treated by resection with the intention to cure (Turnbull 1970). The Turnbull modification of Dukes' staging as defined cannot therefore be used to categorize incurable tumours separately.

The applicability of modified Dukes' staging to both colonic and rectal cancer was confirmed by Shepherd & Jones (1971) in a study of 656 consecutive patients treated by resection at the Middlesex Hospital over the period 1951–61. The 'palliative' cases in this study were analysed separately and were defined as those in which the surgeon considered that there was residual tumour. Not surprisingly, the palliative group of patients had the poorest survival. One problem with this definition of a palliative case is that surgeons are not always able to judge accurately whether they have achieved complete local clearance of tumour. The distinction between tumour and a fibrous reaction around tumour ultimately depends on histological examination.

To this point staging systems had been arbitrarily assembled, based on expectations of tumour behaviour, and then subjected to testing by the accumulation of survival data. A case for analysing the contribution of individual clinical and pathological variables to survival before the formulation of stages was advanced by Spratt & Spjut (1967). In a retrospective study of 1137 patients these authors presented a univariate survival analysis on many individual clinical and pathology variables. However, the limitations of statistical techniques available at the time prevented them from determining the degree of independence of these variables as predictors of survival.

This line of approach was pursued by Watson et al (1976) who used analysis of variance to generate a prognostic score for a range of tumour, host and treatment variables. The expected survival of a particular patient could then be calculated by summing weighted scores for all relevant variables. While this method of prognostication does not fall within the definition of staging, it represents an important initial attempt to develop the concept of a prognostic index, though analysis of variance is an inappropriate statistical method in this context.

The American Joint Committee for Cancer (AJCC) (1977) published recommendations for the staging of colon and rectal cancer which followed the TNM principles established by the Union International Contre Le Cancer (UICC) (1968) for the staging of cancer. The system consisted of five major stages which were dependent on the extent of direct spread of tumour (T), the presence of lymph node metastases (N) and the presence of distant metastases (M) at the time of operation. It therefore incorporated the concept of CP staging. Alphanumeric symbols representing the prognostic variables were used to define each stage. As the system was based on postsurgical treatment information it was designated pTNM staging. The decision to unify the staging of colonic and rectal cancer and to use direct spread, lymph node status and the existence of distant metastases as the prognostic variables was based on a retrospective study of 1826 cases (924 colonic and 902 rectal) from 10 institutions using multiple regression analysis (Wood et al 1979).

The results of testing the system using prospectively collected data (Hermanek 1983) has led to a number of changes to the categories of direct spread and lymph node status. The current version (AJCC 1992) subdivides stage III tumours into N1 (1–3 pericolic or perirectal nodes), N2 (four or more pericolic or perirectal nodes) and N3 (metastases in any lymph node along a named vascular trunk). Cases in which there has been tumour transection can only be separately categorized by the use of an additional residual tumour (R) classification as there is no special provision for them in any pTNM stage. In 1986 agreement was reached between the UICC and the AJCC on a uniform pTNM classification (Hermanek 1986). However, use of the R classification in the unified system remains optional.

As it is clearly important to classify cases in which there has been transection of tumour separately, a recommendation was made by an international working party on CP staging to make this obligatory (Fielding et al 1991a).

When the R classification is used the unified pTNM staging system is comprehensive and has been shown to correlate well with prognosis (Hermanek 1989). Its objective in attempting to achieve uniformity in staging is commendable. The main impediments to its general use lie in its relative complexity and in the additional time required to categorized the level of lymph node spread as described in the current version. Use of the term 'residual tumour' to apply only to the locally incomplete removal of tumour is potentially confusing as any tumour remaining after surgery may be considered residual whether it be due to tumour transection or metastases remaining. Inclusion of the R2 classification for macroscopic residual tumour may encourage the surgeon or even the pathologist to consider that a gross examination is an acceptable means of determining the adequacy of local tumour removal. However, as has been indicated, this should always be determined by histological assessment.

By using various groupings of pTNM defined variables (AJCC 1977) and by adding an additional variable relating to the level of lymph node spread and a category for tumour not resected, Hermanek et al (1980) generated five prognostic groups. Support for this prognostic classification was derived from data on 1439 patients with colorectal cancer recorded by the Erlangen Clinicopathologic Registry of Colorectal Tumours between 1969 and 1977. The greater efficacy of this form of prognostic grouping compared with Dukes' staging in identifying those patients with either a very good or a very poor prognosis was demonstrated.

Hermanek & Altendorf (1981) subsequently published support for the division of pTNM stage III into those with only local node involvement and those with proximal node involvement in which the nodes along major vessels contained metastases. This approach was shown to be of greater value in identifying those with a poor prognosis than a subdivision which distinguished only local and marginal lymph node involvement. The marginal node was defined as the one located most distant from the tumour and most proximal to the resected edge of mesocolon. However, it should be noted that this node does not necessarily correspond with the apical node as used by Dukes to define C2 tumours. The observation was also made that among patients with only local lymph node involvement, the number of nodes containing metastases had no influence on prognosis.

In 1971 a modification of Dukes' staging which included a carefully defined stage D for cases with known metastases remaining after bowel resection (clinical or histological) or histologically proven transection of tumour was used in a prospective study of colorectal cancer at Concord Hospital in Sydney (Table 4.1). Each of the four stages were divided into substages according to the extent of tumour spread. The subdivision of stage C was that originally introduced by Dukes (Gabriel et al 1935). A survival analysis on the first 503 patients was reported and a comparison made with Dukes' staging (Newland et al 1981). The Concord Hospital CP staging system demonstrated a significantly poorer survival of patients with stage C tumours and effectively segregated patients with incurable tumours (stage D) but showed surprisingly little difference in survival between those with stages A or B tumours. This was due to the identification of patients with stage D tumours who would otherwise have been classified in either stage A or stage B. A more detailed evaluation of substaging using the Concord Hospital Staging System based on 1117 cases was published by Newland et al (1987) and is dealt with later in this chapter.

In 1983 following two workshops on staging held in Brisbane and attended by both surgeons and pathologists, recommendations for an Australian clinicopathological staging (ACPS) system were published (Davis & Newland 1983). This system differed from the Concord Hospital method only in that mucosal cancer (Concord substage A1) was classified as stage zero and in the interests of simplicity, substaging was not included.

The staging system developed by the Japanese Research Society for carcinoma of the colon and rectum, which was published in English by Jinnai (1983), incorporated CP staging principles in that it created a separate stage for tumours with liver or remote organ metastases. Another feature of the Japanese system was the definition of three levels of tumour spread to lymph nodes in the operative specimen. This was based on the distance of the involved node(s) from the tumour edge. A classification of bowel resections determined by the extent of lymph node clearance was also described.

During the 1980s there were a number of attempts to assess the relative prognostic importance of a range of histological and clinical variables. Following Broders' initiative (Rankin & Broders 1928), Dukes (1932) histologically graded as well as staged rectal cancer, though details of his grading system were never published. He demonstrated a relationship between stage, grade,

Table 4.1 Concord Hospital staging and substaging definitions

Stage	Substage	Spread
A	A1	Not beyond mucosa
	A2	Into submucosa but not beyond
	A3	Into muscularis propria but not beyond
B	B1	Beyond muscularis propria, free serosal surface not invaded, no lymph node metastases, no tumour in lines of resection, no distant metastases
	B2*	As for substage B1 but with free serosal surface invasion
C	C1	Metastatic spread to local lymph nodes irrespective of depth of direct spread of tumour, no tumour in lines of resection, no distant metastases.
	C2	Metastatic spread to an apical lymph node, irrespective of depth of direct spread of tumour, no tumour in lines of resection, no distant metastases.
D (residual tumour)	D1	Tumour involving a line of resection (histological)
	D2	Distant metastases, i.e. metastases not removed in continuity with the bowel resection specimen (clinical or histological)

* Because the distal portion of the rectum lacks a peritoneal covering, tumours in this region cannot be classified as substage B2.

venous spread and survival (Dukes & Bussey 1958) but regarded grading as subservient to staging (Jass et al 1986). It was subsequently shown using stratified univariate analysis that grade (Newland et al 1981) and venous invasion (Talbot et al 1980) had prognostic effects which were independent of CP stage. The adverse effect of venous invasion was most dramatic when thickwalled extramural veins were involved. The issue as to whether grade and venous invasion contributed effects which were independent of each other remained unresolved.

Using data from 2518 patients in a large British multicentre study of colorectal cancer, an attempt was made to evaluate the independent prognostic effects of a range of pathology variables (Phillips et al 1984). Patients in this prospective study had all undergone curative surgery between 1976 and 1980. Using a form of stratified analysis it was concluded that, despite interrelationships between lymph node status, tumour grade and vascular invasion, each contributed independent prognostic information. Extent of direct spread, apical node involvement and the number of nodes involved also had independent effects on the survival of patients with nodal metastases. One problem encountered by this study was the non-uniformity of histopathology reporting of large bowel cancer (Blenkinsopp et al 1981).

To investigate the independent prognostic effects of a range of clinical and pathology variables, including CP stage, multivariate analysis using the Cox regression model was applied to data from 709 patients in the Concord Hospital series (Chapuis et al 1985a). The results showed CP stage to have by far the most potent independent prognostic effect. Significant but lesser effects were recorded for other pathology variables (grade, venous invasion and direct spread) as well as for some clinical variables (age, sex and obstruction). A similar broad analysis was made using the UK multicentre study database; however, different statistical methods were used and stage was not included as a separate variable (Fielding et al 1986). In addition to pathology variables relating to nodal involvement, vascular invasion and depth of primary penetration, clinical variables including presentation (emergency or routine), obstruction, tumour mobility, cardiopulmonary complications, intraabdominal sepsis and age were shown to exert independent prognostic effects. This study did not detect any independent effect of tumour differentiation.

Data collected as part of a prospective clinical trial which was commenced in the United States in 1977 were also used to study staging. This national project was designed primarily to assess the value of adjuvant therapy in the treatment of large bowel cancer (NSABP Clinical Trial; Wolmark et al 1983a). Only patients treated by curative resection who had tumours assigned to a modified Dukes' B or C stage were included in the study. It should be noted that the results from the study of prognostic factors using this series could, at least theoretically, be influenced by the different forms of treatment employed. Findings relevant to staging were as follows:

1. Tumour size did not correlate with the presence or absence of regional lymph node involvement (Wolmark et al 1983a).
2. Location was a strong prognostic determinant with rectal tumours carrying the worst prognosis (Wolmark et al 1983b).
3. Within Dukes' stage C, depth of tumour penetration had a positive correlation with both tumour size and the number of positive regional lymph nodes; when depth of penetration was controlled statistically there was no correlation between tumour size and the number of positive nodes (Wolmark et al 1984).
4. The prognosis of patients with Dukes' stage C tumours was determined by depth of penetration and the number of involved nodes (1–4 and >4) acting as independent variables. The level of nodal involvement ('near', <2 cm from the bowel wall, or 'far') provided little additional information (Wolmark et al 1986).

In a later study on the NSABP Clinical Trial material to which information on Dukes' stage A cases and cases with proven visceral metastases had been added, it was concluded that the further subdivision of Dukes' stage A tumours was not justified and that Dukes' stage C tumours should be classified according to the level of direct tumour penetration and the number of involved lymph nodes (Fisher et al 1989). When compared with the Astler–Coller and TNM staging systems these authors found Dukes' staging method to be the 'simplest and most consistent algorithm related to prognosis' (Fisher et al 1989).

Another source of data used in the assessment of aspects of staging was that compiled by the Gastrointestinal Tumor Study Group (GITSG) in the United States. As with the NSABP Clinical Trial, the aim was to determine the effects of adjuvant therapy on patients with Dukes' stages B or C tumours who had 'curative' resections. The GITSG trial, which began in 1975, addressed colonic cancer exclusively. The conclusions drawn which were relevant to staging were:

1. Tumour site within the colon was of little prognostic importance (Steinberg et al 1986a);
2. Tumour morphology was an important independent prognostic variable.

Exophytic tumours were found to have a more favourable prognosis than non-exophytic and the greater the maximum tumour dimension the poorer the prognosis (Steinberg et al 1986b).

A new prognostic classification for rectal cancer was proposed by Jass et al (1987) following a retrospective study of patients treated by 'curative' surgery at St Mark's Hospital. As well as the conventional variables relating to stage, a range of histopathological variables defining aspects of tumour grade were included in a multivariate analysis to test for independent prognostic effects. The prognostic classification based on the results of this analysis which included both stage- and grade-related variables was considered by the authors to be superior to Dukes' staging because it allowed the placement of many more patients into groups in which a confident prediction of outcome was possible. This study served to draw attention to the prognostic importance of certain grade-related variables when compared with variables used in staging. The variables related to grade which had significant independent effects were seen as reflecting important aspects of the host/tumour relationship. The practicality of this system for general use has yet to be established.

The case for CP staging was strengthened by the production of a clinicopathological staging booklet by the UK Coordinating Committee on Cancer Research (1989) which provided definitions of non-curative and curative operations. The recommendation was that only curative cases be classified in the manner described by Dukes into A, B or C. The presence of distant metastases, tumour in a margin of excision demonstrated histologically or perforation of the specimen (spontaneously or operatively) were given as the criteria for a non-curative operation. A third category, namely indeterminate for cure, was also recognized. Recommendations contained in the booklet were discussed by Williams et al (1988). The advisability of regarding perforation of the specimen per se as grounds for classifying an operation as non-curative has been questioned (Fielding 1988).

In a pilot prospective study of 597 patients with rectal cancer treated by curative resection Hermanek et al (1989) demonstrated, using multivariate analysis, that the influence of various prognostic factors, including the components of stage, varied between pTNM substages. By recording the number of adverse factors in each tumour substage further prognostic classification was possible. Attention was also drawn to the need to assess prognostic factors for colon and rectum separately because of potential site-related differences.

The concept of prognostic grouping, as distinct from tumour staging, was further developed by Hermanek et al (1990). It was suggested that prognostic grouping should involve the evaluation by multivariate analysis of a wide range of potential prognostic variables and the integration of those with significant independent effects with tumour stage. By this means prognostic accuracy would be enhanced. The need to assess the additional prognostic factors separately for the different tumour stages was again emphasized. The point was also made that a range of clinical and pathological variables with proven independent prognostic effects may be combined using an appropriate mathematical formula to generate a prognostic index. This index is a measure of the risk faced by an individual patient for a particular outcome (e.g. tumour recurrence, survival, etc.).

Since the creation of TNM-based staging systems for colorectal cancer by the UICC and the AJCC, there have been a number of other attempts to achieve uniformity in staging, at least at a national level (Davis & Newland 1983, Williams et al 1988). A committee established by the American Society of Colon and Rectal Surgeons to review 'staging' systems produced a document recommending the recording of a range of stage-related variables which were consistent with the most recent recommendations of the TNM system (Fielding 1988). In 1987 the proceedings of an international symposium on the staging of colorectal cancer were published (Chapuis et al 1987). This symposium explored the strengths and weaknesses of the various staging systems. While there was general support by the participants for an internationally agreed staging system there was no uniformity of opinion on how this might be achieved.

A working party was appointed under the auspices of the 1990 World Congresses of Gastroenterology to report on CP staging for colorectal cancer (Fielding et al 1991a). The eight-member working party was drawn from four countries and included pathologists, surgeons and a statistician. The resulting report included a critical assessment of the six most commonly used staging systems. It also made recommendations for an international documentation system (IDS) and an international comprehensive anatomical terminology (ICAT) for colorectal cancer. The IDS consists of a minimal list of clinical and pathology features for documentation in prospective studies. The ICAT defines the spread of colorectal cancer in a manner which enables the use of any of the six commonly used staging systems. By using the IDS and ICAT recommendations the problems of selecting suitable patients for clinical trials and of comparing results between treatment centres should be minimized.

The Concord Hospital experience in clinicopathological staging

Background

Concord Hospital is a 750-bed teaching hospital attached to the University of Sydney. From its establishment in 1942 until July 1993, Concord was primarily involved in the treatment of war veterans and their dependants. It subsequently became a general community hospital.

As a hospital involved with the care of a predominantly elderly male population, colorectal cancer was a commonly encountered disease. The opportunity for patient follow-up in this veterans' institution was excellent. For these reasons a decision was made in 1970 by the Departments of Surgery and Anatomical Pathology to initiate a long-term prospective study of the disease.

During the planning phase of the study a decision was required on the method of tumour staging. The principles underlying the development of a staging system required a consideration of the possible mechanisms of tumour spread: direct, lymphatic, vascular and transcoelomic. Another consideration was that the stages should be defined by readily identifiable anatomical features.

In 1970 Dukes' staging was the most widely recognized system internationally and was the one most often used in Australia. It had considerable appeal as it was a simple classification which was easy to recall and had a well-established correlation with patient survival. It also complied with a number of the above principles. The intrinsic limitation of the system as defined by Dukes was that it was based exclusively on the findings in the resected specimen. The system therefore could not separately identify patients who had bowel resections but were known to have residual tumour. To issue a pathology report giving the Dukes' stage and to then rely on the clinician(s) receiving the report knowing whether the operation had been curative or palliative seemed to introduce the risk of misinterpretation. Should the clinician receiving the pathology report not know the operative findings, the Dukes' stage could be quite misleading as a guide to prognosis for that particular patient.

Fortuitously, while the issue of staging was under consideration, Rupert Turnbull visited the hospital and described his use of a CP stage D to classify patients with distant metastases and/or locally advanced tumour. As a result of this visit it was decided to develop a CP staging system for use in the Concord Hospital study. The system ultimately accepted was essentially a modification of Dukes' staging in which patients with known residual tumour were separately classified as having stage D tumour (see Table 4.1). Each tumour stage was subdivided into two or more substages according to the extent of tumour spread in order to test for any within-stage difference in prognosis. The subclassification of stage C was that described by Dukes (Gabriel et al 1935). In addition, a range of individual pathology variables was recorded for each case. As the data were to be stored on computer, reclassification into other staging systems and the testing of many pathology variables for their individual prognostic significance were facilitated.

A fundamental requirement for CP staging is the transmission to the pathologist of the operative findings. Without the cooperation of the surgeons required to provide this information, CP staging is not possible. From the beginning of the Concord study use was made of a simple proforma completed by the surgeon at the end of the operation and sent with the specimen to the laboratory. Two essential questions on the proforma were (1) were there metastases remaining and (2) if so, was a biopsy taken? The decision as to whether there was residual tumour due to transection of tumour by the surgeon was always determined by histological means.

To minimize pathologist-related variation in recording findings in the specimen, a standardized approach was used. Surgeons were asked to send unfixed specimens to the laboratory immediately after resections performed during normal working hours. After hours the surgeons were encouraged to open and clean the bowel before placing it in formalin. Specimens opened in the laboratory were immersed in a tank of formalin and kept open by means of a perspex overlay. Specimen dissection was undertaken after a minimum fixation time of 48 hours. Macroscopic variables recorded included site, tumour configuration (polypoid, ulcerating, fungating or stenosing) and maximum surface dimension. Blocks were selected to show the full profile of the tumour through the point of deepest penetration and the relationship of the tumour to the surgical lines of resection and free serosal surface (if present). Blocks to record evidence of adjacent structure or vascular invasion were also taken. The apical lymph node(s), defined as the most proximal of any node(s) found within 10 mm of the level of vessel ligation at the apex of the vascular pedicle, was separately identified. Lymph nodes were harvested using a 'bacon slicer' technique supplemented by palpation. Fat clearing techniques were not used.

Tumours were classified as mucinous or non-mucinous adenocarcinoma and were assessed as either high-grade or other. The presence of venous invasion was recorded only when the findings were unequivocal. Further standardization has been achieved in that more than 90% of specimen dissections were performed by the one pathologist (RN) who also reported or reviewed all of the histology and entered all of the pathology data into the study. Since 1979 all clinical data entry and patient follow-up has been the responsibility of one clinician (PC).

In survival analyses all patients with tumour confined to the mucosa (substage A1) and those who had familial adenomatous polyposis or inflammatory bowel disease were excluded. When synchronous carcinomas were present only data on the tumour with the most advanced stage were used.

Findings

Staging

A key element of CP staging is the accuracy with which tumours are classified as stage D (approximately 20% of all cases). This aspect of CP staging was examined using the first 369 patients in the series so classified (Newland et al 1993). Histological confirmation of distant metastases, though desirable, was obtained in only 37% of cases. However, survival studies demonstrated that a false-positive diagnosis was most unlikely in patients for whom clinical findings alone were used. Survival studies also validated the use of histological demonstration of tumour in a line of resection as a criterion of incurability. The definition of stage D used in this study has therefore been shown to be an acceptable means of identifying patients with known residual tumour.

The comparative results of CP staging versus Dukes' method applied to the same patients have been described previously (Chapuis et al 1985b) and are shown graphically using recent data (Figs 4.1 & 4.2). The following observations are noteworthy:

1. There was no difference in survival between patients with stage A tumours in either system.
2. There was little difference in survival between patients with tumours classified as stage B by the two systems.
3. In relation to stages A and B a pronounced reduction in survival was displayed by patients with stage C tumours in both systems. Thus lymph node metastases, even in the absence of known residual tumour, have a potent prognostic effect. However, patients with CP stage C tumour had noticeably better survival than those with Dukes' stage C tumour. This was a consequence of the CP system having transferred the relatively high proportion of cases in Dukes' stage C with residual tumour (33%) and hence poor survival into stage D.

Substaging

Univariate analysis was used to test for the prognostic importance of finer distinctions of tumour spread within each CP stage (Newland et al 1987). From a more recent survival analysis using 1878 patients the following was noted:

1. The survival of patients with substage A2 tumour was significantly better than for those with substage A3 tumour (p<0.001, Fig. 4.3).
2. The survival of patients with substage A3 was no different to that of those with substage B1 tumour (p = 0.62, Fig. 4.3).
3. The survival of patients with substage B2 tumour was significantly worse than that of those with substage B1 tumour (p = 0.012, Fig. 4.3). Another finding was that the 18 patients with CP stage B tumour who also had invasion of an adjacent structure showed no difference in survival when compared with the remainder of the group (p = 0.388). Only one of these 18 patients had a substage B2 tumour.

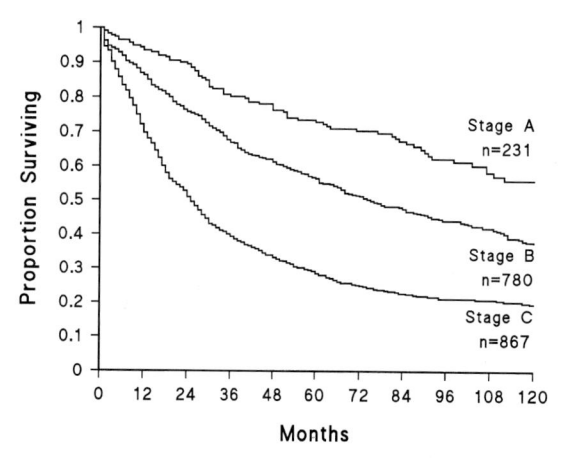

Fig. 4.1 Survival by Dukes' stage (n = 1878).

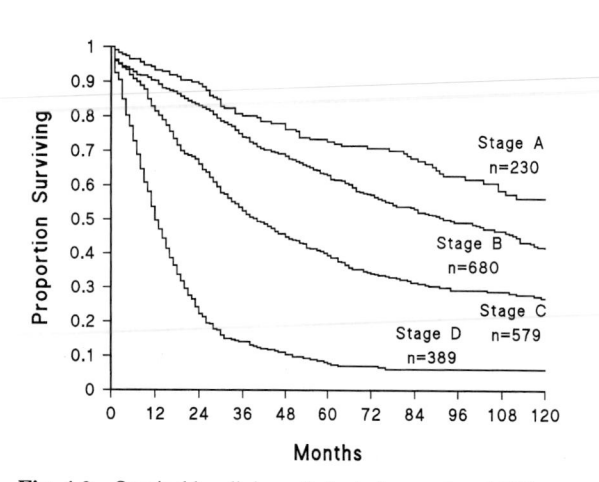

Fig. 4.2 Survival by clinicopathological stage (n = 1878).

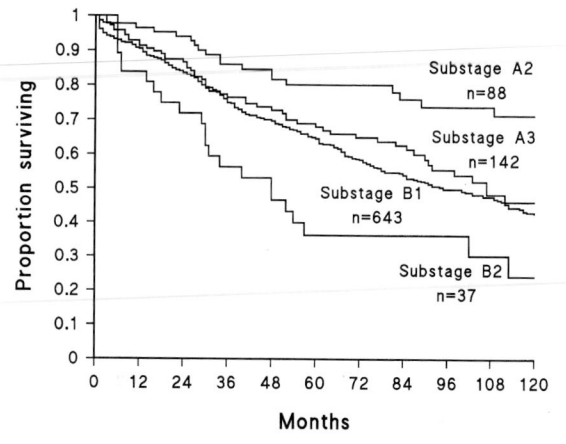

Fig. 4.3 Survival by the substages of clinicopathological stages A (n = 230) and B (n = 680).

4. Patients with substage C2 tumour had a significantly poorer prognosis than those with substage C1 tumour (p<0.001, Fig. 4.4).

5. The survival of patients with substage D2 tumour was significantly poorer than that of those with substage D1 tumour (p = 0.03, Fig. 4.5).

The above findings indicate significant variation in patient survival within all four CP stages when substaging is performed in the manner described. As patients with substage A3 tumour and those with substage B1 tumour made up most of the stage A and stage B cases respectively and there was no survival difference between these two substages, there seems no reason to continue to separate CP stages A and B. Within the composite stage A-B, patients with tumour spread limited to the submucosa and those with spread involving the free serosal surface had a significantly better or worse prognosis respectively than the remainder. It follows from our findings that involvement of a free serosal surface is the only information required on the extent of direct spread beyond the muscularis propria in this composite stage.

Multivariate analysis of pathology variables

The possibility that other pathology variables might add to or modify the prognostic information obtained from CP staging was examined in a series of survival analyses. As it was conceivable that the effects of other variables might vary between stages, a multivariate analysis was performed within each CP stage separately. The confounding variables of age and sex were included in each analysis along with the pathology variables previously referred to.

Stage D Details of the results of an analysis on the first 369 patients in the study with stage D tumour are given elsewhere (Newland et al 1993). Although lymph node metastases, venous invasion, grade, tumour transection and distant metastases exerted significant univariate effects on survival, only the latter two variables had significant independent effects in a multivariate model. Based on these findings, it was suggested that stage D tumours could be further classified as:

- D(1) – tumour transection only
- D(2) – distant metastases only
- D(3) – both tumour transection and distant metastases.

The median survival for each category was 13.8, 11.9 and 7.6 months respectively. A fourth category, D(0), was suggested for those with synchronous distant metastases surgically removed and no known tumour remaining.

Stage C An analysis performed on the first 579 patients with stage C tumour has been reported (Newland et al 1994). Using the Cox proportional

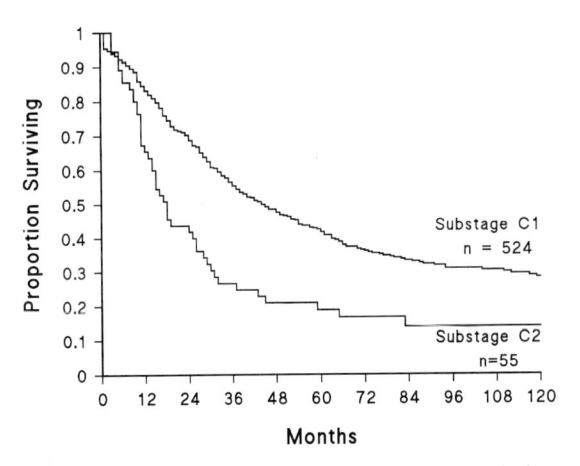

Fig. 4.4 Survival by the substages of clinicopathological stage C (n = 579).

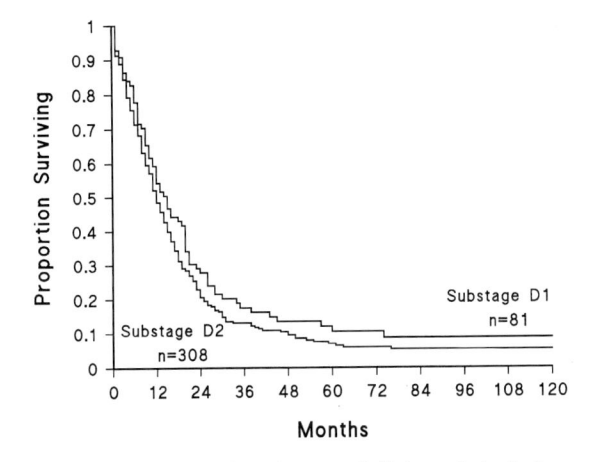

Fig. 4.5 Survival by the substages of clinicopathological stage D (n = 389).

hazards regression model and after controlling for age and sex, significant independent effects on survival in diminishing potency were shown for the following: apical node involvement; spread involving a free serosal surface; spread beyond the muscularis propria; location in the rectum; venous invasion and high tumour grade. In univariate analysis the number of involved lymph nodes had a strong association with prognosis but this disappeared in the multivariate model. Furthermore, replacement of the apical node variable by the number of involved lymph nodes in our trimmed model still did not show a significant independent prognostic effect for this variable. The other variables in the model retained approximately the same coefficients and levels of significance which were recorded in the original trimmed model. It was concluded that the number of involved lymph nodes could not substitute for the apical node variable.

These findings lend support to the use of both the apical node status and the presence of spread beyond the muscularis propria for the prognostic stratification of stage C tumours. These variables were originally used in the Dukes' and Astler–Coller pathologic classifications respectively. For the optimum stratification of stage C tumours, use should be made of all six pathology variables identified as exerting significant independent effects.

Stages A and B A preliminary analysis on stage A and stage B cases combined (n = 910) showed that, after controlling for the effects of age and sex, only spread beyond the submucosa and histological grade had significant independent prognostic effects (unpublished observations). Neither spread beyond the muscularis propria nor involvement of a free serosal surface had a significant independent effect on survival. The failure of the latter to show a significant effect may have been due to the small number of cases (n = 37). Venous invasion was present in 114 cases but was unrelated to survival.

It is noteworthy that tumour site (colon/rectum) and venous invasion exerted significant independent prognostic effects in CP stage C tumours only.

Conclusions

By using a precise definition of the term 'residual tumour' our method of CP staging has enabled the effective segregation of those patients known to have incurable disease at the time of resection (stage D). This process requires cooperation between surgeons and pathologists but has been shown by this ongoing 24-year study to be practicable within a large teaching hospital.

Tumour substages based on clearly identifiable anatomical structures were assessed in terms of their relevance to patient survival. The findings suggested that CP stages A and B should be combined. The only stage-related variables within this composite group which were of prognostic significance were spread beyond the submucosa and spread involving a free serosal surface.

Within CP stage C, the prognostically significant independent stage-related variables were apical node involvement, spread involving a free serosal surface and spread beyond the muscularis propria. Another spread variable, venous invasion, also exerted a significant independent effect. Thus within CP and stage C, independent prognostic influences were recorded for those variables which represented sites from which distant metastases were likely to have developed. As the mechanism of spread linked to each of these variables is different, i.e. lymphatic, venous and transcoelomic, it is understandable that these variables had independent effects.

The only stage-related variables exerting significant independent prognostic effects within stage D were distant metastases and tumour transection.

It should be appreciated that despite the investigation of numerous clinical and laboratory variables, 'a description of the anatomic spread of the tumour remains the most powerful statement of patient survival time of all prognostic factors' (Fielding et al 1991b). It is appropriate therefore that our findings be used for the initial prognostic stratification of patients with colorectal cancer. They have the advantages of being based on the results of multivariate analyses performed on a large series of patients from one institution and of not requiring sophisticated laboratory methods. It is suggested that because the prognostic effects of variables may differ, depending on the stage and site of the tumour, these factors be taken into account when putative prognostic variables are being assessed.

Lack of standardization of clinical assessment has been raised as a problem with CP staging (Williams et al 1988). Obviously the more sensitive the means of detecting distant metastases, the fewer patients with residual tumour will be classified as having CP stage A, B or C tumours. This effect is referred to as 'stage migration' (Feinstein et al 1985) and in this instance it will result in an apparent improvement in the survival of the patients with stage A, B or C tumours. It should be appreciated that methods of detecting distant metastases differ in their effectiveness and in the context of randomized studies uniform methods of assessing the clinical and pathological extent of tumour spread should be employed (Fielding et al 1991a).

The more effective the means of detecting residual tumour, the less will be the differences in survival of patients with tumours staged as having no known residual tumour. The extreme extension of this effect would be to leave only two stages of tumour spread depending on the presence or absence of residual tumour alone. Clearly this ultimate goal of CP staging, if attainable, lies well in the future.

References

American Joint Committee for Cancer 1977 Staging and end results reporting. Manual for staging of cancer. AJCC, Chicago

American Joint Committee for Cancer 1992 Staging and end results reporting. Manual for staging of cancer. AJCC, Chicago

Astler VB, Coller FA 1954 The prognostic significance of direct extension of carcinoma of the colon and rectum. Annals of Surgery 139: 846–851

Blenkinsopp WK, Stewart-Brown S, Blesovsky L, Kearney G, Fielding LP 1981 Histopathology reporting in large bowel cancer. Journal of Clinical Pathology 34: 509–513

Chapuis PH, Dent OF, Fisher R et al 1985a A multivariate analysis of clinical and pathological variables in prognosis after resection of large bowel cancer. British Journal of Surgery 72: 698–702

Chapuis PH, Fisher R, Dent OF, Newland RC, Pheils MT 1985b The relationship between different staging methods and survival in colorectal carcinoma. Diseases of the Colon and Rectum 28: 158–161

Chapuis PH, Dixon MF, Fielding LP et al 1987 Symposium: staging of colorectal cancer. International Journal of Colorectal Disease 2: 123–138

Davis NC, Newland RC 1983 Terminology and classification of colorectal adenocarcinoma: the Australian clinico-pathological staging system. Australian and New Zealand Journal of Surgery 53: 211–221

Dukes CE 1932 The classification of cancer of the rectum. Journal of Pathology and Bacteriology 35: 323–332

Dukes CE, Bussey HJR 1958 The spread of rectal cancer and its effect on prognosis. British Journal of Cancer 12: 309–320

Feinstein AR, Sosin DM, Wells CK 1985 The Will Rogers phenomenon: stage migration and new diagnostic techniques as a source of misleading statistics for survival in cancer. New England Journal of Medicine 312: 1604–1608

Fielding LP 1988 Clinical-pathologic staging of large-bowel cancer: a report of the ASCRS Committee. Diseases of the Colon and Rectum 31: 204–209

Fielding LP, Phillips RK, Fry JS, Hittinger R 1986 Prediction of outcome after curative resection for large bowel cancer. Lancet 2: 904–907

Fielding LP, Arsenault PA, Chapuis PH et al 1991a Clinicopathological staging for colorectal cancer: an International Documentation System (IDS) and an International Comprehensive Anatomical Terminology (ICAT). Journal of Gastroenterology and Hepatology 6: 325–344

Fielding LP, Fenoglio-Preiser CM, Freedman LS 1991b The future of prognostic factors in outcome prediction for patients with cancer. Cancer 70: 2367–2377

Fisher ER, Sass R, Palekar A, Fisher B, Wolmark N 1989 Dukes' classification revisited: findings from the National Surgical Adjuvant Breast and Bowel Projects (Protocol R-01). Cancer 64: 2354–2360

Gabriel WB, Dukes C, Bussey HJR 1935 Lymphatic spread in cancer of the rectum. British Journal of Surgery 23: 395–413

Goligher JC 1976 The Dukes' A, B and C categorization of the extent of spread of carcinomas of the rectum. Surgery, Gynecology and Obstetrics 143: 793–794

Gunderson LI, Sosin H 1974 Areas of failure found at reoperation (second or symptomatic look) following 'curative surgery' for adenocarcinoma of the rectum – clinicopathologic correlation and implications for adjuvant therapy. Cancer 34: 1278–1292

Hermanek P 1983 Prospective study on pTNM classification of colorectal carcinoma. Journal of Experimental and Clinical Cancer Research 3: 277–281

Hermanek P 1986 The new TNM/pTNM classification of colorectal carcinomas – what has changed and why? Coloproctology 10: 6–12

Hermanek P, Altendorf A 1981 Classification of colorectal carcinomas with regional lymphatic metastases. Pathology, Research and Practice 173: 1–11

Hermanek P, Gall FP, Altendorf A 1980 Prognostic groups in colorectal carcinoma. Journal of Cancer Research in Clinical Oncology 98: 185–193

Hermanek P, Guggenmoos-Holzmann I, Gall FP 1989

Prognostic factors in rectal carcinoma: a contribution to the further development of tumour classification. Diseases of the Colon and Rectum 32: 593–599

Hermanek P, Hutter RVP, Sobin LH 1990 Prognostic grouping: the next step in tumour classification. Journal of Cancer Research and Clinical Oncology 116: 513–516

Jass JR, Love SB 1989 Prognostic value of direct spread in Dukes' C cases of rectal cancer. Diseases of the Colon and Rectum 32: 477–480

Jass JR, Atkin WS, Cusick J et al 1986 The grading of rectal cancer: historical perspectives and a multivariate analysis of 447 cases. Histopathology 10: 437–459

Jass JR, Love SB, Northover JMA 1987 A new prognostic classification of rectal cancer. Lancet 1: 1303–1306

Jinnai D 1983 General rules for clinical and pathological studies on cancer of the colon, rectum and anus. Part I: Clinical classification. Japanese Journal of Surgery 13: 557–573

Kirkland JW, Dockerty MB, Waugh JM 1949 The role of the peritoneal reflection in the prognosis of carcinoma of the rectum and sigmoid colon. Surgery, Gynecology and Obstetrics 88: 326–331

Lockhart-Mummery JP 1927 Two hundred cases of cancer of the rectum treated by perineal excision. British Journal of Surgery 14: 110–124

Newland RC, Chapuis PH, Pheils MT, MacPherson JG 1981 The relationship of survival to staging and grading of colorectal carcinoma: a prospective study of 503 cases. Cancer 47: 1424–1429

Newland RC, Chapuis PH, Smyth EJ 1987 The prognostic value of substaging colorectal carcinoma: a prospective study of 1117 cases with standardized pathology. Cancer 60: 852–857

Newland RC, Dent OF, Chapuis PH, Bokey EL 1993 Clinicopathologically diagnosed residual tumour after resection for colorectal cancer: a 20-year prospective study. Cancer 72: 1536–1542

Newland RC, Dent OF, Lyttle MNB, Chapuis PH, Bokey EL 1994 Pathologic determinants of survival associated with colorectal cancer with lymph node metastases: a multivariate analysis of 579 patients. Cancer 73: 2076–2082

Nicholls RJ, Ritchie JK, Wadsworth J, Parks AG 1979 Total excision or restorative resection for carcinoma of the middle third of the rectum. British Journal of Surgery 66: 625–627

Phillips RKS, Hittinger R, Blesovsky L, Fry JS, Fielding LP 1984 Large bowel cancer: surgical pathology and its relationship to survival. British Journal of Surgery 71: 604–610

Polk HC 1972 Extended resection for selected adenocarcinomas of the large bowel. Annals of Surgery 175: 892–896

Rankin FW, Broders AC 1928 Factors influencing prognosis in carcinoma of the rectum. Surgery, Gynecology and Obstetrics 46: 660–667

Shepherd JM, Jones JSP 1971 Adenocarcinoma of the large bowel. British Journal of Cancer 25: 680–690

Simpson WC, Mayo CW 1939 Mural penetration of the carcinoma cell in the colon: anatomic and clinical study. Surgery, Gynecology and Obstetrics 68: 872–877

Spratt JS, Spjut HJ 1967 Prevalence and prognosis of individual clinical and pathologic variables associated with colorectal carcinoma. Cancer 20: 1976–1985

Steinberg SM, Barkin JS, Kaplan RS, Stablein DM 1986a Prognostic indicators of colon tumours. Cancer 57: 1866–1870

Steinberg SM, Barwick KW, Stablein DM 1986b Importance of tumour pathology and morphology in patients with surgically resected colon cancer: findings from the Gastrointestinal Tumor Study Group. Cancer 58: 1340–1345

Talbot IC, Ritchie S, Leighton MH, Hughes AO, Bussey HJR, Morson B C 1980 The clinical significance of invasion of veins by rectal cancer. British Journal of Surgery 67: 439–442

Turnbull RB 1970 Cancer of the colon. The five-and ten-year survival rates following resection utilizing the isolation technique. Annals of the Royal College of Surgeons of England 46: 243–250

Turnbull RB, Kyle K, Watson FR, Spratt J 1967 Cancer of the colon: the influence of the no-touch isolation technique on survival rates. Annals of Surgery 166: 420–425

UK Coordinating Committee on Cancer Research 1989 Clinicopathological staging booklet. UKCCCR, London

Union Internationale Contre Le Cancer 1968 TNM classification of malignant tumours. UICC, Geneva

Watson FR, Spratt JS, LeDuc RJ 1976 Analysis of variance and covariance for colorectal adenocarcinomas in man as a logical prelude to 'staging'. Journal of Surgical Oncology 8: 155–163

Williams NS, Jass JR, Hardcastle JD 1988 Clinicopathological assessment and staging of colorectal cancer. British Journal of Surgery 75: 649–652

Wolmark N, Cruz I, Redmond CK, Fisher B, Fisher ER 1983a Tumour size and regional lymph node metastasis in colorectal cancer: a preliminary analysis from the NSABP clinical trials. Cancer 51: 1315–1322

Wolmark N, Wieand HS, Rockette HE et al 1983b The prognostic significance of tumour location and bowel obstruction in Dukes B and C colorectal cancer. Annals of Surgery 198: 743–752

Wolmark N, Fisher ER, Wieand HS, Fisher B 1984 The relationship of depth of penetration and tumour size to the number of positive nodes in Dukes C colorectal cancer. Cancer 53: 2707–2712

Wolmark N, Fisher B, Wieand HS 1986 The prognostic value of the modifications of the Dukes' C class of colorectal cancer. Annals of Surgery 203: 115–122

Wood DA, Robbins GF, Zippin C, Lum D, Stearns M 1979 Staging of cancer of the colon and cancer of the rectum. Cancer 43: 961–968

5 Sphincter-saving resection and total reconstruction for low rectal cancer

N. S. WILLIAMS

The last 20 years have seen an explosion in sphincter-saving resection for carcinoma of the rectum. There are several factors that have been responsible for this. The introduction of mechanical circular stapling devices is one of the most important reasons. Since Fain et al (1975) returned from Moscow with the Russian SPTU gun and demonstrated the feasibility of the technique to surgeons in the West, there has been a gradual improvement in design and technique. With the disposable instrument and its detachable head, it is now possible to perform a sphincter-saving resection (SSR) for most low rectal cancers (Fig. 5.1). Even if a stapled anastomosis cannot be performed for technical reasons, the surgeon can often resort to a transanal coloanal anastomosis (Parks 1972) (Fig. 5.2). The latter expertise has become more widespread as a result of greater experience with restorative proctocolectomy and local transanal procedures.

Not only do we now have the expertise to perform these low colorectal and coloanal anastomoses, but there is abundant evidence that such techniques can be performed as safely as the gold standard operation, which is abdominoperineal excision of the rectum (APER) (Williams 1984). Thus morbidity and mortality rates are remarkably similar for the two operations (Table 5.1). Operative mortality in a study of patients with similar rectal carcinomas sited between 0–12 cm from the anal verge was 4% following APER and 7% following SSR (Williams et al 1985) which was not significantly different.

Another important factor which has led to the boom in sphincter preservation has been the

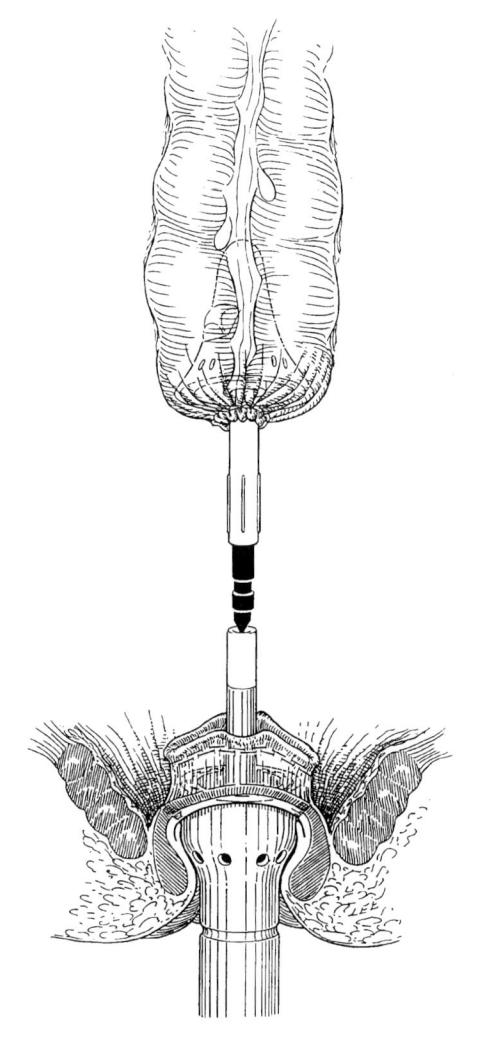

Fig. 5.1 Low colorectal anastomosis. Double stapling technique utilizing Premium CEEA gun. (From Williams N 1993. Surgery of the Anus, Rectum and Colon. WB Saunders, with permission.)

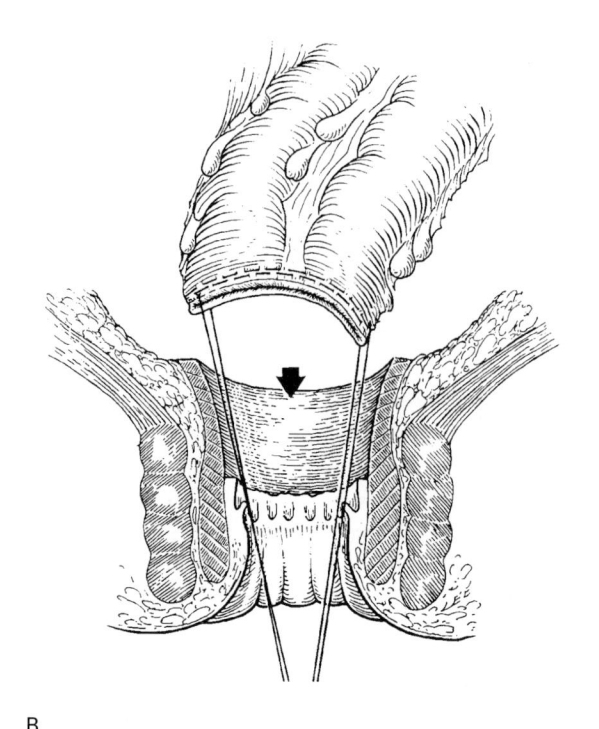

Fig. 5.2 Abdominotransanal technique to achieve coloanal anastomosis. (A) The abdominal phase, during which the rectum is transected at the level of the pelvic floor with a minimum of 2 cm of normal rectum below the tumour. (B) The stapled end of colon is brought down through the denuded anorectal cuff. (C) The coloanal anastomosis is constructed transanally. (From Williams N 1993. Surgery of the Anus, Rectum and Colon. WB Saunders, with permission.)

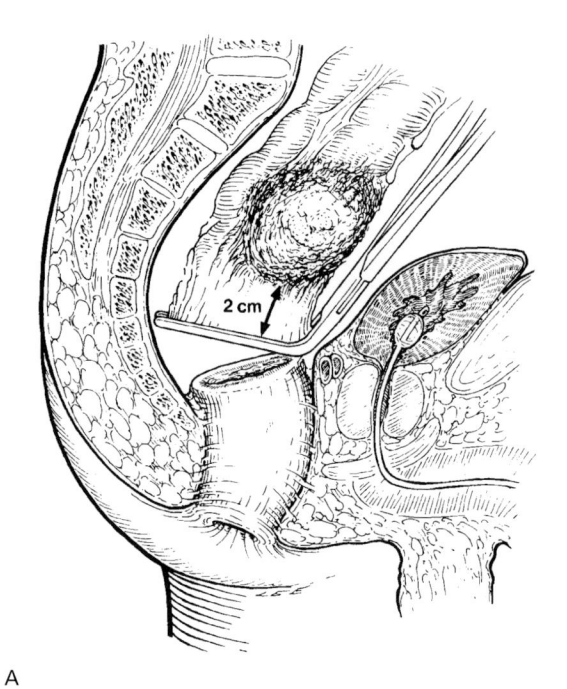

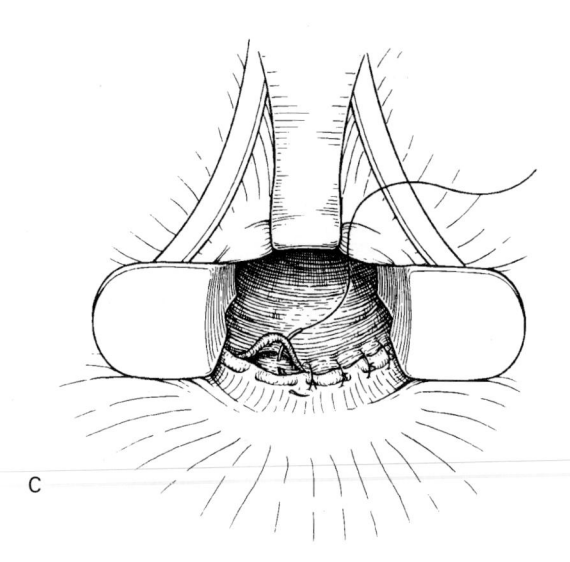

realization that it is no longer necessary to resect the tumour with a minimum margin of 5 cm of macroscopically normal rectum. Histopathological studies (Pollett & Nicholls 1983, Williams et al 1983) have demonstrated that distal intramural spread is rare, but when it does occur the tumour is advanced and patients are highly likely to die from distant metastases long before they develop local recurrence, no matter how much distal rectum has been excised. Retrospective studies comparing recurrence and survival in patients in whom the tumour was resected with a margin of greater or less than 5 cm have also shown no significant differences (Table 5.2).

Despite the change in philosophy and move away from an operation which leaves the patient with a permanent colostomy, there is no room for complacency. It is now clear that controlled trials comparing APER and SSR for low rectal cancers are not feasible. Nevertheless, the onus is to carefully collect prospective data to ensure that this change in philosophy is well-founded. Thus, we have to be convinced that recurrence and survival are not impaired and that anorectal function is reasonable. However, we must not stand still and we need to investigate ways in which the results, both in terms of survival and function, can be improved.

Table 5.1 Mortality and anastomotic leak rate after stapled low colorectal anastomosis

Authors	Total no. of patients	Height of tumour or anastomosis from anal verge (cm)	Mortality	Clinical leak rate
Fain et al (1975)	165	7–16	4 (2.4)	6 (3.6)
Goligher et al (1979)	24	Low	1 (4)	0
Ling et al (1979)	18	Below 5	0	3 (17)
Adolff et al (1980)	26	Mean 12	1 (3.8)	2 (7.7)
Bolton & Britton (1980)	22	Mean 14	0	1 (4.5)
Kirkegaard et al (1981)	30	7–12	1 (3.3)	2 (6.7)
Beart & Kelly (1981)	35*	Mean 13	1 (2.9)	1 (2.9)
	10	Below 6	0	1 (10)
Cade et al (1981)	32	Below 8	NS	3 (9.4)
Heald & Leicester (1981)	73*	2.5–12	NS	13 (17.8)
Kirwan (1981)		Mean 8	1 (3.3)	NS
Shahinian et al (1981)	29*	Low	0	1 (3.4)
Blamey & Lee (1982)		8–14	NS	3 (6)
Brennan et al (1982)	10	Low	0	1 (10)
Lazorthes et al (1986)	57	Below 8	NS	3 (5.3)
Fazio et al (1985)	79	Low	NS	1 (1.3)
Antonsen & Fronberg (1987)	178	Low	NS	27 (15)
Belli et al (1988)	74	Low	NS	3 (4)
Griffen et al (1989)	75	Low	NS	2 (2.7)

*Includes some patients with diverticular disease.
NS – not stated.
Figures in parentheses are percentages.

Table 5.2 Comparison of distal margin of clearance with local recurrence and 5-year survival rates

Authors	<4 cm	>4 cm	<5 cm	>5 cm
Recurrence				
Deddish & Stearns (1961)	4/62 (6.5%)	4/39 (10%)		
Monson et al (1976)			9/76 (11.8%)	3/30 (10%)
Wilson & Beahrs (1976)			56/400 (14%)	20/156 (13%)
Pollett & Nicholls (1983)			15/32 (6.5%)	8/102 (7.8%)
Williams et al (1983)			7/48 (15%)	3/31 (10%)
Crude 5-year survival rates				
Copeland et al (1968)			46/141 (32.6%)	86/206 (41.8%)
Pollett & Nicholls (1983)			159/232 (68.5%)	71/102 (69.6%)
Williams et al (1983)			33/48 (69%)	18/31 (58%)

From Keighley & Williams (1993).

Recurrence and survival

There are a number of inherent difficulties associated with studies which attempt to compare the results of the two operations. Until recently, there were no prospective studies, most being retrospective. It is impossible in studies of this nature to obtain groups of patients with identical characteristics. Surgeons have often been selective in the procedure they have performed. The decision has usually involved several factors. The patient's build and sex and the surgeon's previous experience were obviously important and the extent of local spread has often been a factor. A tumour which exhibited extensive local spread on clinical and radiological assessment was more likely to have been treated by APER. However, as more expertise has been gained with sphincter-preserving techniques, so less bias has been introduced in selection criteria. Thus, the more recent studies

Local recurrence

Studies which attempt to examine recurrence rates are fraught with difficulties. Patients may have silent metastases which cannot be detected by clinical or even by modern radiological techniques. Even after death it may not be possible to determine the extent and pattern of spread unless a meticulous post-mortem examination is performed and clearly the latter is impossible. Modern radiological modalities such as CT scan, MRI and in particular endoluminal ultrasound will assist detection, but even now there are very few studies which have utilized these methods in a prospective manner in all patients who have undergone surgery.

With these reservations in mind, examination of the comparative data (Table 5.3) shows that overall there is no significant difference in local recurrence rates between the two operations. Nevertheless, there are two studies which demonstrate a higher rate of local recurrence after APER. Thus Phillips et al (1984) found an 18% local recurrence rate after SSR compared with 12% after APER. More alarmingly, however, Neville et al (1987) found a 32% incidence after SSR and a 13% rate after APER. These two studies bear closer inspection. Both reviewed the experience of a large number of surgeons in many different types of hospitals. Many of these were general surgeons who did not specialize in colorectal surgery. It is also not clear whether irrigation of the rectal stump to prevent the implantation of free tumour cells was routinely employed in the sphincter-saving group. Nor is it clear whether there was any difference in the local spread of the tumour between the two groups.

Of particular concern, however, is the high incidence of local recurrence in the SSR group, particularly in Neville et al's paper (32%). This rate is far higher than that recorded for SSR in the other series in Table 5.3. Similarly if one examines all the recent data on recurrence rates after SSR from non-comparative series (Table 5.4), Neville's data are at the upper end of the scale. Indeed, their nearest rival is the study from Hurst et al (1982), who recorded a local recurrence rate of 33% in a small number of patients operated on early in their experience with the stapling gun. This wide discrepancy in recurrence rates in our view suggests that the difference is surgeon-related and eloquently makes the point for specialization. Differences in case mix are unlikely to be the explanation. One aspect of technique which might account for surgeon variability, and which has recently been highlighted, is the avoidance of

Table 5.3 Incidence of local recurrence after abdominoperineal and low anterior resection

		No. of patients		Local recurrence	
Reference	Year	APR	Anterior resection	APR	Anterior resection
Morson et al	1963	1596	177	155 (9.7)	13 (7.3)
Slanctz et al	1972				
Dukes' B			–	(25)	(23)
Dukes' C		–		(38)	(33)
Patel et al	1977	326	142	52 (16.0)	23 (16.2)
Williams & Johnston	1984	83	71	7 (8)	8 (11)
Phillips et al	1984	478	370	57 (12)	67 (18.1)
Neville et al	1987			(13)	(32)
Fick et al	1990	27	31	4 (15)	4 (13)
Amato et al	1991	69	78	7 (10)	9 (12)
Dixon et al	1991	61	150	3 (5)	6 (4.0)

Values in parentheses are percentages.
APR – Abdominoperineal resection.
From Abulafi & Williams 1994.

Table 5.4 Incidence of local recurrence after sphincter-saving resection for carcinomas of the low rectum since 1980

Author	Operative method*	Period of follow-up (years)	Number of cases treated	Number with recurrence
Keighley & Matheson (1980)	Abd-transanal	1–3	7	3 (43)
Hurst et al (1982)	Ant resection with stapler	0.5–2	34	11 (32)
Parks & Percy (1982)	Abd-transanal	1–5	73	6 (8)
Anderberg et al (1983)	Ant resection with stapler	?	39	9 (24)
Luke et al (1983)	Ant resection with stapler	2.5–5	44	10 (22.7)
Goligher (1984)	Abd-transanal	2–5	18	2 (11)
Lasson et al (1984)	Ant resection with stapler	0.5–3	40	8 (20)
Reid et al (1984)	Ant resection with stapler	2–6	29	8 (28)
Oates (1985)	Ant resection with stapler	0.5–4	60	4 (7)
Heald & Ryall (1986)	Ant resection with stapler	0.5–6.5	115	3 (2.6)

Values in parentheses are percentages.
* Abd – abdomino, Ant – anterior.
From Keighley & Williams 1993.

'coning' where the plane of dissection during SSR may be closer to the rectum than in APER (Anderberg et al 1983, Reid et al 1984). Coning leaves behind elements of the mesorectum which may contain micrometastases which, if left, will lead to local recurrence. Such a risk can be considerably reduced if the dissection is carried out in the so-called 'holy plane' described by Heald (1988), which also allows the whole of the mesorectum to be excised en bloc with the rectum (Fig. 5.3).

Another surgeon-related factor which undoubtedly influences recurrence rates is inadvertent tumour perforation. Patel et al (1977) noted the seriousness of this complication – of 57 patients with a rectal tumour perforation, 34 (60%) developed local recurrence. Phillips et al (1984) noted a recurrence rate of 28% when tumour perforation was present versus 11% in its absence. A retrospective study by Zringibl et al (1990) reported that the incidence of local recurrence following tumour perforation was 51% (46 of 91 patients) compared with 20.6% (219 of 1062 patients) when perforation did not occur. It may be argued that a low sphincter-saving resection is more prone to perforation of the rectum or tumour since part of the dissection may not be as well visualized as during APER. Similarly, leakage from an anastomosis carries a high risk of recurrence. Thus, Akyol et al (1991) found that of those patients undergoing an SSR, 46.9% who leaked developed recurrence compared with 18.5% who did not. These data once again highlight the

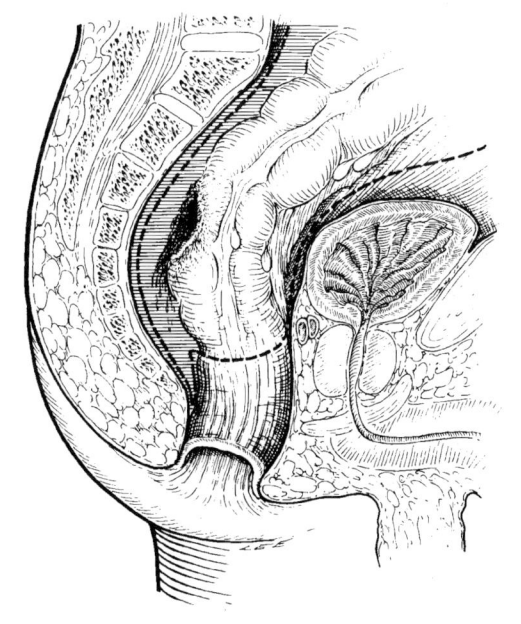

Fig. 5.3 Plane of dissection for total mesorectal excision. (From Williams N 1993. Surgery of the Anus, Rectum and Colon. WB Saunders, with permission.)

importance of the skill factor in reducing local recurrence and prolonging survival.

Surgical technique is clearly very important and perhaps paramount in reducing the incidence of local recurrence after low sphincter-saving surgery. Nevertheless, it is clear that even in the best hands patients recur and therefore we need to consider what else can be done to prevent this complication. Adjuvant radiotherapy, chemotherapy and immunotherapy may have a role and these are considered in detail in Chapter 9 and 10. However, there are modalities which may be useful when applied by the surgeon to the tumour bed at the time of surgery. One such modality is photodynamic therapy (PDT). A study by our group (Quirke et al 1986) demonstrated how it is possible to leave microscopic tumour deposits behind in the pelvis as a result of lateral spread no matter how careful the surgical technique. In addition, as mentioned above, others have highlighted the risk of leaving micrometastases in the mesorectum (Cawthorn et al 1990).

Adjuvant intraoperative PDT is a strategy devised to deal with this residual disease, which can be controlled by the surgeon at the time of the operation. The treatment involves injection of a photosensitizing agent that is retained in the tumour in higher concentrations than in surrounding normal tissue. Following resection and before the anastomosis is constructed, the tumour bed, which may contain microscopic disease, is illuminated with visible light of an appropriate wavelength, usually generated from a laser. The light activates the drug within these deposits, causing oxidative necrosis with little or no damage to surrounding normal tissues. Early reports (Abulafi et al 1991, Allardice et al 1992) suggest that this approach is safe and possibly effective. The only side-effect is transient skin photosensitivity. Potential advantages of PDT over conventional adjuvant treatment include direct application at the time of operation, dealing with residual disease without risk to other structures and minimum discomfort and toxicity. Furthermore, it is given as a one-off treatment and so, unlike other methods, further patient compliance and attendance at hospital are not required. At present haematoporphyrin derivative (HpD) is the photosensitizer that is used most frequently and is the subject of a prospective controlled trial. However, it is now being replaced by second and even third generation photosensitizers which have a far superior tumour to normal tissue ratio and are likely to be more effective. Furthermore, these photosensitizers can theoretically be activated by non-laser light, thus making the therapy cheaper and more readily available. It remains to be seen whether adjunctive intraoperative PDT will become a routine procedure in the course of a sphincter-saving resection for rectal cancer, but the omens are favourable.

Another innovation which may have an impact on local recurrence and which could be under the control of the surgeon is radioimmunoguided surgery. Thus, a radiolabelled monoclonal antibody is administered preoperatively (Dawson et al 1991, Sardi et al 1989, Sickle-Santanello et al 1987). During the surgery, a handheld gamma probe is used to identify areas of increased activity which are presumed to be tumour deposits. A biopsy specimen may be taken from these areas for histological examination. If the findings are positive or suspicious, the resection may be extended to include the affected area.

Early results have been encouraging with frequent identification of tumour sites that might have been otherwise missed. However, the specificity and sensitivity of the monoclonal antibodies continue to be a problem with significant false-positive and false-negative results. Very early spread will not be detected, as the minimum tumour size that can be detected is 0.1 g. Also, the antibodies may be localized to areas of inflammation, such as a duodenal ulcer or the uterus. Despite these difficulties, there is optimism that monoclonal antibodies will be developed which are more specific and sensitive and hence make this approach more feasible.

Survival

Survival data tend to mirror recurrence data. Table 5.5 lists series in which survival after low SSR and APER have been compared for tumours of similar pathological characteristics below 15 cm from the anal verge. The earlier SSRs that were performed were anterior resections with a

Table 5.5 FIve-year survival rates for abdominoperineal excision of the rectum (APER) and sphincter-saving resection (SSR) when used to treat midrectal tumours

Authors	Distance of tumour from anal verge (cm)	APER % (n)*	SSR % (n)*
Mayo et al (1958)	6–9	69 (108)	72 (46)
Deddish & Stearns (1961)	6–10	62 (106)	65 (33)
Williams et al (1966)	6–15	57	46
Slanctz et al (1972)	8–13	47 (106)	56 (61)
Patel et al (1977)	<10	56 (279)	64 (105)
Strauss et al (1978)	7–15	44 (34)	55 (49)
**Nicholls et al (1979)	8–12	57 (106)	73 (81)
Jones & Thomson (1982)	<15	52 (73)	67 (125)
**McDermott et al (1981)	6–11	71 (141)	68 (170)
**Williams & Johnston (1984)	7.5–12	62 (78)	74 (66)
Dixon et al (1991)	Low	52 (215)	64 (224)

*n – number of patients who survived operation.
**Indicates cancer – specific survival rates; the remainder are crude 5-year survival rates.

manual anastomosis of either one or two layers. The later studies consist primarily of stapled anastomoses. Our own study (Williams et al 1985) compared our low SSR results with those of an age- and sex-matched group of patients with low rectal cancer who had undergone APER prior to 1975. The SSR group were composed of patients who had undergone surgery according to our change of philosophy. Thus, the aim of the new policy was to perform a SSR for all rectal cancers wherever possible either by a manual or a stapling technique. A minimum distal margin of clearance of 5 cm was always the goal, but if by taking such a margin an anastomosis was not possible, this was reduced to 2 cm. If an anastomosis could not then be achieved per abdomen and conditions were favourable, a transanal coloanal anastomosis was constructed. As can be seen in Figure 5.4, the corrected five-year survival rates were not significantly different between the two groups. Nor was the incidence of local recurrence after 2 years – 13.6% after SSR and 18.8% after APER.

Function after sphincter-saving resection

Although various techniques including abdominotranssacral resection and abdominotransphincteric procedures have been described, the two most common techniques of sphincter preservation nowadays are anterior resection with a stapled anastomosis and, less commonly, the abdominotransanal anastomosis originally described by Parks (1972). There is abundant evidence that both procedures can be performed with a reasonable chance that eventually normal function will be retained. Nevertheless, in some patients the outcome from the functional point of view may not be satisfactory. It is therefore necessary to assess

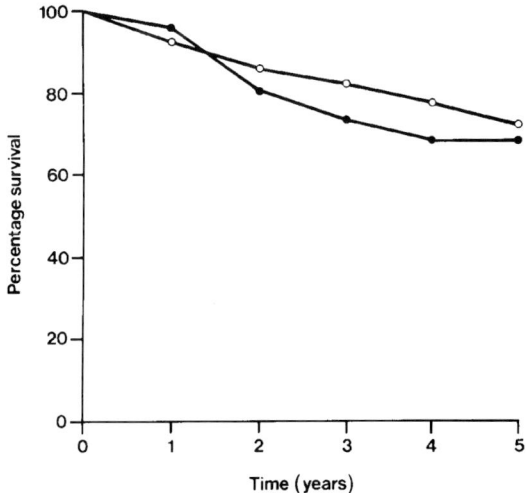

Fig. 5.4 Comparison of cumulative 5-year survival rates between patients who had undergone sphincter-saving resection and those who had undergone abdominoperineal excision for low rectal cancer (Williams et al 1985). o———o SSR, •———• APER. (From Williams N 1993. Surgery of the Anus, Rectum and Colon. WB Saunders, with permission.)

what technical modifications have been introduced to improve function and how progress may be advanced.

When the concept of low sphincter-saving resection was first mooted, many pundits considered that the result for many patients would be an incontinent perineal colostomy. It was thought that the sensory receptors required for continence lay in the rectal wall and that at least 6–8 cm of rectum must remain for continence to be preserved. Early suggestions that the sensation of reservoir fullness may not be entirely due to sensory receptors in the rectal wall were derived from studies in children which showed that patients with rectal agenesis who underwent pull-through procedures often retained the sense of rectal filling (Scharli and Kiesewetter 1970). These were followed by physiological evidence from the postoperative assessment of adult patients in whom the rectum was almost totally removed in operations for low rectal cancer (Lane and Parks 1977, Williams et al 1980). These patients seemed to retain their awareness of reservoir filling. In addition, most of them retained their rectoanal distension reflex and, provided enough time had elapsed for adaptation to occur, they were continent with reasonable anorectal function. Their function was also enhanced by the retention of the anal mucosa, which allowed discrimination of rectal contents to be retained. This discriminatory ability is thought to reside in the nerve-rich transitional zone in the upper anal canal. As rectal filling occurs, the rectoanal inhibitory response is initiated, which induces relaxation of the proximal anal canal by inhibition of internal sphincter tone (Duthie & Gairns 1960). This inhibition allows rectal contents to come into contact with the sensory anal canal mucosa and allows the individual to determine whether it is safe to release contents or it is wise to suppress the desire for evacuation.

This early work therefore demonstrated that virtual complete rectal excision and restoration of gastrointestinal continuity was compatible with normal function and that some receptors necessary for continence must lie outside the rectal wall, presumably in the fascia and muscles of the pelvic floor. Nevertheless, this and subsequent work also demonstrated that defects in function do occur and the impetus in recent years has been to identify these problems and to try and rectify them.

Function after low anterior resection (LAR)

The functional results from several series of low colorectal anastomoses performed using a circular stapling instrument are reviewed in Table 5.6. It might be expected that the loss of the rectum with its reservoir and accommodative functions would result in some frequency of defaecation. This is supported by the findings of a reduced maximum tolerable volume and rectal compliance, which correlates with a frequent bowel habit (Pedersen et al 1986, Suzuki et al 1980, Williams et al 1980). This, however, tends to improve with time. Continence may also be impaired to some degree in the immediate postoperative period. This again improves with time and most problems occur within 2 years following the operation (Williams et al 1980). Any major continence problem tends to result from a documented intraoperative injury or major postoperative complication, particularly sepsis from anastomotic leaks (Horgan et al 1989).

Manometric studies of the anal sphincter are difficult to assess. Resting anal pressure, which is a measure of internal anal sphincter function, has been found in some studies not to be significantly affected by LAR (Pedersen et al 1986, Suzuki et al 1980), whereas in others it has been found to be significantly reduced postoperatively (Williams et al 1980, Horgan et al 1989). These discrepancies may indicate an increasing tendency in some centres to tackle very low lesions with consequential effects on the internal anal sphincter mechanism. This is compatible with McDonald & Heald's (1983) data which have demonstrated how function becomes more impaired the closer the anastomosis is to the anal verge. Thus, 62% of patients in whom the anastomosis lay below 5 cm from the anal verge had some degree of impairment of their continence. With regard to the rectoanal inhibitory reflex, some patients seem to retain the reflex after LAR, whereas others do not (Horgan et al 1989, Pedersen et al 1986, Williams et al 1980). However, surprisingly

Table 5.6 Functional outcome after low anterior resection

Author	No. of patients	FU (months)	Distance of tumour* or anastomosis from anal verge (cm)	Perfect	Continence Minor defects	Poor	Bowel frequency/ 24 h	Comments
Cade et al (1981)	50		8–13	48	–	2		
Goligher et al (1979)	24		5–10	19	3	2		Minor and poor results re continence were in group of 10 with anastomosis below 7 cm
Heald (1980)	32	3	3–8 (includes some colo-anal)	30	2	0		
Williams & Johnston (1983)	40	39.6±18	5–12*	30	10	0	65% 3/day	Of 10 with minor incontinence 4 had problems with flatus only
Kirkegaard et al (1981)	29	3	7–12*	29	0	0	86% 2/day (others had 3–4/day)	
Williams et al (1980)	20	6–180	3–7	14 (all 2 years FU) Not specified (no major problems)	6	0	75% 3/day	10 patients had coloanal (no distinction made)
Pedersen et al (1986)	13	12	6–12*				92% 3/day	2 had endoanal coloanal anastomosis
McDonald & Heald (1983)	22	3–34 (20.5)	10	20	2	0	Not specified	
	32	3–31 (19.5)	5.10	23	8	1		
	21	5–28 (16)	5	8	12	1		
Horgan et al (1989)	15	6	5–12*	12	2	1	Not specified	Poor outcome, had poor preop anal pressures

(i.e. *relates to heading above these parameters, not to comparisons of data)
From Waldron 1991.

the presence or absence of the reflex does not correlate with continence. Most studies do not indicate any deleterious effect on the external sphincter musculature after this procedure.

It should be realized that most studies on this subject have been retrospective in nature and rarely have patients been studied pre- and postoperatively. A substantial proportion of patients in this age group have impaired anorectal function to begin with and this should be taken into account when assessing the data. It also highlights the need to test patients preoperatively to determine if their sphincter function is adequate for a sphincter-saving resection. Thus Horgan et al (1989) found that one of 20 patients could have been predicted to have poor function following surgery on the basis of a significantly diminished anal sphincter pressure preoperatively.

Function after transanal coloanal anastomosis

As previously emphasized, this procedure is now

only used when it is not possible to use a stapling instrument, yet it is deemed that the sphincter mechanism can be preserved. However, for some time in the late 1970s and early 1980s the technique was more widespread as this was a time when staplers had just been introduced and were not as refined as they are now. Consequently, the interpretation of data relating to transanal coloanal anastomosis must take this factor into consideration.

Table 5.7 presents an overview of the functional outcome of this procedure from a variety of centres. Most reports suggest that frequency of bowel action combined with urgency and soiling often pose problems in the first 3–6 months following surgery, although Parks, who developed the technique, reported 69 of 70 patients as having normal continence at the first outpatient visit, with approximately half having a frequency of 4–5 stools per day, the other half being normal in this respect (Parks and Percy 1982). The variability in the functional results may be influenced by the level of the anastomosis as measured from the anal verge in different series (Keighley and Matheson 1980).

Despite early problems, most patients do seem to return to more normal function within 1 year, although a significant minority do still have problems with bowel frequency. Physiological studies have demonstrated internal sphincter weakness and often the rectoanal inhibitory reflex is lost initially, but returns in time (Lane and Parks 1977). Perhaps these imperfections in internal anal sphincter function account for some of the problems with continence. The potential for direct damage to the internal anal sphincter during stretching by the retractor to allow visualization of the anastomosis in a transanal approach was thought to be the cause of this damage. This view was supported by Keighley's data (1988) from his restorative proctocolectomy studies. Thus, he found improved function following total abdominal mucosectomy without anal retraction. Studies to determine whether the use of a stapling instrument would overcome this problem have similarly come from work on restorative proctocolectomy. Thus, Johnston et al (1987) and we (Williams et al 1989) found that, although there was some impairment of internal anal sphincter after a stapled anastomosis, this was less than after a transanal anastomosis. These findings suggest that, whereas some damage may be inflicted from the abdominal dissection, more is inflicted by stretching the sphincter during the transanal procedure.

The reduction in rectal compliance and capacity that occurs after a transanal coloanal anastomosis

Table 5.7 Functional outcome after transanal coloanal anastomosis

Author	No. of patients	FU (months)	Perfect	Continence Minor defects	Poor	Bowel frequency/ 24 h	Comments
Parks & Percy (1982)	70	3	69	0	1	56% 3 (others had 4–5)	
Keighley & Matheson (1980)	6	12	4	1	1	3–4/day	Poor result associated with local recurrence
Castrini et al (1985)	17	22 (mean)	17	0	0	1	
Enker et al (1985)		12					
Drake et al (1987)	25	20±3	21	4	0	3±1	
Lane & Parks (1977)	12	12	10	1	1	60% approx 'normal'; others had 2–3/day	One poor outcome due to ascending colon used in anastomosis with overflow incontinence
Hautefeuille et al (1988)	31		30			2	
Bernard et al (1989)	30	6	26	2	2	63% 3 (mean 3.8)	

From Waldron 1991.

is, not surprisingly, similar to that which occurs after a stapled procedure. Problems with bowel frequency do seem to correlate with this reduction in 'neorectal' capacity. It was this finding that encouraged various centres to improve the storage capacity of the neorectum by creating a colonic pouch.

Colonic pouch–anal anastomosis

As a result of the success achieved with the ileal pouch in the surgical treatment of inflammatory bowel disease and familial adenomatous polyposis and the relatively persistent problems of frequency of bowel action even after 1 year following the transanal coloanal anastomosis, both Lazorthes et al (1986) and Parc et al (1988) described the use of a colonic J pouch anastomosed directly to the anal canal (Fig. 5.5). Subsequently, Nicholls et al (1988) described their experience with the same procedure. One report used the transphincteric approach (Lazorthes et al 1986) while the other two utilized Parks' endoanal route for the anastomosis. All these reports demonstrated reduced bowel frequency (Table 5.8). Parc et al (1988) noted a frequency of 1.1/day after 3 months, but problems with continence were present in up to 33% of patients at 1 month. However, as with the straight coloanal technique, continence improved with time and all patients were continent at 3 months.

Lazorthes et al (1986) and Nicholls et al (1988) compared outcome with a similar group of patients who had undergone the straight coloanal anastomosis and included tests of anorectal

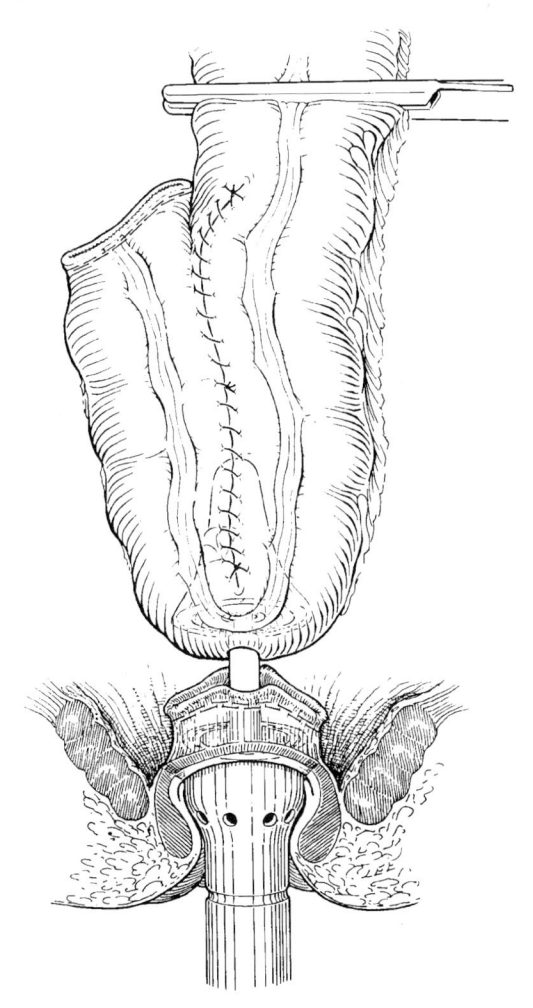

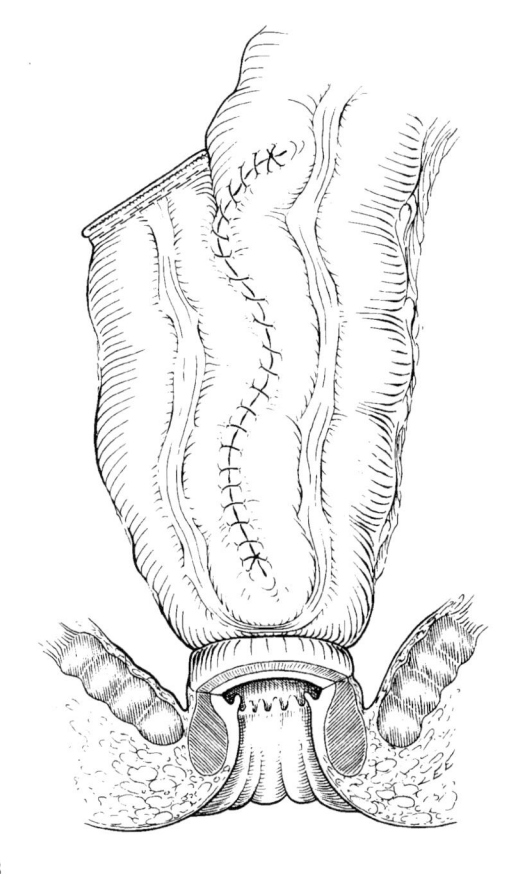

Fig. 5.5 (A) Construction of J-colonic pouch. (B) Stapled pouch anal anastomosis. (From Williams N 1993. Surgery of the Anus, Rectum and Colon. WB Saunders, with permission.)

Table 5.8 Functional outcome after colonic pouch—anal anastomosis

Author	No. of patients	FU (months)	Perfect	Continence Minor defects	Poor	Bowel frequency/ 24 h	Comments
Lazorthes et al (1986)							
Coloanal	15	20 (mean)	12	3	0	33%*2 (mean 3±1.2)	No problems with evacuation of pouch
Pouch	36	36 (mean)	28	8	0	87% 2 (mean 1.7±0.7)	
Nicholls et al (1988)							
Coloanal	15	47±23	9	6	1	1–6.5 (mean 2.3)	All patients with a pouch had 2 BM/day. Only 1 patient had difficulty evacuating the pouch
Pouch	13	7±4	10	3	0	0.5–2 (mean 1.4)	
Parc et al (1988)	24	3	24	0	0	1–3 (mean 1.1)	All colonic pouches. 25% needed suppository to aid emptying every other day (no sense of desire to evacuate)

*$p = 0.01$
From Waldron 1991.

function in their follow-up. Lazorthes et al (1986) demonstrated a direct correlation between a much diminished frequency of bowel action and a significantly increased neorectal capacity. A significantly greater number of pouch patients had a stool frequency of less than two per day, as opposed to the straight coloanal group. While the pouch group had slightly better continence levels in the first year, both groups were very satisfactory in this regard in the second year. Similar findings were found by Nicholls et al (1988). However, one problem which emerged particularly from Parc et al's data was difficulty in evacuation; 25% of their patients required suppositories or enemas to aid emptying of the pouch.

A study from our own group has shed some light on the evacuation of colonic pouches. However, this study must be interpreted in the knowledge that our operative technique has been different from those previously described. Instead of using the Parks' transanal anastomosis technique, we have stapled a J colonic pouch to the anorectal stump after first transecting it with the transverse stapling instrument.

Using integrated dynamic proctography (Womack et al 1985), Marzouk (1990) has been able to associate two aspects of colonic pouch design with evacuation difficulties. Initially, like Parc (1988) and Lazorthes (1986), we used long colonic limbs measuring 10–12 cm. This led to too large a pouch and this design was more often associated with evacuation problems. Secondly, as with the ileal pouch, the presence of a residual rectal 'spout' between the pouch and the anal canal was associated with emptying abnormalities. We found that both the preceding factors caused the pouch to fall back into the sacral hollow and interfere with the opening of the anoneorectal angle during attempted evacuation. It seems advisable, therefore, to recommend fashioning a colonic pouch from approximately 6 cm limbs of colon and reestablishing continuity at the level of the upper anal canal. It would also seem beneficial to use a stapled technique as opposed to an endo-anal technique to form the pouch anal anastomosis. In this way, the internal anal sphincter is less likely to be damaged.

The evidence to date does suggest that the addition of a colonic pouch will improve anorectal function by reducing frequency. It also appears that there is no increase in mortality or postoperative morbidity. However, it will be necessary to await the results of various ongoing prospective trials to confirm that the addition of a colonic pouch is worthwhile.

Total anorectal reconstruction

Despite the considerable advances that have been made in sphincter preservation, particularly with the introduction of stapling guns, there remain patients in whom colorectal or coloanal anastomosis and preservation of continence is impossible. These are usually patients in whom the cancer is locally advanced and is involving the sphincter mechanism or is so low in the rectum that cancer clearance is not compatible with sphincter preservation. If such patients are to avoid a permanent colostomy, they require a total anorectal reconstruction.

For many years, there has been considerable interest in such techniques. The emphasis until recently has been to replace the sphincter mechanism. Thus, following the abdominoperineal excision of the rectum, the colon has been pulled down to the perineum and a coloperineal anastomosis has been constructed. A neosphincter of some form has then been constructed or implanted. Such neosphincters can be classified into three types:

1. implantable sphincter prosthesis
2. smooth muscle cuff
3. transposed striated muscle.

Implantable sphincter prosthesis

The prosthesis which has received most attention is that which has been developed from the one used to treat urinary incontinence. The urinary prosthesis was designed by Scott and colleagues (1974) and in essence consists of an inflatable silastic cuff which surrounds the urethra. The cuff is inflated from a reservoir which is activated by the patient squeezing a balloon and by so doing fluid is transferred to the cuff, which inflates, thus obstructing the urethra.

Szinicz (1980) modified this device and, after experiments in animals, implanted it around an end colostomy in seven patients who had undergone an abdominoperineal excision of the rectum (Fig. 5.6). It appears that most patients required revisional surgery and there were problems with device failure. Nevertheless, continence was finally achieved in several patients. The pressure required for occlusion and continence to be achieved was a minimum of 120 cmH$_2$O. Subsequently, AMS (American Surgical) manufactured a similar device which was implanted around the anal canal in patients who were incontinent. Christiansen & Lorentzen (1987) reported a successful outcome with this device in a man with neurogenic faecal incontinence. Wong and colleagues from Minneapolis have also used the same device in incontinent patients (Wong and Rothenberger 1993). Of 11 patients so treated, two developed an infection and mechanical failure occurred twice. In 10 patients who had their covering colostomy closed, eight reported excellent continence to gas, liquid and solid stool, follow-up being a mean of 15 months.

As yet, there has not been a report of the prosthesis being used around pulled-through colon as part of a total reconstruction. However,

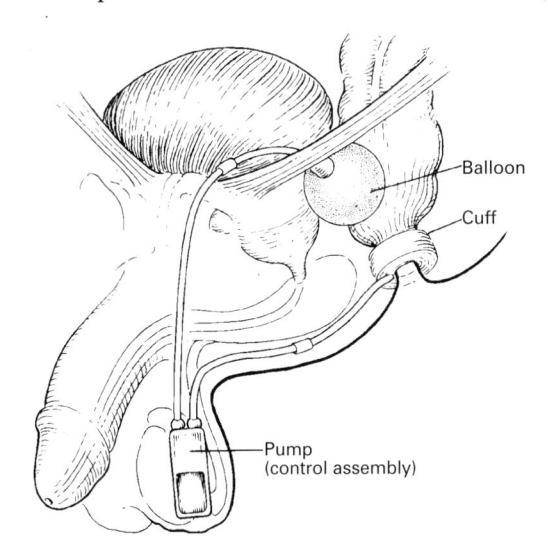

Fig. 5.6 Implantable artificial sphincter. The cuff is placed around the neoanal canal. An inflatable pump control assembly is placed in the scrotum and the balloon reservoir is positioned under the symphysis pubis. (From Williams N 1993. Surgery of the Anus, Rectum and Colon. WB Saunders, with permission.)

the long-term future of such a device when used in this way must remain problematical. Any foreign body applied so close to the colon is likely eventually to erode through into the bowel lumen.

Another prosthesis which has been tried is that adapted from the Erlangen magnetic occlusion device used to produce continence in colostomies. The colostomy device consisted of a magnetic ring, which was implanted into the anterior abdominal wall either at the time of abdominoperineal excision or as a secondary procedure. The colon was passed through the centre of the ring and a mucocutaneous suture was performed. After healing, the patient used a cap which had a central spigot which fitted into the lumen of the colostomy and achieved a constant force of attraction with the implanted ring of 10–13 mmHg, thus producing occlusion (Fig. 5.7). This prosthesis enjoyed a brief period of popularity in the late 1970s, but after longer follow-up the success rate was approximately only 25% (Alexander-Williams et al 1977). Despite these findings, Schier and others (1986) used a similar device in the perianal region in children with neuropathic incontinence. Not surprisingly, only nine of 25 patients achieved acceptable results and sepsis was a common problem.

Smooth muscle neosphincter

Schmidt (1982) described placing a smooth muscle collar around the end of the colon to produce continence in colostomies. The smooth muscle was obtained from the descending colon during abdominoperineal excision of the rectum. The mucosa was dissected from the smooth muscle, which was then stretched in its transverse axis to 100% of its breadth. The smooth muscle segment was then sutured around the distal segment of the colon as a collar (Fig. 5.8). The theory behind the procedure was that smooth muscle acted as a free smooth muscle graft and, being denervated, remained contracted to occlude the colonic lumen. The free graft was said to develop a secondary blood supply from the colon and electron microscopy studies suggested that the muscle architecture was maintained (Schmidt 1981, Schmidt et al 1979). Patients were taught how to irrigate through their colostomy and in 509 patients reported by Schmidt (1982), the results were said to be excellent. However, most

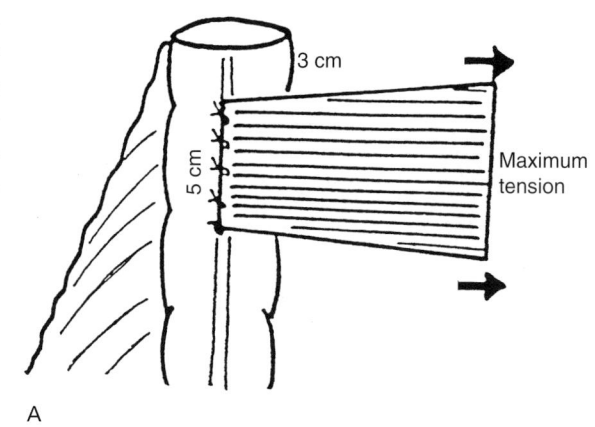

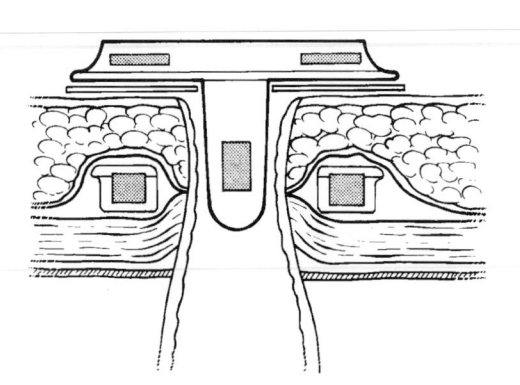

Fig. 5.7 Erlangen magnetic ring for continent colostomy which has been used as part of total reconstruction. (From Williams N 1993. Surgery of the Anus, Rectum and Colon. WB Saunders, with permission.)

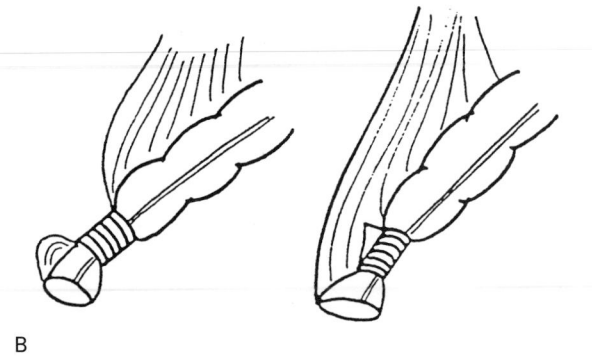

Fig. 5.8 Schmidt procedure to create smooth muscle sphincter. (A) Colonic smooth muscle taken from a separate colonic segment is stretched to 100% of its length and then (B) wrapped around the distal colon. (From Williams N 1993. Surgery of the Anus, Rectum and Colon. WB Saunders, with permission.)

other investigators who have used this technique suggest that any continence that is achieved results from the irrigation rather than the neosphincter (Schwemmle et al 1982).

The same technique has also been used as part of total reconstruction following APER, the colostomy together with its smooth muscle collar being implanted into the perineum (Elias et al 1993, Torres & Gonzalez 1988). Elias et al (1993) recently described their experience with this technique. Between 1989 and 1992, 23 patients underwent the operation. Two patients developed severe complications, leaving 21 patients for evaluation. Ten patients were incontinent to flatus but did not require a pad, whereas 11 patients had minor soiling and did need a pad. None of the patients suffered major incontinence requiring conversion to an end-colostomy. Interestingly, 6 months after operation the muscular transplanted ring had disappeared in half the patients, but this did not seem to have any repercussions on the quality of the functional results.

Fedorov and his colleagues in Moscow performed a similar procedure (Fedorov et al 1989). However, they modified the sphincter reconstruction in the following way. The smooth muscle graft after stretching was wrapped round the terminal colon so that each wrap overlapped the preceding one by one-third. Each wrap of the flap was sutured along its upper end to the intestinal wall with interrupted sutures. In this way, a spiral of smooth muscle cuff was created measuring 5–6 cm in length. Satisfactory functional results were reported in 22 of the 26 patients who were available for evaluation 6 months after surgery. In addition, a high pressure area was shown to be present in the neosphincter region, which was maintained for at least 6 months. No indication was given in this report as to whether the patients had to irrigate on a regular basis, although this seems likely.

Transposed striated muscle

Transposition of striated muscle to create a neosphincter has been tried frequently, but mainly for the treatment of faecal incontinence. Such patients have a relatively normal anorectum and therefore the results are likely to be better than those when the neosphincter is combined with a coloperineal anastomosis. Chittenden in 1930 was perhaps the first to create a striated muscle neosphincter following a rectal excision and coloperineal anastomosis. He used muscle slips from the glutei to reconstruct a sphincter following a Kraske operation.

Since then, other muscles, notably the gracilis and adductor longus, have been tried and the gracilis seems to be the most popular. Pickrell first described the use of the gracilis for young patients with incontinence in 1952. Other reports by him (1954, 1955 and 1956) established transposition of this muscle as being the optimum method to construct a neosphincter. The gracilis is a long muscle with its principal blood and nerve supply situated proximally and this allows it to be detached from its insertion into the tibia and transposed to the perineum.

Although Pickrell and others since have used the gracilis in children and young adults with rudimentary sphincters, it was Simonsen et al (1976) who adapted the technique for adults who had undergone reconstruction following abdominoperineal excision of the rectum for cancer. Twenty four patients with ages ranging from 22 to 70 years underwent the procedure. Following a standard abdominoperineal resection, the descending colon was mobilized sufficiently to reach the perineum. The gracilis was then transposed and its aponeurotic borders were sutured to the remaining structures of the pelvic floor, i.e. to the posterior border of the deep perineal transverse muscle, to the ischial tuberosity anteriorly, to the gluteal muscles laterally and to the presacral aponeurosis posteriorly. The transposed gracilis muscle was then incised and 6–8 cm of colon was brought through the incision. This part of the colon was then encircled by the gracilis and its distal tendon and the latter was sutured to the contralateral ischial tuberosity. Fifteen days after the procedure the excess colon was resected and the mucosal border was sutured to the skin around the colostomy. The patient was then taught to exercise the gracilis muscle for 30 days after surgery.

Of the 22 patients who were followed up for periods ranging from between 45 days to 9 years,

17 were described as having an excellent or good result. Furthermore, perception for solid stools was preserved in 86.4% of patients and for flatus in 22.7% of patients. These findings are quite remarkable as in objective studies carried out by our own group, both neorectal and neoanal sensation were absent in all patients who had undergone total anorectal excision and a coloperineal anastomosis. Furthermore, patients were totally incontinent unless the gracilis muscle was electrically stimulated (Abercrombie et al 1994).

However, it must be stated that Chinese surgeons were successful in using the same technique as Simonsen et al (1976). Wu et al (1986) described 41% of 31 patients who had normal function following total anorectal reconstruction using the Simonsen technique.

Wong & Wee (1984) approached the problem in a similar manner. However, they considered that transposition of the gracilis muscle in the manner described by Pickrell was inefficient. The angulation of the gracilis at the neurovascular hilum made contraction less effective. As a consequence, they detached the gracilis from its origin and reattached it to the pubic arch. The distal end of the gracilis was then applied around the colon in an alpha loop configuration and reattached to a similar point on the opposite pubic arch. This configuration was thought to mimic the circular sphincter effect of the external anal sphincter and also to simulate the puborectalis sling by restoring the 80° angulation of the lower colon. Although an interesting concept, they only described one case and furthermore when we attempted to perform the same manoeuvre, the gracilis became ischaemic because it received a blood supply from its origin, which in our patient was crucial to its viability.

Fedorov and Shelygin (1989), from the Research Institute of Proctology in Moscow, utilized the adductor longus instead of the gracilis to fashion a neoanal sphincter after rectal excision and coloperineal anastomosis. The procedure was carried out in 67 patients, but unfortunately it is impossible to determine from the paper the exact technique that was used or the results.

Cavina et al (1987) described a technique of reconstruction which utilized both gracilis muscles. The rectal excision and coloperineal anastomosis were performed in the usual way. One gracilis was applied around the colon simulating a posterior sling and the other gracilis was applied in a more superficial layer around the colon as a circular sphincter. The technique also differed from previous ones in that temporary electrical stimulation was applied to the muscles to prevent 'atrophy'. Through small separate incisions, electrodes were placed close to the nerves of the muscles and these were stimulated for 10 minutes each day for several weeks via an external generator. Using the technique, 17 of 27 patients in whom follow-up was possible were considered to have 'very good continence for stool and flatus'.

Our own group have sought to improve neosphincter function by continuous electrical stimulation. Our concept is that all methods that use striated muscle as a neosphincter are likely to fail since striated muscle is in the main composed of fast twitch muscle fibres which will fatigue rapidly when contracted. The normal anal sphincter is primarily composed of slow twitch fibres, which are more fatigue-resistant. Work in experimental animals (Salmons & Henriksson 1981) has demonstrated that if fast twitch muscle is continually electrically stimulated, it can convert to slow twitch muscle, which is relatively fatigue-resistant. Thus, we have applied this concept to the gracilis neosphincter and incorporated it into a method for total anorectal reconstruction.

Electrically stimulated neoanal sphincter

Much of our initial work has concentrated on providing a neoanal sphincter for patients who are incontinent but still have a rectum and anal canal and a deficient anal sphincter. Once experience was gained with these patients, we moved on to use the technique as part of total reconstruction. It should be stated at the outset that this is still developmental work and we are continuing to modify the procedure.

Experiments in dogs demonstrated that a neoanal sphincter could be constructed from hind limb muscle and that chronic low-frequency electrical stimulation converted the muscle from fast twitch fatiguable muscle to slow twitch fatigue-resistant muscle (Hallan et al 1990). Utilizing this technique in incontinent patients, we found that continence could be restored in approximately 65% of patients (Williams et al 1991). Interestingly, a similar improvement was found by colleagues in Holland who used the same principle, although employing a different technique (Baeten et al 1991).

The technique of total reconstruction was initially performed in the following way. Two types of patients underwent the procedure. In one the abdominoperineal excision had been performed several years previously and in the other the first stage of the operation was performed at the time of the APER. In both groups it was considered that all patients were likely to have been cured by the APER. The first stage of the procedure consisted of a coloperineal pull-through and division of the distal blood supply to the gracilis muscle. The left colon was divided at the level of the distal descending colon and, in order for it to reach the perineum, the colon was mobilized round to the mid transverse colon. The distal colon was then sutured to the perineal skin at the position previously occupied by the anal orifice (Fig. 5.9). The remaining perineal muscles were repaired as well as possible and sutured where indicated to the serosa of the pulled-through colon. A covering loop ileostomy was then constructed to defunction the colon. The division of the distal blood supply to the gracilis was next performed.

The second stage was performed approximately 6–8 weeks after the first when all wounds had healed (Fig. 5.10). This consisted of transposing the gracilis muscle from the thigh to the perineum and wrapping the muscle in a gamma configuration around the pulled-through colon. The tendon of the muscle was sutured to the contralateral ischial tuberosity. The main nerve to the gracilis was then identified as it lay on the adductor magnus muscle beneath the adductor longus. An electrode was then carefully sutured over the main nerve and its lead was connected to a purpose-designed electrical generator (NICE Inc, Ft Lauderdale, USA) which was positioned in a subcutaneous pocket either on the left lower chest wall or in the left upper quadrant of the abdomen.

The muscle was then intermittently stimulated, gradually increasing the stimulus until it was continuous and conversion of the muscle from fast twitch to slow twitch was evident on physiological testing. After conversion had taken place, the covering ileostomy was closed. When the

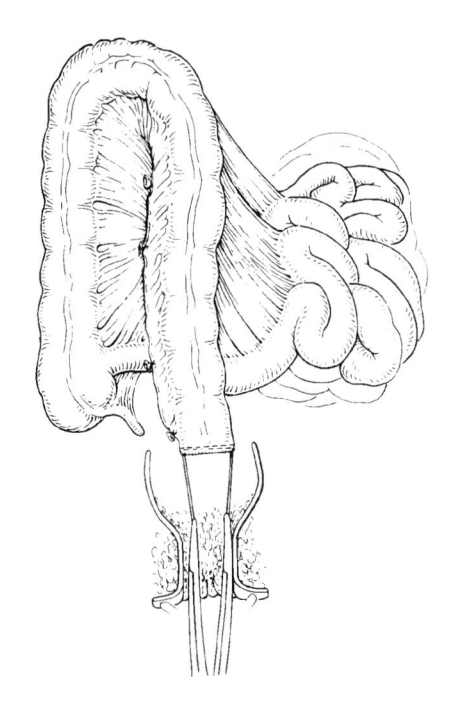

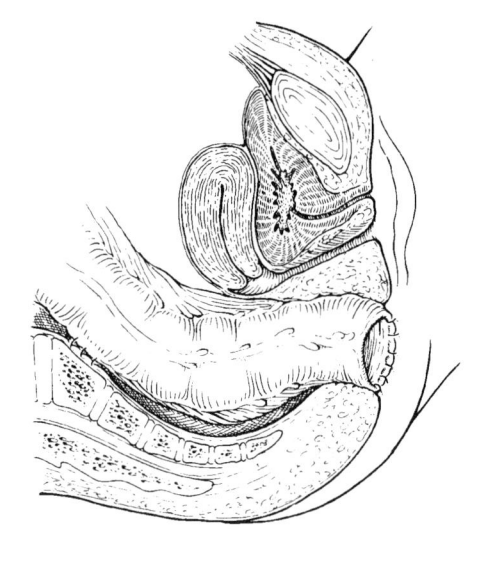

Fig. 5.9 Total anorectal reconstruction. Coloperineal anastomosis: (A) The proximal colon is brought down into the pelvis and (B) is sutured to the perineal skin.
(From Williams N 1993. Surgery of the Anus, Rectum and Colon. WB Saunders, with permission.)

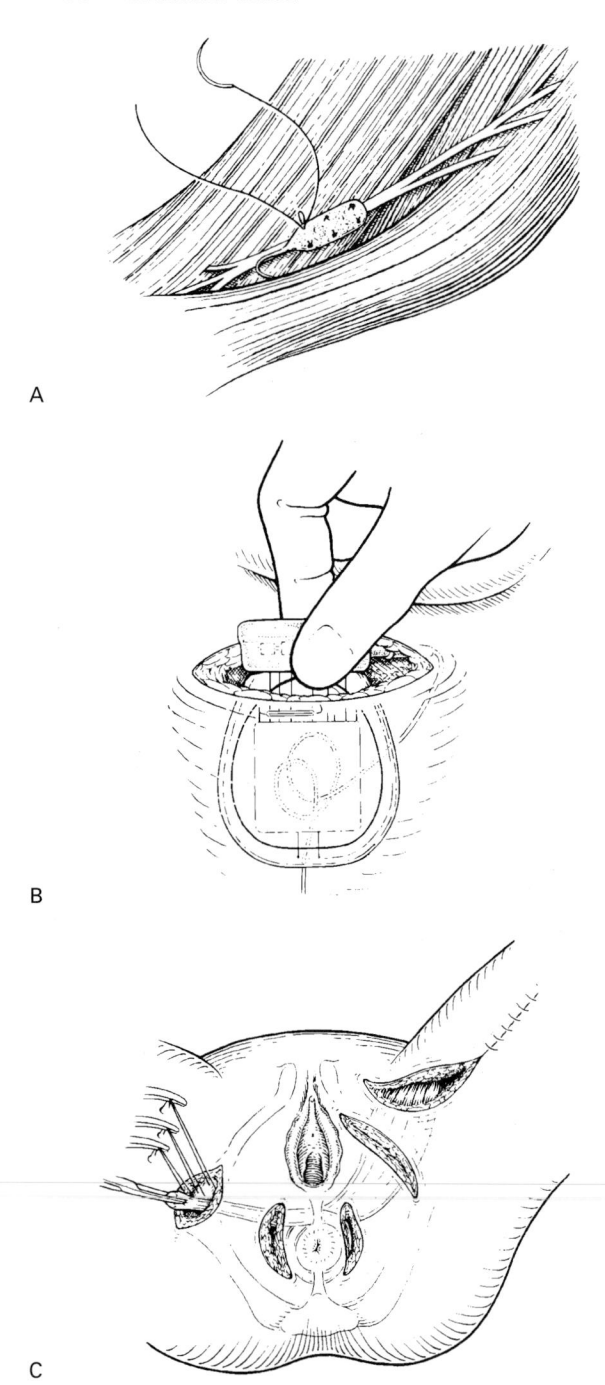

Fig. 5.10 Total anorectal reconstruction. Electrically stimulated gracilis neosphincter. (A) An electrode is placed on the nerve to the gracilis muscle and is in turn (B) connected to a totally implanted stimulator, which is implanted in a subcutaneous pocket. (C) The gracilis muscle is mobilized from the thigh and transposed around the neoanal canal. (From Williams N 1993. Surgery of the Anus, Rectum and Colon. WB Saunders, with permission.)

patient wished to evacuate, the stimulator could be turned off by moving the magnet over the overlying skin; after evacuation was complete, the stimulator could be switched on by a similar manoeuvre. The patient was encouraged to evacuate the neorectum every 3–4 hours and gradually to increase this period.

Results

Since 1990, 11 patients have undergone total anorectal reconstruction following abdominoperineal resection using an electrically stimulated gracilis neosphincter. Two successfully reached the stage when the covering stoma was due to be closed, but one decided not to proceed and one patient died due to a sudden myocardial infarction. Of the nine patients remaining who went on to the final stage, three failed due to sepsis (n=2) and neoanal stenosis (n=1). Five patients have acceptable function in that on most occasions they are able to control solid motion and their quality of life is preferable to that with a colostomy. In the remaining patient, function was initially acceptable but he developed a local recurrence of an amelanotic melanoma. Function deteriorated and after 4 years he required conversion to a permanent colostomy.

It is clear from this initial experience that, whereas a neosphincter which generates reasonable pressures in the neoanal canal can be constructed, the loss of other functions following abdominoperineal resection need to be addressed. These include:

1. anal sensation
2. rectal sensation
3. evacuation
4. anorectal reflexes.

As a consequence, we have introduced modifications to the original technique in an attempt to mimic some of these lost functions. It will be appreciated that not all of these modifications have been used in all patients and the ideal procedure has yet to be defined. Nevertheless, progress has been made and useful function has been restored to some patients.

The modifications used and the reasons for their introduction are as follows.

Anoplasty

A coloperineal anastomosis alone may lead to ectropion and mucus discharge. To remedy this problem, and in an attempt to provide neoanal sensation, we have created skin flaps from the perineal skin in order to fashion a skin tube to which the distal colon can be anastomosed. Not only might this improve sensation, but it should prevent stenosis.

Colonic pouch

In order to restore neorectal capacity, a J-colonic pouch with 6 cm limbs is created from the distal colon using a 90 mm GIA stapler.

Two gracilis muscles

In two patients in whom continence was unsatisfactory, the other gracilis was utilized and wrapped around the distal colon in the opposite direction. Using the purpose-designed stimulator, both muscles could be stimulated continuously. This modification in these patients improved their continence. Whether both muscles should be used de novo in all cases remains to be determined.

Continent colonic conduit

A few patients have had their continence restored but have been unable to evacuate satisfactorily. As a consequence, we have provided them with a colonic conduit through which they could irrigate the distal half of the colon to effect evacuation. This technique has been developed from our work with patients who have suffered from severe idiopathic constipation and have either had delay in transit through the left side of the colon or who have had a rectal evacuation disorder (Williams et al 1994). The conduit consists of a segment of narrowed colon incorporating an intussusception which acts as a non-return valve. The intussusception is stabilized with a mixture of staples and sutures (Fig. 5.11). The conduit tends to be continent for liquids and solids, but rarely for flatus. Patients seem to readily accept the modification in preference to a permanent colostomy. Once again, it remains to be determined whether the conduit should be used routinely.

Conclusions

Clearly total anorectal reconstruction is at an early stage in development and is only indicated in highly motivated, fit patients whose prognosis is excellent. Even at its most basic, it requires patients to undergo several procedures which must still be considered experimental. Nevertheless, there seems to be a need to provide patients with an alternative to a permanent colostomy and there is no shortage of patients who readily

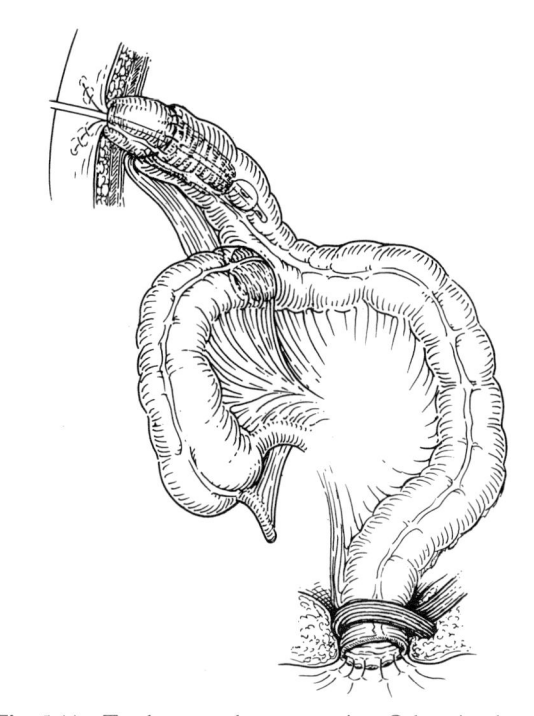

Fig. 5.11 Total anorectal reconstruction. Coloperineal anastomosis, electrically stimulated neosphincter and transverse colonic conduit. The neosphincter maintains continence, whilst antegrade irrigation via the conduit achieves evacuation.

submit themselves to these types of procedure whilst appreciating their experimental nature.

Most attention until recently has centred around restoring a functioning sphincter, the most promising of which seems to be the electrically stimulated gracilis neosphincter. However, it is obvious that the combination of such a sphincter with a straight coloperineal anastomosis is but a crude attempt to restore what is a very sophisticated mechanism. It has now been realized that other functions need to be replaced after excisional surgery and the modifications described above are attempts to do this. There is no doubt that further refinements will be introduced in the future which hopefully will offer patients a more acceptable alternative to what many regard as an unacceptable burden on their lives.

Acknowledgements

I am grateful to Mr John Abercrombie for his suggestions relating to the anorectal reconstruction section and to Miss Janet Mutch for typing the chapter.

References

Abercrombie JF, Rogers J, Williams NS 1994 Complete anorectal sensory loss following total anorectal reconstruction. British Journal of Surgery 81: 761

Abulafi AM, Williams NS 1994 Local recurrence of colorectal cancer: the problem, mechanisms, management and adjuvant therapy. British Journal of Surgery 81: 7–19

Abulafi AM, Allardice JT, Dean R, Grahn MF, Williams NS 1991 Adjunctive intra-operative photodynamic therapy for colorectal cancer. Gut 32 (suppl): 2

Adolff M, Arnoud JP, Bee Hary S 1980 Stapled vs sutured colorectal anastomosis. Archives of Surgery 115: 1436–1438

Akyol AM, McGregor JR, Galloway DJ, Murray G, George WD 1991 Anastomotic leaks in colorectal cancer surgery: a risk factor for recurrence? International Journal of Colorectal Disease 6: 179–183

Alexander-Williams J, Amery AH, Devlin HB et al 1977 Magnetic continent colostomy device. British Medical Journal 2: 1269–1270

Allardice JT, Grahn MF, Rowland AC et al 1992 Safety studies for intra-operative photodynamic therapy. Lasers in Medical Science 7: 133–142

Amato A, Pescatori M, Buti A 1991 Local recurrence following abdominoperineal excision and anterior resection for rectal carcinoma. Diseases of the Colon and Rectum 34: 317–322

Anderberg B, Enblad P, Sjödahl R, Wetterfors J 1983 The EEA-stapling device in anterior resection for carcinoma of the rectum. Acta Chirurgica Scandinavica 149: 99–103

Antonsen HK, Fronberg O 1987 Early complications after low anterior resection for rectal cancer using the EEA stapling device. A prospective trial. Diseases of the Colon and Rectum 30: 579–583

Baeten CGMI, Konsten J, Spaans F et al 1991 Dynamic graciloplasty for treatment of faecal incontinence. Lancet 338: 1163–1165

Beart RW Jr, Kelly KA 1981 Randomised prospective evaluation of the EEA stapler for colorectal anastomoses. American Journal of Surgery 141: 143–147

Belli L, Beati CA, Frangi M, Aseni P, Rondinara GF 1988 Outcome of patients with rectal cancer treated by stapled anterior resection. British Journal of Surgery 75: 422–424

Bernard D, Morgan S, Tasse D, Wassef R 1989 Preliminary results of coloanal anastomosis. Diseases of the Colon and Rectum 32: 580–584

Blamey SL, Lee PW 1982 A comparison of circular stapling devices in colorectal anastomoses. British Journal of Surgery 69: 19–22

Bolton RA, Britton DC 1980 Restorative surgery of the rectum with circumferential stapler. Lancet 1: 850–851

Brennan SJ, Pickford IR, Evans M, Pollock AV 1982 Staples or sutures for colonic anastomosis – a controlled trial. British Journal of Surgery 69: 722–724

Cade D, Gallagher P, Schofield PF, Turner L 1981 Complications of anterior resection of the rectum using the EEA stapling device. British Journal of Surgery 68: 339–340

Castrini G, Pappalardo G, Mobarhan S 1985 A new technique for ileoanal and coloanal anastomosis. Surgery 97: 111–116

Cavina E, Seccia M, Evangelista G et al 1987 Construction of a continent perineal colostomy by using electrostimulated gracilis muscle after abdominoperineal resection: personal technique and experience with 32 cases. Italian Journal of Surgical Sciences 17: 305–314

Cawthorn SJ, Parums DV, Gibbs NM et al 1990 Extent of mesorectal spread and involvement of lateral resection margin as prognostic factors after surgery for rectal cancer. Lancet 335: 1055–1059

Chittenden AS 1930 Reconstruction of anal sphincter by muscle slips from the glutei 1930. Annals of Surgery 92: 152

Christiansen J, Lorentzen M 1987 Implantation of artificial sphincter for anal incontinence. Lancet i: 244–245

Copeland EM, Miller LD, Jones RS 1968 Prognostic factors in carcinoma of the colon and rectum. American Journal of Surgery 116: 875–881

Dawson PM, Blair SD, Begent RHJ, Kelly AMB, Boxer GPI, Theodorou NA 1991 The value of radio-immunoguided surgery in first and second look laparotomy for colorectal cancer. Diseases of the Colon and Rectum 34: 217–222

Deddish MR, Stearns MW 1961 Anterior resection for carcinoma of the rectum and rectosigmoid area. Annals of Surgery 154: 961–966

Dixon AR, Maxwell WS, Holmes J, Thornton R 1991 Carcinoma of the rectum: a 10-year experience. British Journal of Surgery 78: 308–311

Drake DB, Pemberton JH, Beart RW Jr, Dozois RR, Wolff BG 1987 Coloanal anastomosis in the management of benign and malignant rectal disease. Annals of Surgery 206: 600–605

Duthie HL, Gairns FW 1960 Sensory nerve endings and sensation in the anal region of man. British Journal of Surgery 47: 585–595

Elias D, Lasser P, Leroux A, Rougier P, Comandella MG, Deraco M 1993 Colostomies périnéales pseudo continentes après amputation rectale pour cancer. Gastroenterology and Clinical Biology 17: 181–186

Enker WE, Stearns MW Jr, Janov AJ 1985 Perianal coloanal anastomosis following low anterior resection for rectal carcinoma. Diseases of the Colon and Rectum 28: 576–581

Fain SN, Patin S, Morganstern L 1975 Use of mechanical apparatus in low colorectal anastomosis. Archives of Surgery 110: 1079–1082

Fazio VW, Jagelman DG, Lavery IC, McGonagle BA 1985 Evaluation of the Proximate-ILS circular stapler. A prospective study. Annals of Surgery 201: 108–114

Fedorov VD, Shelygin YA 1989 Treatment of patients with rectal cancer. Diseases of the Colon and Rectum 32: 138–145

Fedorov VD, Odaryuk TS, Shelygin YA, Tsarkov PV, Frolov SA 1989 Method of creation of smooth muscle cuff at the site of the perineal colostomy after extirpation of the rectum. Diseases of the Colon and Rectum 32: 562–566

Fick TE, Baeten CG, von Meyenfeldt MF, Obertop H 1990 Recurrence and survival after abdominoperineal and low anterior resection for rectal cancer without adjunctive therapy. European Journal of Surgical Oncology 16: 105–108

Goligher JC 1984 Surgery of the anus, rectum and colon. Baillière Tindall, London

Goligher JC, Lee PWR, Macfie J et al 1979 Experience with the Russian model 249 suture gun for anastomosis of the rectum. Surgery, Gynecology and Obstetrics 148: 517–524

Griffen FD, Knight CD Sr, Whitaker JM, Knight CD Jr 1989 The double stapling technique for low anterior resection. Results, modifications and observation. Annals of Surgery 211: 745–751

Hallan RI, Williams NS, Hutton MRE et al 1990 Electrically stimulated sartorius neosphincter: canine model of activation and skeletal muscle transformation. British Journal of Surgery 77: 208

Hautefeuille P, Valleur P, Perniceni T et al 1988 Functional and oncological results after coloanal anastomosis for low rectal cancer. Annals of Surgery 207: 61–64

Heald RJ 1980 Towards fewer colostomies – the impact of circular stapling devices on the surgery of rectal cancer in a district hospital. British Journal of Surgery 60: 198–200

Heald RJ 1988 The 'holy plane' of rectal surgery. Journal of the Royal Society of Medicine 81: 503–508

Heald RJ, Leicester RJ 1981 The low stapled anastomosis. Diseases of the Colon and Rectum 68: 333–337

Heald RJ, Ryall RDH 1986 Recurrence and survival after total mesorectal excision for rectal cancer. Lancet 1: 1479–1482

Horgan PG, O'Connell PR, Shinkwin CA, Kirwan WO 1989 Effect of anterior resection on anal sphincter function. British Journal of Surgery 76: 783–786

Hurst PA, Prout WG, Kelly JM, Bannister JJ, Walker RT 1982 Local recurrence after low anterior resection using the staple gun. British Journal of Surgery 69: 275–276

Johnston D, Holdsworth PJ, Nasmyth DG et al 1987 Preservation of the entire anal canal in conservative proctocolectomy for ulcerative colitis: a pilot study comparing end-to-end ileo-anal anastomosis without mucosal resection with mucosal proctectomy and endo-anal anastomosis. British Journal of Surgery 74: 940–944

Jones PF, Thomson HJ 1982 Long term results of a consistent policy of sphincter preservation in the treatment of carcinoma of the rectum. British Journal of Surgery 69: 564–568

Keighley MRB 1988 Abdominal mucosectomy reduced the incidence of soiling and sphincter damage after restorative proctocolectomy and J pouch. Diseases of the Colon and Rectum 30 (suppl): 386–390

Keighley MRB, Matheson D 1980 Functional results of rectal excision and endo-anal anastomosis. British Journal of Surgery 67: 757–761

Keighley MRB, Williams NS 1993 Surgery of the anus, rectum and colon. WB Saunders, London

Kirkegaard P, Christiansen J, Hjartrup A 1981 Anterior resection for mid rectal cancer with the EEA stapling instrument. American Journal of Surgery 140: 312–314

Kirwan WD 1981 Integrity of low colorectal EEA-stapled anastomosis. British Journal of Surgery 68: 539–540

Lane RHS, Parks AG 1977 Function of the anal sphincters following colo-anal anastomosis. British Journal of Surgery 64: 596–599

Lasson ALL, Ekelund GR, Lindstrom CG 1984 Recurrence risks after stapled anastomosis for rectal carcinoma. Acta Chirurgica Scandiniavica 150: 85–89

Lazorthes F, Fages P, Chiotasso P, Lemozy J, Bloom E 1986 Resection of the rectum with construction of a colonic reservoir and colo-anal anastomosis for carcinoma of the rectum. British Journal of Surgery 73: 136–138

Ling L, Broom A, Ryden S 1979 Low anterior resection using stapling instrument. Acta Chirurgica Scandinavica. 145: 487–489

Luke M, Kirkegaard P, Lendorf A, Christiansen J 1983 Pelvic recurrence rate after abdominoperineal resection and low anterior resection for rectal cancer before and after introduction of the stapling technique. World Journal of Surgery 7: 616–619

McDermott FT, Hughes ES, Pihle E, Milne BJ, Price AB 1981 Comparative results of surgical management of single carcinomas of the colon and rectum: a series of 1939 patients managed by one surgeon. British Journal of Surgery 68: 850–855

McDonald PJ, Heald RJ 1983 A survey of post-operative function after rectal anastomosis with circular stapling devices. British Journal of Surgery 70: 727–729

Manson PN, Carmen ML, Collar JA, Veidenheimer MC 1976 Anterior resection for adenocarcinoma. Lahey Clinic experience. American Journal of Surgery 131: 434–441

Marzouk D 1990 Investigation of colonic and ileo-anal pouch function. Thesis, University of Cairo, Egypt

Mayo CW, Fly OA 1956 Analysis of five years survival in carcinoma of the rectum and rectosigmoid. Surgery, Gynecology and Obstetrics 103: 94–98

Morson BC, Vaughn EG, Bussey HJR 1963 Pelvic recurrence after excision of the rectum for carcinoma. British Medical Journal 2: 13–15

Neville R, Fielding LP, Amendola C 1987 Local tumour recurrence after curative resection of rectal cancer – a ten-hospital review. Diseases of the Colon and Rectum 30: 12–17

Nicholls RJ, Ritchie JK, Wadsworth J, Parks AG 1979 Total excision or restorative resection for carcinoma of the middle third of the rectum. Journal of Surgery 66: 625–627

Nicholls RJ, Lubowski DZ, Donaldson DR 1988 Comparison of colonic reservoir and straight colo-anal reconstruction after rectal excision. British Journal of Surgery 75: 318–320

Oates GC 1985 Cited in Goligher JC 1985 Neoplasms: surgical treatment. Current Opinions in Gastroenterology: 1: 43

Parc R, Tiret E, Frileux P, Moszkowski E, Loygue J 1988 Resection and colo-anal anastomosis with colonic reservoir for rectal carcinoma. British Journal of Surgery 73: 139–141

Parks AG 1972 Transanal technique in low rectal anastomosis. Proceedings of the Royal Society of Medicine 65: 975–976

Parks AG, Percy JP 1982 Resection and sutured colo-anal anastomosis for rectal carcinoma. British Journal of Surgery 69: 301–304

Patel SC, Tovee EB, Langer B 1977 Twenty-five years experience with radical surgical treatment of carcinoma of the extra-peritoneal rectum. Surgery 82: 460–465

Pedersen IK, Hint K, Olsen J, Christiansen J, Jensen P, Mortensen PE 1986 Anorectal function after low anterior resection for carcinoma. Annals of Surgery 204: 133–135

Phillips RKS, Hittinger R, Blesovsky L, Fry JS, Fielding LP 1984 Local recurrence followng 'curative' surgery for large bowel cancer – the rectum and rectosigmoid. British Journal of Surgery 71: 17–20

Pickrell KL, Broadbent TR, Masters F, Metzger JT 1952 Construction of rectal sphincter and restoration of anal continence by transplanting the gracilis muscle; report of 4 cases in children. Annals of Surgery 135: 853–862

Pickrell K, Masters F, Georgiade N, Horton C 1954 Rectal sphincter reconstruction using gracilis muscle transplant. Plastic Reconstructive Surgery 13: 46–55

Pickrell K, Georgiade N, Maguire C, Crawford H 1955 Correction of rectal incontinence; transplantation of gracilis muscle to construct a rectal sphincter. American Journal of Surgery 90: 721–726

Pickrell K, Georgiade N, Crawford N, Maguire L, Boone A 1956 Gracilis muscle transplant for correction of urinary incontinence in male children. Annals of Surgery 143: 764–779

Pollet WG, Nicholls RJ 1983 The relationship between the extent of distal clearance and survival and local recurrence rates after curative anterior resection for carcinoma of the rectum. Annals of Surgery 198: 159–163

Quirke P, Durdey P, Dixon MF, Williams NS 1986 Local recurrence of rectal adenocarcinoma due to inadequate surgical resection: histopathological study of lateral tumour spread and surgical excision. Lancet ii: 996–999

Reid JD, Robins RE, Atkinson KG 1984 Pelvic recurrence after anterior resection and EEA stapling anastomosis for potentially curable carcinoma of the rectum. American Journal of Surgery 147: 629–632

Salmons S, Henriksson J 1981 The adaptive response of skeletal muscle to increased use. Muscle and Nerve 4: 94–105

Sardi A, Workman M, Mojzisik C, Hinkle G, Nieroda C, Martin EW Jr 1989 Intra-abdominal recurrence of colorectal cancer detected by radio-immunoguided surgery (RIGS system). Archives of Surgery 124: 55–59

Scharli AF, Kiesewetter WB 1970 Defaecation and continence: some new concepts. Diseases of the Colon and Rectum 13: 81–107

Schier F, Schneiger W, Wittal GH 1986 Anal incontinence in childhood: psychological development after sacral sphincter replacement. Coloproctology 8: 115–118

Schmidt E 1981 Sphincter kontinenz-plastik indikation technik und Ergebnisse. Dtsch Med Wochenschr 1: 12–14

Schmidt E 1982 The continent colostomy. World Journal of Surgery 6: 805–809

Schmidt E, Bruch HP, Genlich N, Rothhammer A, Rowen W 1979 Kontinente colostomie durch freie transplantation autolager. Diek dormmuskalactic Chirurg 50: 96–100

Schwemmle K, Kuaze HH, Padberg W 1982 Management of the colostomy. World Journal of Surgery 6: 554–559

Scott BF, Bradley WE, Timm G 1974 Treatment of urinary incontinence by an implantable prosthetic urinary sphincter. Journal of Urology 112: 75

Shahinian TK, Bowen JR, Dorman BA, Soderberg CH Jr, Thompson WR 1980 Experience with the EEA stapling device. American Journal of Surgery 139: 549–553

Sickle-Santanello BJ, O'Dwyer PJ, Mojzisik C et al 1987 Radio-immunoguided surgery using the monoclonal antibody B73.2 in colorectal tumours. Diseases of the Colon and Rectum 30: 761–764

Simonsen OS, Stolf NAG, Aun F, Raia A, Habra Gama A 1976 Rectal sphincter reconstruction in perineal colostomies after abdominoperineal resection for cancer. British Journal of Surgery 63: 389–391

Slanctz CA, Horter FP, Grinnell RS 1972 Anterior resection versus abdominoperineal resection for cancer of the rectum and rectosigmoid: an analysis of 524 cases. American Journal of Surgery 123: 110–117

Suzuki H, Matsumoto K, Amano S, Fujioka M, Honzumi M 1980 Anorectal pressure and rectal compliance after low anterior resection. British Journal of Surgery 67: 655–657

Szinicz G 1980 A new implantable sphincter prosthesis for artificial anus. International Journal of Artificial Organs 3: 358–362

Torres RA, Gonzalez MA 1988 Perineal continent colostomy: report of a case. Diseases of the Colon and Rectum 31: 957–960

Waldron DJ 1991 Colo-anal anastomosis. In: Kumar D, Waldron DJ, Williams NS (eds) Clinical measurement in coloproctology. Springer Verlag, London, p 189–200

Williams NS 1984 The rationale for preservation of the anal sphincter in patients with low rectal cancer. British Journal of Surgery 71: 575–581

Williams NS, Johnston D 1983 The quality of life after rectal excision for low rectal cancer. British Journal of Surgery 70: 460–462

Williams NS, Johnston D 1984 Survival and recurrence after sphincter saving resection and abdominoperineal resection for carcinoma of the middle third of the rectum. British Journal of Surgery 71: 278–282

Williams NS, Price R, Johnston D 1980 The long-term effect of sphincter preserving operations for rectal carcinoma on function of the anal sphincter in man. British Journal of Surgery 67: 203–208

Williams NS, Dixon MF, Johnston D 1983 Reappraisal of the 5 cm rule of distal excision for carcinoma of the rectum: a study of distal intramural spread and of patients' survival. British Journal of Surgery 70: 150–154

Williams NS, Durdey P, Johnston D 1985 The outcome following sphincter-saving resection and abdominoperineal resection for low rectal cancer. British Journal of Surgery 72: 596–598

Williams NS, Marzouk DEMM, Hallan RK, Waldron DJ 1989 Function after ileal pouch and stapled pouch-anal anastomosis for ulcerative colitis. British Journal of Surgery 76: 1168–1171

Williams NS, Patel J, George BD, Hallan RI, Watkins ES 1991 Development of an electrically stimulated neo-anal sphincter. Lancet 338: 1166–1169

Williams NS, Hughes SF, Stuchfield B 1994 Continent colonic conduit for rectal evacuation in severe constipation. Lancet 343: 1321–1324

Williams RD, Yurko AA, Kerr G, Zollinger RM 1966 Comparison of anterior and abdominoperineal resection for low pelvic colon and rectal cancer. American Journal of Surgery 111: 114–119

Wilson SM, Beahrs OH 1976 The curative treatment of carcinoma of the sigmoid, rectosigmoid and rectum. Annals of Surgery 183: 556–565

Womack NR, Williams NS, Holmfield JHM, Morrison JFB, Simpkins KC 1985 New method for the dynamic assessment of anorectal function in constipation. British Journal of Surgery 72: 994–998

Wong WD, Rothenberger DA 1993 Artificial anal sphincter. In: Fielding LP, Goldberg SM (eds) Robb and Smith's operative surgery surgery of the colon, rectum and anus, 5th edn. Chapman and Hall, London

Wong SKC, Wee JTK 1984 Reconstruction of an orthotopic functional anus after abdominoperineal resection. Australian and New Zealand Journal of Surgery 54: 575–578

Wu F, Xie RB, Zhang DW 1986 Abdominoperineal resection and anosphincteroplasty in carcinoma of the lower rectum and anal canal. Chung-Hua Wai Ko Tsa Chih 24: 387–388, 444

Zringibl H, Husemann B, Hermanek P 1990 Intra-operative spillage of tumour cells in surgery for rectal cancer. Diseases of the Colon and Rectum 33: 610–614

6 Local procedures, including endoscopic resection

G. F. BUESS

Introduction

Local excision of rectal cancer has for a long time been looked upon mainly as a palliative treatment. The extensive work of two pathologists, Morson (1966, 1984) and Hermanek (1994, Hermanek et al 1983), has demonstrated that there are early stages of rectal cancer which show a low rate of lymph node metastases. Experience of local excision from various centres for colorectal cancers could prove these theoretical facts as relevant (Whiteway et al 1985, Köckerling et al 1994, Nicolls 1994, Staimmer 1994). New technological developments and the introduction of endoscopic surgical techniques have widened clinical experience with local excision significantly (Salm et al 1994). Local excision can be accepted today for resection of T1 low-risk cancers according to Hermanek. In the future the combination of pre- or postoperative irradiation with local excision might indicate the use of local excision for more advanced tumour stages. The results of future prospective clinical trials for evaluation of these treatment modalities have to be critically analysed.

The indication for local excision

Local excision is indicated for resection of tumours in the lower rectum and, by the application of the endoscopic controlled procedure, tumours of favourable pathology in the upper rectum and lower sigmoid can be dealt with in a similar manner.

The main indication for local tumour excision is the resection of adenomas. Large sessile adenomas are frequently found on histological evaluation of the resected specimen to have carcinoma present within them. Conventional transanal resection is indicated when the adenoma is localized in the lower half of the rectum within the reach of the palpating finger.

Using Transanal Endoscopic Microsurgery (TEM), resection of adenomas is possible in the middle and upper rectum and the lower sigmoid, within the reach of a conventional rigid rectoscope. Only very large or circumferential adenomas situated at a high level need to be resected by a conventional open technique.

Resection of early carcinomas with curative intent should be restricted to T1 low-risk cancer according to Hermanek et al (1983). In conventional transanal procedures the location should be limited to the lower rectum, and the upper margin of the tumour should be within reach of the palpating finger. Using TEM, the location should be confined to the area of the rectum where full thickness resection is possible, i.e. the extraperitoneal region of the rectum; this limits the maximal distance from the anal verge at the anterior wall to 12 cm, at the side walls to 15 cm and the posterior wall to 20 cm.

More advanced carcinomas can be resected within the described areas with palliative intent using the same surgical techniques. This can be acceptable in old patients and other patients who are at high risk from more extensive conventional surgical procedures.

Transanal approach for local excision

Different types of mechanical retraction can be used. The use of conventional mechanical retractors is inconvenient for the surgeon and the assistant. Mechanical retractors have been in use for thousands of years and interesting devices have been found for example in Pompeii. Today retractors of the Parks or similar type are used (Parks & Stuart 1973). These retractors can have two or three different blades.

When using retractors, conventional surgical instruments are used for the surgical task. The area is infiltrated with saline, to reduce bleeding. Excision is performed using either scissors or long high-frequency electrodes, to reduce the blood loss during dissection. In adenomas most authors use the technique of submucosectomy. In resection of carcinomas full thickness excision is mandatory. Using mechanical retractors the view is restricted and also manipulation of conventional instruments is limited because of the lack of degrees of freedom during dissection. The retractor blades can act as mechanical obstacles and prevent tension-free approximation of the wound edges, especially during suturing of the wall defect.

Dorsal approaches

The first cancer resections of the rectum were performed using the technique of Kraske (1885). This type of approach was reactivated by Mason (1974). If the tumour is located close to the sphincter a sphincter splitting approach is performed. In higher located tumours the sphincter is preserved. An oblique incision is performed alongside the lateral sacral rim. The muscular wall of the rectum is dissected free and a full thickness excision of the tumour bearing area is performed. Segmental resection and end to end anastomosis are also possible. Postoperative pain is frequent and wound healing problems are typical and can result in septic problems in a significant number of cases (Thompson & Tucker 1987, Staimmer 1994).

Endoscopic procedures – transanal endoscopic microsurgery (TEM)

Transanal Endoscopic Microsurgery (TEM) was the first endoscopic procedure to be developed for operations on the gastrointestinal tract. Development started in 1980, and the first clinical application was in 1983 (Buess et al 1984, Buess 1994). The reasons for the development of this technique were the invasiveness of dorsal approaches to the rectum and the limited view given by the conventional transanal approaches, followed by high recurrence rates of adenomas due to the limited view during the procedure.

The technique of TEM is rather complex and needs substantial training. Via a rigid rectoscope of 40 mm diameter the rectum is inflated. Under constant CO_2 insufflation the endoscopic view is stable and the steroscopic technique gives an excellent view of the rectum and lower sigmoid. With the use of new combination devices usually only two instruments are used. The tumour is excised by high frequency diathermy and the wall defect closed by endoscopically controlled continuous suturing. After 11 years of clinical application there has been a low complication rate with a mortality of 0.5%. Postoperative recovery is fast, with minimal postoperative functional defects and low recurrence rates due to the preciseness of the procedure.

Technology for TEM

Complex new technology was developed for TEM in the years between 1980 and 1983. In the last few years only slight modifications have been made to the instrumentation, except for the significant development of a new combination instrument by ERBE company in Tübingen.

The TEM system consists of a 10 or 20 cm long rectoscope with a 40 mm diameter. For introduction a glass window is used which allows the passage of the instrument into the rectum under direct view and CO_2 insufflation. Before starting the operation itself, the rectoscope is connected to a retractor which is attached to the operating table.

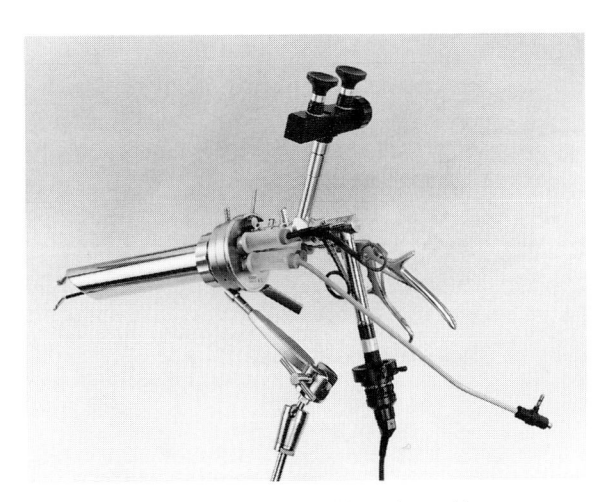

Local procedures, including endoscopic resection 95

Fig. 6.1 Operative rectoscope with optics and instruments introduced via different channels.

A working insert is then introduced which allows the insertion of up to three operating instruments and a stereoscopic optical system (Fig. 6.1). The instruments (Fig. 6.2) have a similar design to laparoscopic instruments: the angulations give more freedom of movement and allow better access to the sacral cavity.

The stereoscopic optics give an excellent view over the operative field. The direct view provides a much sharper image and real colours, as well as a precise three-dimensional view with the possibility of accommodation, which is at present not possible with the use of video techniques.

Together with ERBE (Tübingen, Germany), a new complex instrumentation technique was designed for the dissection of the rectal wall, which allows combinations of different functions, so that only two instruments are necessary for all functions. This instrumentation (Fig. 6.3) has four integrated functions (Farin 1993):

- Bipolar cutting. When the cutting mode is activated via the foot pedal a needle is automatically driven forward by an integrated pneumatic drive and precise dissection is possible.
- Monopolar coagulation. In case of bleeding, activation of the coagulation mode pulls the cutting needle backwards automatically. Monopolar coagulation via the blunt tip of the instrument is performed while the integrated

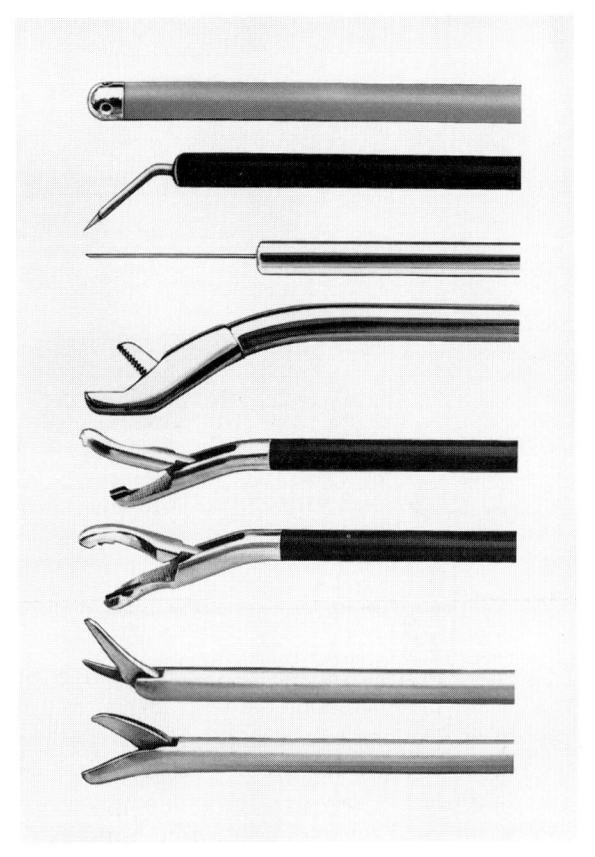

Fig. 6.2 Operative instruments for TEM.

suction channel is used to keep the area dry.
- Suction. The suction channel is connected with a roller pump, which is constantly working with defined suction volumes.
- Rinsing. This is activated to clean the working field.

Preoperative examination

Precise preoperative evaluation of the local situation is mandatory before using TEM. The location of the tumour, distance from the anal verge and the precise position on the circumference is mandatory knowledge, in order to decide whether the tumour can be reached with the operative rectoscope and which positioning of the patient is necessary to perform the operation. To answer this question, the examination has to be

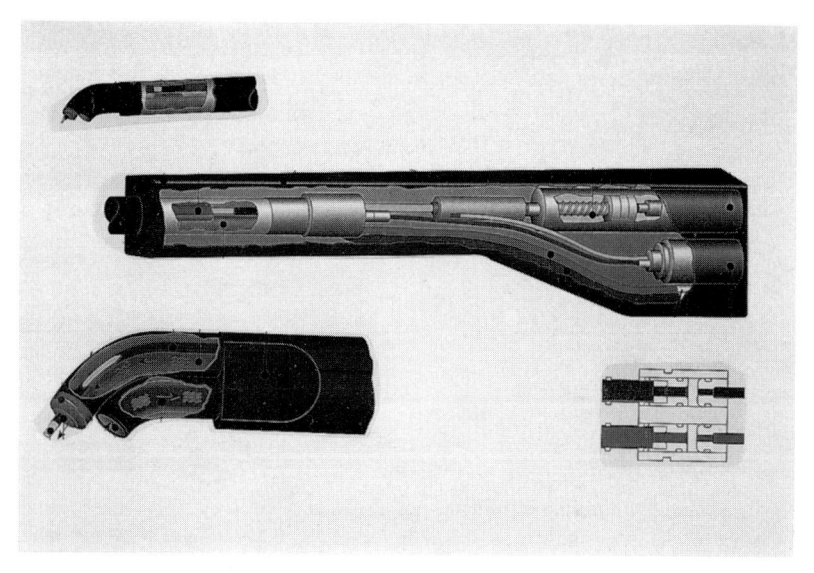

Fig. 6.3 ERBE combination instrument, electronically controlled for bipolar cutting, monopolar coagulation, rinsing and suction.

performed with a rigid scope. The upper tumour margin for the operation is around 20 cm, but in case of angulations in a narrow sigmoid it might be difficult to reach this area. A basic rule is that a tumour which is easy to reach with a rigid scope can be operated on by TEM. Large tumours in this area which are difficult to reach should be resected transabdominally.

It is difficult and in many cases impossible to decide whether the tumour is benign or malignant. Clinical staging by palpation can only be performed for tumours in the lower rectum, which can be reached with the palpating finger. Endoluminal ultrasound examination cannot detect small cancers in the area of the submucosa and in case of angulations T2 tumours can also be missed by ultrasound.

Positioning of the patient and anaesthesia

Depending on the location of the tumour the patient is positioned so that the tumour lies at the bottom. This is because the instruments and the optics are designed to work downwards. General anaesthesia is mandatory. We have experienced problems with the patient starting to move after one hour of regional anaesthesia. The reason for this may have been that because of sedation the CO_2 was not expired sufficiently.

The type of dissection

Two different types of dissection are possible. In small adenomas, in adenomas close to the sphincter and in adenomas in the intraperitoneal portion of the rectum and sigmoid, excision of the mucosa and submucosa is performed directly, leaving the circular muscular layer intact. In adenomas excised close to the sphincter we want to prevent impairment of the sphincter function which might result from resection of parts of the internal sphincter muscle. In tumours located in the intraperitoneal part of the rectum and sigmoid, a full thickness excision would open the peritoneum, which would cause leakage of CO_2 into the peritoneum and consequently restrict the view. However, in most cases the technique used is full thickness excision. Full thickness excision should be performed for all local excisions of carcinoma and in our opinion it is also the best technique for excision of adenomas. This is because around 20% of all tumours diagnosed preoperatively as adenomas show the presence of cancer within the adenoma on final histological evaluation. Mucosectomy has the disadvantage that the specimen tends to tear from the safety margin, which means that the pathologist is not able to define whether the specimen has been removed in toto and in case of cancer whether the margin of clearance is sufficient.

Operative steps

- Introduction of the rectoscope and after localization of the lesion, positioning of the instruments (Fig. 6.4).
- Definition of the safety margin. The margin of clearance is defined by marking dots using the high frequency device. In adenoma we advise a 5 mm margin, and in the case of proven or suspected cancer a 10 mm margin of clearance is desirable (Fig. 6.5).
- Start of dissection. Usually we start at the lower edge of the defect by circumcising the lower circumference.
- Control of bleeding. In mucosectomy smaller bleeders result from small vessels in the plane of the muscular wall. These vessels are visualized by use of suction, the bleeder is stopped by compression of the vessel and coagulated in the monopolar mode.

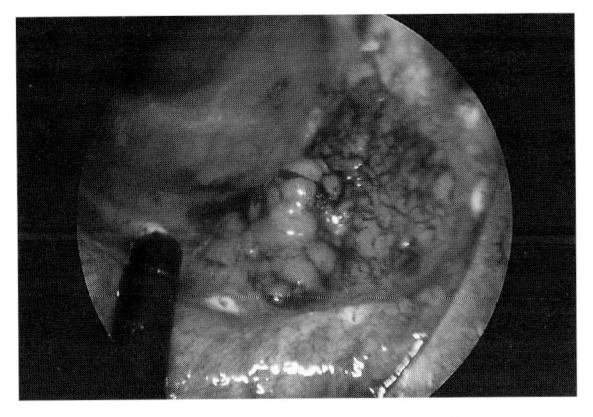

Fig. 6.5 Definition of the margin of clearance by coagulation dots.

- Dissection of the central part. The tumour is folded upwards (Fig. 6.6), so that the base is well exposed for dissection. Larger vessels in the perirectal area can be dissected and coagulated before transection. In most cases the vessels are not seen before transection, so that major bleeding can result. Spurting vessels should be grasped with a forceps, so that the walls of the vessel are compressed before coagulation. Coagulation of large vessels with the suction can result in retraction and increased difficulties in stopping the bleeding. The plane of dissection in full thickness excision is directly on the dorsal plane of the muscular layer. In the case of cancer on the dorsal circumference, parts of the perirectal fat, including the regional lymph nodes, can be resected with the specimen.

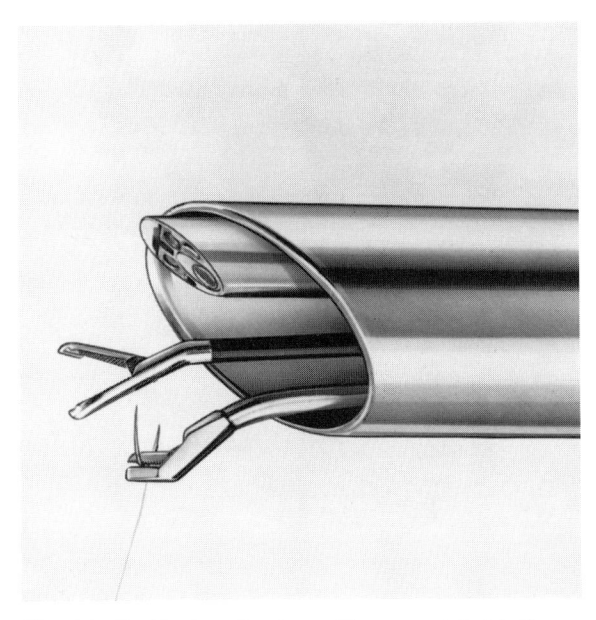

Fig. 6.4 Positioning of optics and instruments inside the rectoscope.

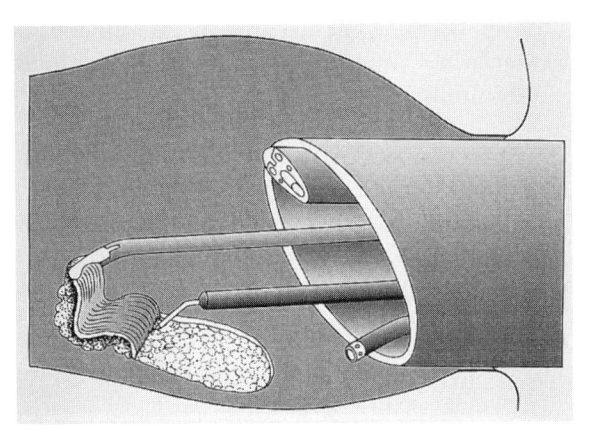

Fig. 6.6 Dissection at the base of a full thickness resection by folding the bowel wall upwards.

98 Colorectal cancer

- Dissection of the upper part. At this stage in larger tumours the view can be restricted due to the tumour mass. A precondition for precise work at this stage is the exact positioning of the marking dots as a guideline for transection, because the border of the tumour is not always exactly visible, so that cuts are performed from marking dot to marking dot.
- Haemostasis during the procedure. Small capillary bleeders may substantially restrict the view, so that it is essential to coagulate each small vessel and to keep the working field completely dry. Dissection should only be continued once complete haemostasis has been attained.
- Tumour cell spillage. Theoretically, during the procedure tumour cells from superficial tumour areas (often small parts of cancer which may be embedded within an adenoma and do not reach the surface of the tumour) can be embedded into the rectal wall defect. In case of cancer or suspected cancer we therefore rinse the defect with β-iodine before suture closure is started.
- Suture closure. In all cases we close the resulting defect with a transverse continuous suture. In case of mucosectomy, suture is not always performed in conventional transanal dissection. We believe that this is because suturing is sometimes restricted by the retractor blades. In contrast to this, TEM offers ideal conditions for suturing, so that stenoses, which can result after mucosectomies without suture, can be prevented. In cases of high located mucosal defects without suture a secondary perforation might occur, when an area of muscular wall which has been coagulated might perforate some time after the operation. In all cases of full thickness excision we are convinced that local infection can be reduced by suture closure.

The suture starts with a PDS suture in SH needle size. The suture should be shortened to a maximum of 10 cm. As in conventional surgery, the suture is performed with needle holder and forceps (Fig. 6.7). Due to the restricted degrees of freedom of movement of the needle holder some tricks are necessary to master the suture. In some positions, for example, the needle holder is kept in position and the bowel tissue is pulled over the needle with the forceps.

After a number of stitches (five to eight) the thread is put under tension and a silver clip is pressed on it. The silver clip holds the suture absolutely safely, so that knotting, which is difficult with parallel positioned instruments as in TEM, is not necessary. Semicircumferential

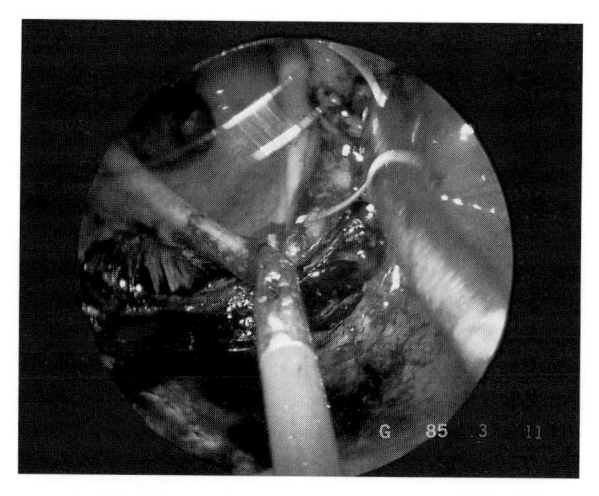

Fig. 6.7 Suturing of a full thickness defect with needle holder and forceps.

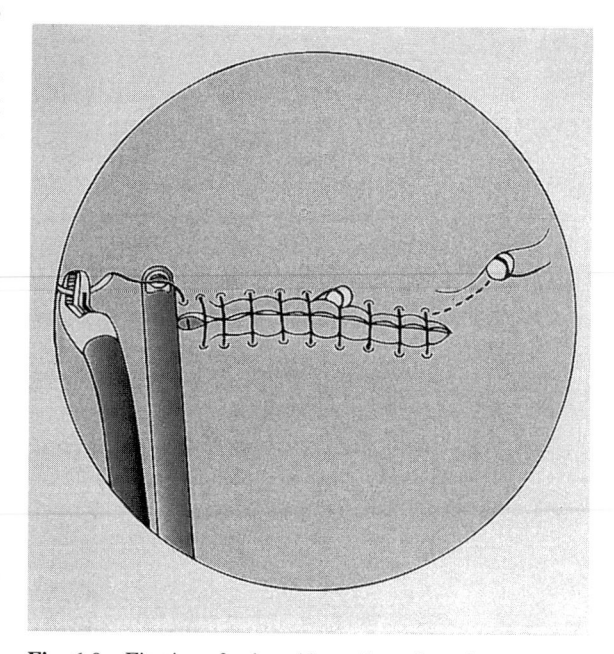

Fig. 6.8 Fixation of a thread by a silver clip as knot substitute.

defects need around three continuous sutures, complete segmental resections need sometimes up to eight sutures.

The postoperative course

Patients can mobilize as soon as anaesthesia allows. Postoperative pain only occurs when the excision is performed close to the dentate line and the suture includes the mucosa of the sensitive anal canal. Higher located excisions are completely pain free, although sometimes a sense of pressure results in the area of the sphincter because of the moderate dilatation of the sphincter due to the introduction of the 40 mm rectoscope. In this context it should be mentioned that the use of a Parks retractor needs much more dilatation than 40 mm to achieve a sufficient view.

Postoperative diet depends on the type of procedure performed. In the case of mucosectomy or a small full thickness excision, complete oral nutrition can start on the second postoperative day. In segmental resection we start complete oral nutrition as in conventional operations on the fifth postoperative day.

Postoperative problems

Postoperative pain

As explained above, local pain is only seen after resection of lesions located close to the anal canal. Medication in such patients is only necessary on the first and second postoperative days. In all higher located excisions, which are the majority, there is no pain at all in the area of operation and only in some patients a certain feeling of slight pressure in the area of the sphincter, which needs no analgesia.

Postoperative incontinence

Within the first postoperative days incontinence may occur, especially following operations close to the sphincter region and in old patients with preoperative existing continence problems. Prospective studies show that after 3 months the vast majority of patients show nearly normal sphincter function (Jehle et al 1992) and after one year show normal sphincter function (to be published). Studies of sphincter function after transanal surgery or after dorsal approaches to the rectal cavity are unavailable. When compared with sphincter function following anterior rectal resection, TEM results are favourable (Jehle et al 1995).

Micturition

A common postoperative problem is difficulty in micturition. This is more often seen in older male patients. The reason for this problem when it starts directly after the operation and disappears on the second postoperative day is most likely the mechanical trauma induced by the compression of the urethra by the operative rectoscope during the procedure.

In a few cases micturition problems can continue after this period and occur in combination with septic symptoms. In such patients a suture dehiscense with infection of the perirectal space might be the reason for the problem and should be excluded by careful rectoscopy.

Typical postoperative temperature rise following TEM

A rise in temperature of up to 38° is seen in most patients in the first two to three days after the operation. This could be induced by bacterial contamination of the perirectal tissue during full thickness excision. In most cases the pyrexia reduces after two days. Our nurses label this rise in temperature 'TEM temperature'.

Dehiscence of suture line

The second most frequent problem is related to suture dehiscence. Depending on the size of the excision, tension may result on the suture line, which can be followed by suture dehiscence.

Routine rectoscopy in a number of patients has shown that most suture dehiscences are without any clinical symptoms. This finding has clinical relevance when septic problems arise. In patients with a postoperative temperature of more than 38°C lasting more than three days, suture dehiscence should be suspected. Careful rectoscopic examination without performing an enema to prevent additional local trauma is indicated.

In case of suture dehiscence oral nutrition should cease and i.v. infusion and antibiotics should commence. In the majority of cases the temperature settles within a few days and oral nutrition may then recommence.

In 1% of patients septic problems continue despite these measures. In this situation a temporary colostomy may be necessary to assist the local healing process.

Postoperative bleeding

Discharge of a few millilitres of blood in the first few postoperative days is typical. The source of bleeding can be either the suture line or more likely from mucosal tears in the anal canal. Sudden discharge of larger amounts of blood, mostly after the second postoperative day, is a typical sign of suture dehiscence. In the area of local infection in the perirectal tissue, small vessels are eroded and tend to bleed for a certain period. In most patients bleeding stops spontaneously after one episode. In 1% of patients there is more severe bleeding which needs intervention. This can be performed using a rigid rectoscope. The bleeder is localized with a suction tube and the area of bleeding is coagulated.

Results

The latest results from the Tübingen Clinic include data for 190 adenomas and 75 carcinomas operated on between 1989 and 1993 (Mentges et al 1994). The mortality was 0.3% and complications forcing reintervention were 3% following resection of adenomas and 8% following resection of carcinomas. Thirty four patients had pT1 tumours with local resection, two of these patients developed recurrent cancer during follow-up. In both patients a radical resection with curative intent could be performed. Salm et al (1994) published a survey covering the experiences of 44 clinics in Germany. In 1900 patients, 1411 adenomas and 433 carcinomas were resected. Of patients with cancer 246 were resected with curative intent and 147 with palliative intent. Complications were found in 6.3% of patients and 4% recovered with conservative treatment. Surgical reintervention was needed by 2.3% (including transanal interventions). The specific problems seen in the learning phase of TEM were analysed by Salm et al (1994), who stated that TEM shows lower complication rates compared to conventional surgical procedures and that the mortality rate of 0.2% is also lower.

Conclusion

The highest incidence of colorectal cancer occurs in the rectum and lower sigmoid. Endoscopic diagnosis and ultrasound examination are easy to perform in this area. The conventional procedure for tumour resection with transabdominal surgical access is a major intervention, especially in tumours situated close to the sphinter region. The quality of life, including sphincter function, after these operations is significantly impaired (Jehle et al 1995), so less invasive procedures should be preferred, if the outcome for the patient shows no disadvantages.

The clinical data available today are valid arguments for the acceptance of local excision of a T1 low risk cancer when resected using a full thickness technique with a clear safety margin.

In the lower half of the rectum, resection by the use of retractors is the standard treatment. TEM offers some additional benefits. The dilatation of the sphincter region is less compared to retractor techniques and the gas insufflation in combination with the stereoscopic optics give an optimal view. Compared to techniques using retractors, TEM gives a better operative view in the middle part of the rectum and also allows precise procedures in the upper rectum. The relatively high recurrence rate after transanal resection of adenomas with the use of mechanical retractors (Wunderlich & Parks 1983) results in our view from the reduced vision of the operative area, especially in high located tumours.

All surgical techniques of rectal wall resection which can be performed with the use of the dorsal approach can also be performed with TEM. In the clinics where the author has been working in the last 10 years, in no patient was a dorsal approach necessary. We are convinced that dorsal approaches, because of their high complication rates (Thompson & Tucker 1987, Staimmer 1994), should not be performed any more and that patients who have an indication for a dorsal approach should be referred to a TEM centre.

Low complication rates after TEM and the extremely low mortality in combination with the low recurrence rates indicate that, in experienced hands, TEM should be the most precise surgical procedure for local excision. From the functional side the results following TEM are excellent (Jehle et al 1992). The disadvantages of the procedure are the high costs of the complex technology and the need for special training, which our centre offers. The surgeon and his team need a case load of at least two interventions per month in order to gain sufficient experience of routine operations. This is available at the major centres, which means that TEM is an excellent technique for these major colorectal centres.

References

Buess G 1994 Endoluminal rectal surgery (TEM), In: Buess G, Cuschieri A, Périssat, J. (eds) Operative Manual of Endoscopic Surgery (1). Springer-Verlag, Heidelberg, pp 303–325

Buess G, Hutterer F, Theis J, Böbel M, Isselhard W, Pichlmaier H 1984 Das System für die transanale endoskopische Rektumoperation Chirurg 55: 677–680

Farin G 1993 Pneumatically controlled bipolar cutting instrument. Endoscopic Surgery and Allied Technologies 4: 97–101

Hermanek P, 1994 Onkologische und histopathologische Grundlagen einer lokalen Therapie in kurativer Intention. In: Hermanek P, Marzoli GP (eds) Lokale Therapie des Rektumkarzinoms. Springer-Verlag, Heidelberg, pp 7–14

Hermanek P Frühmorgen P, Guggenmoos-Holzmann I, Altendorf A Matek W 1983 The malignant potential of colorectal polyps – a new statistical approach. Endoscopy 15: 16–20

Jehle EC, Haehnel T, Starlinger MJ, Becker HD 1995 Level of the anastomosis does not influence functional outcome after anterior rectal resection for rectal cancer. American Journal of Surgery 169: 147–154

Jehle EC, Starlinger MJ, Kreis ME et al 1992 Alterations of anal sphincter functions following transanal endoscopic microsurgery (TEM) for rectal tumors. Gastroenterology 102: 365

Köckerling F, Hermanek P, Gall FP 1994 Ergebnisse der lokalen Therapie in Erlangen. In: Hermanek P, Marzoli GP (eds) Lokale Therapie des Rektumkarzinoms. Springer-Verlag, Heidelberg, pp 121–130

Kraske P 1885 Zur Exstirpation hochsitzender Mastdarmkrebse. Verh. Dtsch. Gs. Chir. 14: 464–474

Mason AY 1974 Trans-sphincteric surgery of the rectum. Progress in Surgery 13: 66–97

Mentges B, Buess G, Raestrup H, Manncke F, Becker HD 1994 TEM results of the Tubingen group. Endoscopic Surgery and Allied Technologies 5: 251–254

Morson BC 1966 Factors influencing the prognosis of early cancers of the rectum. Proceeding of the Royal Society of Medicine 59: 607–608

Morson BC, Whiteway JE, Jonas EA, MacRae FA, Williams CB 1984 Histopathology and prognosis of malignant colorectal polyps treated by endoscopic polypectomy. Gut 25: 437–444

Nicholls RJ 1994 Results at St. Mark's Hospital. In: Hermanek P, Marzoli GP (eds) Lokale Therapie des Rektumkarzinoms. Springer-Verlag, Heidelberg, pp 137–139

Parks AG, Stuart AE 1973 The management of villous tumours of the large bowel. British Journal of Surgery 9: 688–695

Salm R, Lampe H, Bustos A, Matern U 1994 Experience with TEM in Germany. Endoscopic Surgery and Allied Technologies 5: 251–254

Staimmer D 1994 Ergebnisse der lokalen Therapie in der SGKRK-Studie und in München-Neuperlach. In: Hermanek P, Marzoli GP (eds) Lokale Therapie des Rektumkarzinoms. Springer-Verlag, Heidelberg, pp 131–136

Thompson BW, Tucker WE 1987 Transsphincteric approach to lesions of the rectum. Southern Medical Journal 80: 41–43

Whiteway J, Nicholls RJ, Morson DC 1985 The role of surgical local excision in the treatment of rectal cancer. British Journal of Surgery 72: 694–697

Wunderlich M, Parks AG 1983 Peranale Exzision villöser Rektumadenome Acta Chir Austriaca Suppl. 51

7 Laparoscopic surgery in colorectal cancer

T. A. TEOH   S. D. WEXNER

Introduction

Laparoscopic surgery has gained much popularity in the last few years. The use of the laparoscope as a therapeutic tool has escalated from a diagnostic tool used by gynaecologists to an instrument that can be used in many facets of modern-day surgery. Amidst much controversy, it soon became apparent that the benefits of laparoscopic cholecystectomy were significant, especially relative to the postoperative course. Now, laparoscopic cholecystectomy is generally the procedure of choice for uncomplicated gall bladder disease.

Laparoscopic colorectal surgery, however, does not share the same place as its predecessor. Its development was fuelled largely by industrial sources and by certain entrepreneurial laparoscopic colorectal 'institutes'. Soon after, it was apparent that unlike conventional surgery, the skills required for laparoscopic cholecystectomy and even appendectomy were very different than those required for laparoscopic bowel surgery (SAGES 1991). Tedious and technically demanding surgery was followed by high complication rates in initial experiences (Altman 1992, Hoffman et al 1994, Jacobs et al 1991). Moreover, the purported advantages of laparoscopic colorectal surgery were not as apparent, as length of hospitalization and costs were similar to the results noted after standard surgery. 'Should laparoscopic colorectal surgery be done?', 'Are curative cancer operations possible laparoscopically?', 'Are there real benefits with the laparoscopic approach?'. There presently do not exist any scientifically valid answers to these questions. However, we will discuss the issues shrouding the controversy in laparoscopic colorectal surgery and its role in colorectal cancer.

Why is learning and performing laparoscopic surgery different?

The 'learning curve' is an intrinsic part of any procedure. There is a learning phase not only for new techniques but also for established operations. For established techniques, preceptorship is an excellent means to ascend the learning curve and there exist many surgeons capable of imparting needed skills to the surgeon under training.

Traditionally, the continent ileostomy and the ileoanal reservoir were known to have steep learning curves and the popularity of these procedures waned in the beginning. More than 10 years of experience, refinements and, simplification of techniques achieved by high-volume inflammatory bowel disease centres paved the way for the ileoanal reservoir to be undertaken safely and efficaciously by many smaller volume practices. The laparoscopic procedures that are taught have not stood the test of time nor application for general usage. Techniques that are routinely undertaken by the advanced laparoscopist are not so easily performed by a surgeon whose laparoscopic experience is limited to cholecystectomy, appendectomy and herniorrhaphy.

There exist several differences between laparoscopic colorectal surgery and most other laparoscopic procedures including fundoplication and splenectomy.

Anatomical site

All other laparoscopic procedures involve one main anatomical region. The large bowel traverses all the quadrants of the abdominal cavity and the procedure often requires dissection in more than one region. To obtain the best operating angle, surgeons often have to change their position relative to the patient and change the position of equipment during the procedure. Dissection is extremely difficult when undertaken with the video monitors facing in the opposite direction.

Retraction and countertraction

As dissection of the gall bladder or appendix progresses, mobility of the organ usually aids further dissection. In laparoscopic colon surgery, however, the dissected bowel hinders vision. The laxity of mobilized bowel does not aid easy retraction within the confined space of the peritoneal cavity. Certain ports dedicated to retraction have to be designated or alternating manoeuvres like high Trendelenburg, marked right or left tilt and low reverse Trendelenburg positions have to be employed throughout the procedure. The principle of countertraction, so often employed in surgery, is also important in laparoscopic dissection. However, these manoeuvres are, again, progressively more difficult as more bowel is mobilized.

Location of lesion or pathological segment

Most other laparoscopic operations have a defined site of pathology. Cholelithiasis requires removal of the gall bladder, fundoplication requires wrapping of the gastric fundus, operations for hernia require repair of the hernia orifices. Colonic resections, however, require resection of the correct segment of bowel. In conventional surgery, preoperative diagnostic colonoscopy and contrast studies, complemented with careful palpation and visualization of the bowel, enables accurate localization of the correct site of pathology. The tactile ability is severely compromised in laparoscopic surgery and the potential for incorrect segment removal is increased. Numerous cases reported document the gravity of this problem.

Vascular control and ligation

Some procedures, such as herniorrhaphy or fundoplication, do not entail vascular division. Most other organs have a single vessel or vessels relatively fixed in position to ligate. With experience, these arteries and veins can be rapidly, safely and inexpensively ligated and divided. Mesenteric vessels, however, run in a layer of often thick mesenteric fat. Laparoscopically isolating these pedicles and subsequently ligating and dividing them can be much more difficult than in conventional surgery. Once bleeding occurs, the field of view is marred and laparoscopic vision is severely compromised. To effect safe ligation and division of mesenteric vessels, meticulous and somewhat difficult dissection of the pedicle and subsequent safe ligation with clips or endoscopic loops can be substituted only by expensive vascular stapling devices. Even with modern technology, this step also can be difficult especially in obese patients with thickened, fatty mesentery or in patients with inflammatory bowel disease in whom the mesentery is friable.

Removal of specimen

Gall bladders can almost always be removed through a 10–12 mm port. Fundoplications and hernia repairs do not even require specimen removal. Being an appreciably larger organ, retrieval of the resected colon requires a larger portal of removal. To effect removal of specimens in colorectal surgery, larger incisions have to be made. Technology has offered an alternative with larger ports which obviate the need for an incision, but rather stretch the fascia to enable the specimen to be delivered. Specimen bags have been devised to placate surgeons who are concerned with contamination by bacteria or tumour when the specimen is negotiated through the small wound.

Fashioning of anastomoses

An integral part of most colonic resections is fashioning an anastomosis. This step is in contrast to other procedures where extirpation of the organ marks the end of the procedure. Although the skills required to perform the other procedures are well recognized, they are vastly different from those attributes necessary to effect a well-vascularized, tension-free, circumferentially intact anastomosis. To achieve this goal laparoscopically is a challenge which requires technical prowess, often infinite patience and experience.

Cancer procedures

Resection of malignancy is unusual in most other laparoscopic operations. In contrast, the same principles of cancer 'curing' operations practised in conventional colorectal surgery must be maintained in laparoscopic resections. Dissection must then be extensive with resection of all appropriate vascular and lymphatic drainage. Furthermore, when rectal resections are undertaken, adequate distal and lateral margins are mandatory. (Cawthorn et al 1990) Lastly, the results of laparoscopic colorectal cancer resections are still unknown. Specifically, no 5-year distant recurrence or survival data are available and no prospective randomized trials have assessed 2-year local recurrence rates. All other laparoscopic procedures can be considered as having been successful if the patient leaves the hospital soon after surgery without having suffered any morbidity. Late recurrence of an inguinal hernia, although potentially distressing, is not in the same realm as local recurrence of a rectal carcinoma.

Laparoscopic procedures in colon and rectal surgery

Currently, benign conditions and palliation for metastatic disease are the most widely accepted indications for laparoscopic bowel resections (Bauer et al 1994, Etienne et al 1993, Franklin et al 1993, Milson et al 1993). Laparoscopic resections for cancer 'curing' are still highly controversial and by no means standard care. In light of this controversy, many surgeons have suggested that laparoscopic cancer resections should only be performed in the setting of prospective randomized trials.

Almost all colon and rectal surgical procedures have been attempted or are being performed with varying degrees of assistance from the laparoscope (Franklin 1993, Puente et al 1994, Quattlebaum et al 1993, Sosa et al 1994, Tucker et al 1994, Wexner & Johansen 1992, Wexner et al 1992). We shall address in this section an outline of currently performed procedures.

General considerations

Laparoscopic surgery should only be performed by surgeons who are adequately trained. (Weiss & Wexner 1995a, 1995b). 'Experienced' surgeons have often only performed a few cases more than have the novices. Preceptorship with a more experienced surgeon should be the rule in the initial phase. The entire surgical team should be similarly trained. A basic feature of laparoscopy, particularly in more complicated procedures like bowel resections, is that the surgeon relies heavily on the team, so much so that single surgeon endeavours are almost impossible.

See and associates (1993) surveyed 297 urologic surgeons who completed a laparoscopy training course. At 3 months, surgeons who performed clinical procedures without additional training were 3.39 times more likely to have had at least one complication compared with surgeons who sought additional training ($p=0.03$). At 12 months, surgeons who had attended the training course alone, were in solo practice or performed laparoscopic surgery with a variable assistant were 4.85, 7.74 and 4.80 times more likely, respectively, ($p=0.004$, $p=0.0008$, $p=0.0015$) to have had a complication than their counterparts who attended the course with a partner, were in group practice or operated with the same assistant. At both time intervals, there was a significant inverse correlation between laparoscopic complication rates and the number of procedures performed. Although data like these do not exist for laparoscopic colorectal surgery, there is no reason to suppose that different conclusions would be reached. Specifically, the rate of complications along the learning curve can be decreased by additional education. It therefore seems wise to make such a schema compulsory.

The patient and pathology and not the technology or technique should dictate the type of resection or procedure to be performed. Only after the decision to operate is made on these grounds should the mode of surgery (open or laparoscopic) be considered. The eagerness to perform laparoscopy must not compromise basic surgical principles. The same operation should be performed whether laparoscopically or open. Since colotomy and excision of tumour is unacceptable in conventional surgery, the laparoscopic approach cannot and must not justify such woefully inadequate procedures merely because they are easier (Morson & Bussey 1985, Morson et al 1984).

Contraindications to the laparoscopic approach depend largely on surgical expertise; dissection in patients with morbid obesity, liver cirrhosis and multiple adhesions requires advanced skills and should be contraindications for surgeons with little experience. Relative contraindications include acute inflammatory bowel disease, advanced sepsis and bowel obstruction.

It is important that basic surgical data and common sense prevail over the ego of the surgeon. Skills that are evident in some may not be similar in others. Failure to complete the laparoscopic procedure does not constitute a failure in treatment. Conversion to laparotomy should not be considered a defeat but rather invocation of sound surgical judgement. Anecdotal reports of 6–9-hour long laparoscopic colectomies are legion and the wisdom of these herculean feats must be questioned. Similarly, surgeons have utilized 8–11 ports to perform a completely intracorporeal resection and anastomosis for carcinoma. Following these lengthy pursuits, an often generous incision is made for delivery of the specimen. Again, a 'successful' outcome means long-term cure of the patient's disease, not short-term boosting of the surgeon's ego. In general, if 'significant' progress is not made either with the entire procedure within 2 hours of insufflation or with an individual phase of the procedure within 30 minutes, the procedure should be converted to a laparotomy.

Preoperative preparation

The patient should be advised of the risks, benefits, potential complications and alternatives available. An informed consent must always include a possible laparotomy and possible intraoperative colonoscopy. Routine preoperative preparation as for open procedures should be undertaken.

Patient positioning and initiation of procedure

Patients should be supine with the lower limbs in the modified lithotomy position within Allen stirrups (Allen Medical, Bedford Heights, Ohio). The hips and knees are flexed gently at a 10–15° angle so as not to impede movement of the long laparoscopic instruments. This position allows access to the anus for the passage of stapling devices for low anastomosis, for insertion of the colonoscope for intraoperative localization of the lesion or for colonoscopic retraction of the flexures (Reissman et al 1995b). Furthermore, the space between the legs is an excellent position in which to place either the camera operator or assistant. In that space, their activities will facilitate rather than compromise the motions of the surgeon.

The patient should be endotracheally intubated, with a nasogastric tube and urinary catheter in situ. Ureteric stents are sometimes used to help in identification of the ureter. This manoeuvre is especially useful in pelvic dissections in patients who have had prior pelvic surgery or radiation. However, it is important not to routinely employ additional costly invasive procedures which would not be utilized during laparotomy just to facilitate laparoscopy.

It is important that equipment be strategically and ergonomically placed to allow easy access and vision by the surgical team. Two video monitors are placed in the line of dissection on the side of the surgical field. The surgeon stands on the opposite side so that this eyes and hands are working in the same direction. When a different sector of the abdomen is operated on, it is important that a few moments are taken to adjust the position of the monitors or for the surgeon to move either to the contralateral side or between the patient's legs. This latter location is especially useful during flexure mobilization.

Port placement

An extremely popular question that frequently arises in most discussions in laparoscopy is the number and the sites of port placement. Novices at laparoscopy courses and lectures are often seen frantically taking notes on exact port positions.

Experience has shown that port positioning should be tailored to each procedure, patient and surgeon. There are, however, several basic guiding principles. Generally, port sizes should be a minimum of 10–12 mm to allow maximal surgical flexibility by easy interchangeability of most instruments and the camera. In initiating the procedure, the first port, which is for the camera, is usually through or adjacent to the umbilicus. Subsequent port sites are placed under vision after inspection of the anatomy of the patient.

Although it is important that adequate ports be placed to effect the safe and efficient conduct of the procedure, careful planning and familiarity with the procedure are required to ensure optimum usage. Most major procedures can be performed with no more than 4–5 ports. Knowledge of available technology and different manufacturers' products is also essential and planning port sizes and sites should take these differences into account. Body habitus will also affect the exact placement of ports. Standard laparoscopic instruments, from the midabdominal ports, will not reach the pelvis in a person with a long or broad torso. It is important to place ports close enough to reach the operative field and yet not cross and obstruct each other. In general, ports are placed in fluid motion throughout the procedure. Also, in general, one port can be placed in each quadrant and one at the umbilicus. However, contingent upon the patient's anatomy, the identical pathology can be approached with three, four or five ports. Thus, routine placement of five ports is both wasteful and often unnecessary.

The placement of incisions for specimen removal or stoma creation should also be taken into consideration. Often, these incisions can incorporate one or two port sites, thus reducing the number of scars. In anterior resections or sigmoid colectomies, the left mid or lower abdominal port can be enlarged for removal of the specimen and introduction of the anvil of the circular stapling device. In abdominoperineal resections, the left lower port may be used as the site for the stoma and the right lower port for the drain (Reissman et al 1944a). In laparoscopic-assisted right colectomies, the umbilical port can be enlarged to effect the extracorporeal phase of the procedure. Laparoscopic-assisted total colectomies can be extracorporeally completed through a Pfannensteil incision (Wexner et al 1992, Lointier et al 1993).

Cosmesis, at present, is the only universally accepted advantage of laparoscopic bowel surgery. Surgeons should thus be conscious of this benefit and, within limits of safety and efficacy, maximize this effect. Incisions for trocar placement can be hidden in natural creases and lines or made in the direction of Langers' lines to enhance the cosmetic effect (Teoh et al 1995).

Mobilization of bowel

Most procedures usually start with mobilization of bowel. As with open surgery, gentle traction and countertraction aid in visualization of the correct planes. It is important to be familiar with the technique of sharp dissection with electrocautery in laparoscopic surgery. This method facilitates accurate and haemostatic dissection. Positioning of the patient contributes significantly to aid retraction by using the gravity effect to move the bowel away from the field of vision. When mobilizing the flexures, a reverse Trendelenburg position is adopted with a tilt contralateral to the side being mobilized. A steep Trendelenburg position aids in pelvic dissection (Nogueras & Wexner 1992).

The actual dissection is no different to that in open surgery. The white line of Toldt is incised along the colon up to the flexures. With experience, the entire colon and its mesentery can be completely mobilized as in conventional surgery. Some difficulty is encountered when omentum has to be mobilized from the transverse colon, especially in obese patients. However, adhering to the technique of electrocautery of smaller vessels and clipping or ligating larger vessels, it can be safely accomplished.

Confirmation of site of lesion

Unlike open surgery, the tactile ability to localize the tumour or lesion is lost. Large bulky tumours can sometimes be seen, but smaller tumours and large polyps that do not have serosal signs indicative of their location need additional localization techniques. Postcolonoscopy preoperative barium enema, although used by some surgeons, adds cost, discomfort, and potential morbidity. Other surgeons include with the initial colonoscopy marking of the lesion with Indian ink, indigo carmine, indocyanine green or methylene blue to allow visualization during laparoscopy. If the site of lesion is in doubt, an intraoperative colonoscopy to confirm the site of the lesion is performed and the serosal surface is marked with clips. These manoeuvres help to reduce the rate of incorrect segment removal (Cohen and Wexner 1994, Corbitt 1992, Larach et al 1993a, Monson et al 1992).

Ligation of vessels

Once the colon is mobilized, attention is directed to ligation of vessels which can be done either extra- or intracorporeally. When extracorporeal ligation is performed, an incision is made, the bowel is eviscerated with the mobilized mesentery and the vessels are ligated in the normal fashion. The incision required to perform this phase is much smaller than that required without laparoscopic mobilization and this is the only proven advantage of laparoscopic assistance.

If intracorporeal ligation is preferred or mandated because of a shortened mesentery, several methods are available. A vascular stapling device, similar to that used for bowel, with modified clip sizes, can be applied to ligate the vessels. This procedure, however, adds to the cost and operating time. To save costs, meticulous dissection of the vascular pedicles and subsequent clipping or ligation with an endoscopic loop obviates the need for the stapler. This dissection, however, is significantly more difficult and time-consuming. Ligation of vessels at the origin can be routinely effected with experience. Technically, the resection margins, mesenteric excision and height of vascular ligation, when properly performed, can equal that of open surgery.

Resection and anastomosis of bowel

Again, the surgeon has the option of performing this phase either extra- or intracorporeally. If extracorporeal resection and anastomosis is performed, conventional methods are applied. The mesenteric defect can also be easily closed. Right-sided anastomoses can be performed with an endoscopic linear cutting and anastomotic device. However, one must question the rationale behind utilization of several hundred pounds (sterling) worth of staplers to effect a totally intracorporeal anastomosis, only to subsequently make an incision to remove the resected bowel. Such intracorporeal extravaganzas represent a triumph of technology over common sense.

Conversely, left-sided lesions lend themselves well to an intracorporeal anastomosis, facilitated by a circular stapler (Knight & Griffen 1980). The port site can be incised to the fascia or the port can be exchanged for a 33 mm port (Ethicon Endosurgery Inc, (Cincinnatti, Ohio USA) through which the specimen can be removed. It is important at this juncture to estimate the length of bowel that needs to be resected and to ensure that the proximal resected end comfortably reaches the distal end for a tension-free anastomosis. This manoeuvre can be effected through the laparoscope by marking the proximal edge of resection prior to transcutaneous delivery of the bowel. Debate continues as to whether the mode of removal influences wound complications like tumour implantation and wound infection. Thus, specimen bags to prevent soilage of the wound and port-sized wound protectors are available. Although in theory tissue morcellators can reduce the size of the incision, in practice pathologists cannot at the present time stage a morcellated tumour.

After resection of the specimen, the detachable head of the circular stapler is inserted, secured with a purse string and reintroduced into the peritoneal cavity. After the 33 mm port is reinserted, pneumoperitoneum is reestablished and under laparoscopic guidance, the detachable head is replaced onto the shaft of the transanally introduced stapler. After the stapler is fired both the anastomosis and the doughnuts are tested for integrity.

Alternative approaches to effect the anastomosis have been practised by some surgeons. Enthusiasts have performed intracorporeal handsewn purse strings and endoscopic loop purse strings. The distal rectal stump can also be everted through the anus and transected and either a purse string is sewn or a stapled closure is performed. The stapling device is then introduced and the anastomosis fashioned as described above. A triple stapling technique has been described which decreases the potential for contamination as well as the need for an incision.

Critics of these techniques are concerned with potential sphincter injury when the specimen is delivered or the stump is everted through the anus. These criticisms arise from sound scientific evidence that transanal manipulation has resulted in transient, if not permanently decreased internal sphincter pressures. Horgan and associates (1989) showed that even appropriate controlled use of a 31 mm circular stapling device led to a significant decrease ($p<0.05$) in maximal resting pressure. Other authors have demonstrated similar deleterious effects after mucosectomy (Choen et al 1991, Keighley 1987, Lavery et al 1989, Liljeqvist et al 1988) and even after non-mucosectomy (double-stapled) restorative proctocolectomy (Chindasub et al 1994, Jorge & Wexner 1993, Liljeqvist et al 1988, Luukkonen & Jarvinen 1993, McIntyre et al 1994, Reissman et al 1995a, Wexner et al 1991) with a 28 mm circular stapler. Thus, if even controlled rapid use of a circular stapler causes these problems, what effect might prolonged uncontrolled extirpation of the left colon and its attendant mesentery have (Beck & Wexner 1992, Horgan et al 1989)?

To date, none of the proponents of this technique have offered either objective physiologic or subjective functional proof that the sphincter mechanism is not damaged during specimen removal. Preoperative, intraoperative and postoperative manometric pressures with incontinence scores are necessary to dispel otherwise sound evidence of the inadvisability of this manoeuvre. Another concern with this transanal manoeuvre is the intraluminal seeding of malignant cells when the anvil is pushed proximally past the tumour. One must question whether the avoidance of a 3 cm incision is worth the extra cost, extra effort, extra operative time, the risk of tumour implantation and the risk of injury to the sphincter. Once again, common sense must prevail and one must justify at every step the benefit of the next step.

If an abdominoperineal excision is being performed, then delivery of the sigmoid should be through an 18 mm rather than a 33 mm port to avoid creation of too large a stoma. However, the fascia should be scored to prevent a postoperative fascial ileal obstruction (Teoh et al 1994). The remainder of the procedure can be effected from the perineal approach as it would be without laparoscopic facilitation.

Termination of procedure

After assurance of a tension-free, well-vascularized and circumferentially intact anastomosis, a careful check for haemostasis is performed. Drains, if required, can be brought out through one of the port sites. The pneumoperitoneum is released and the port sites and incisions closed. Care must be taken with closure of port sites as hernias have been reported (O'Donovan & Larach 1994, Reissman et al 1994b). An instrument with a J-shaped hollow threading needle may facilitate full-thickness, all-layered closure.

The Cleveland Clinic Florida experience

To assess the potential value of laparoscopic surgery and, specifically, its role in colorectal surgery, a three-phase programme to introduce laparoscopy to the institution was commenced (Wexner et al 1993). Phase I included a 6-month extensive training period in animal models. Phase II included a 3-month programme performing laparoscopic cholecystectomies in humans. When laparoscopic skills were fairly well developed, Phase III was initiated with performance of laparoscopic colorectal surgery in humans.

A prospective registry was established according to the guidelines of the American Society of Colon and Rectal Surgeons (1991). The registry included information pertaining to morbidity, mortality, duration of surgery, duration of ileus, length of hospital stay, age, sex, diagnosis, indication for surgery and surgical procedure performed. From initiation of the registry in August 1991 to February 1994, 100 cases of laparoscopic or laparoscopic-assisted colorectal procedures were performed by two surgeons working as a team. The mean age of patients was 49 (12–88) years and there were

60 males. Procedures that were performed included 37 total abdominal colectomies (TAC), 25 with ileoanal reservoirs, seven with ileorectal anastomosis and five with end ileostomies. A further 47 patients had segmental colonic or bowel resections, including five anterior resections of the rectum, three with abdominoperineal resections, 14 right colectomies, 10 sigmoid colectomies, seven reversal of Hartmann's procedure, seven ileocaecectomies and one transverse colectomy. Sixteen other patients had other procedures including stoma creation and rectopexy. Twenty two patients (22%) sustained 26 intraoperative or postoperative complications and there was no mortality.

The complication rate was further assessed at each phase of development of laparoscopy. The first one-third of patients (n=33) and second one-third of patients (n=33) had significantly higher complication rates (42% and 27%, respectively) than did the last one-third (12%; $p<0.05$). Interestingly, complication rates in each group were proportional to the number of TAC performed (18 in the first third, 13 in the second third and six in the last third). Throughout the study, the complication rate of TAC was significantly higher when compared to the other procedures (42% and 17% respectively, $p<0.01$). The mean length of hospital stay for all 100 patients was 7.1 (2–40) days. This morbidity compares favourably with rates reported by other authors (Table 7.1).

In this series, 15 patients had resections for malignancy. Five tumours were in the rectum, two in the left colon, one in the transverse and seven in the right colon. The average age was 67.4 (40–84) years. All patients received preoperative preparation similar to that described above. For right-sided lesions, laparoscopic assistance was used to mobilize the required bowel. A 2–4 cm transumbilical incision was then made for vessel ligation, specimen resection and anastomosis. For left-sided lesions, the inferior mesenteric artery and vein were divided at their origins either with clips, endoloops or with the endoscopic vascular stapling/cutting device. When rectal dissection was performed, care was taken to ensure total mesorectal excision with wide lateral margins. Distal resection was facilitated with the application of the vascular cutting/stapling device. Subsequently, either an incision was made

Table 7.1 Mean length of stay, morbidity and mortality of recent series

Author	Year	Patients (n)	Mean stay (days)	Range (days)	Morbidity %	Mortality %
Lointier et al	1993	6	10	7–16	16	0
Bauer et al	1994	8	6.7	5–10	0	0
Milsom et al	1993	9	7	5–12	0	0
Chindasub et al	1994	10	8	NS	20	0
Tate et al	1993	11	12.3	NS	45	0
Van Ye et al	1994	14	9.1	4–9	7	0
Jacobs et al	1991	14/20	4	NS	15	0
Corbitt	1992	18	4	3–6	0	0
Larach et al	1993a	18	8.4	4–25	39	
Vara-Thorbeck et al	1994	18	7.6	4–12	34	0
Sosa et al	1994	14	6.3	4–10	14.3	
Franklin et al	1993	19	7.4	NS	16	0
Quattlebaum et al	1993	20	4.4	2–12	30	0
Scoggin et al	1993	20	5	2–31	20	
Peters & Bartels	1993	24	4.8	NS	13	0
Musser et al	1994	24	8.5	NS	28	0
Etienne et al	1993	35	9	5–23	26	0
Senagore et al	1993	38	7	NS	15	0
Puente et al	1994	38	4.8	3–14	24	0
Monson et al	1992	40	8	NS	15	2.5
Phillips et al	1992	51	4.6	1–30	8	2
Zucker et al	1994	65	4.4	3–8	6	0
Wexner et al	1993	74	7	2–40	34	0
Tucker et al	1994	114	4.8	NS	7	0
Mean		618	7.1	1–40	18.8 (0–39)	

or one of the ports was exchanged for the 33 mm port and the specimen was delivered. The tumour-bearing segment was then excised and anastomosis effected with the detachable head circular stapling device in the manner described earlier. The surgical resection margins and lymph node harvest were identical to those achieved during our routine procedures for malignancy.

Two patients required conversion to laparotomy – one for an iliac artery injury sustained during dissection, another for two enterotomies in the rectum during anterior resection. Morbidity in two patients was due to prolonged ileus in one and heart block requiring a pacemaker in another. For cancer resections, the mean length of surgery was 2.7 (1–4.5) hours, mean length of postoperative ileus 3 (0–5) days and mean length of hospital stay 6.8 (5–16) days. Pathology review revealed five Dukes' A, eight Dukes' B and two Dukes' C tumours. The mean number of lymph nodes harvested was 19 (3–84).

Controversies in laparoscopic colorectal surgery

At present, there exist no prospective, randomized clinical trials comparing laparoscopy with conventional surgery. Most trials compare either historical controls or non-randomized patients. Long-term follow-up studies addressing cancer recurrence and disease-free periods will not be available at least for the next few years. Available literature progressed from case reports and technical notes to the present comparative series (Table 7.2).

The advantages purportedly offered by laparoscopy include earlier return of bowel function, reduced postoperative pain, shorter hospital stay, early return to activity, enhanced cosmesis and the often quoted 'exact same operation' as in conventional open surgery. The learning curve effect is evident in many series. There are specific complications relating to the use of the laparoscopic approach. From insertion of the veress needle, damage to the major vessels and underlying structures may occur. Specific to colorectal procedures, ureteral injury has been reported (Dunlop et al 1993). Phillips, in his report of 51 laparoscopic colectomies, noted that the circular

Table 7.2 Intraoperative time

Author	Year	Time (h)	Range (h)
Chindasub et al	1994	4	(NS)
Guillou et al:	1993		
Right colectomy		3.9	(2.3–5.7)
Sigmoid colectomy		2.6	(1.5–3.3)
Jacobs et al:	1991		
Right colectomy		2.5	(1.8–4.3)
Sigmoid colectomy		2.8	(1.6–4.25)
Larach et al	1993a	3.5	(1.0–8.5)
Monson et al:	1992		
Right colectomy		3.5	(2.0–5.2)
Sigmoid colectomy		4.0	(2.5–5.5)
Musser et al	1994	2.8	(2.6–3.0)
Phillips et al	1992	2.3	(1.5–6.5)
Puente et al	1994	4.5	(2.4–6.3)
Senagore et al	1993	2.9	(2.7–3.1)
Sosa et al	1994	2.8	(2.4–4.8)
Tucker et al	1994	2.8	NS

stapled anastomosis was incomplete in 18% of cases (Phillips et al 1992). This extraordinarily high rate of incomplete anastomosis compares poorly with the 2–8% rate during laparotomy (Lazorthes & Chiotasol 1986). The development of the endoscopic linear cutting device, subsequently, would have reduced the need for this step but at a greater cost.

As outlined above, the tactile ability in laparoscopy is compromised. Corbitt (1992) converted three out of 18 procedures due to inability to identify the colonic lesion. Larach et al (1993a) and Monson et al (1992) have also reported incorrect segment removal. In a recent postal survey of members of the American Society of Colon and Rectal Surgeons, 18 additional instances of incorrect segment removal have surfaced (Cohen & Wexner 1994). Sixty nine percent of 635 responders advocated routine use of additional manoeuvres such as intraoperative colonoscopy or preoperative lesion marking to overcome this problem.

In our series, the complication rate reduced remarkably from 39% in the first 28 cases that we performed to 12% in the last 44 cases (Cohen & Wexner 1994). Overall complication rates from initial series range from 0 to 39% (see Table 7.1) Tate et al (1993) compared the morbidity rate with a non-randomized group of patients who underwent open surgery and found similar proportions of morbidity in both groups (5/11 vs 4/14 respectively). Other authors reached similar conclusions (Musser et al 1994, Senagore et al 1993). Van Ye et al (1994), when assessing with historical controls, actually found less morbidity in the laparoscopic group (1/14 vs 10/20 patients). The difference in morbidity rates is theorized to be due to less insult to the body in the minimally invasive approach. The smaller abdominal wound translates to less pain, earlier postoperative recovery and mobilization. However, a 'small' incision is a relative concept; whereas Caushaj et al (1994) consider conversion as the need for an incision >6 cm, Senagore et al (1993) consider the procedure successful if performed through a 10 cm incision.

Length of hospital stay and hence reduced cost have been major driving factors for the development of laparoscopic surgery. Authors have reported length of hospitalization with means ranging from 4.4 days to 12.3 days (see Table 7.1) The ranges reported in determining these means, however, ranged from 1 to 40 days. While it is easy to explain the upper limit of the range, one would be hesitant to rationalize the lower end of the scale. Criteria for determining hospital discharge are very varied. Indications for extended hospital stay range from medically related reasons of prolonged morbidity or the need for stoma therapy education to social reasons like family members being unable to transport patients home. Not only the subjective practice preferences of different surgeons but also the idiosyncrasies of patients all contribute to length of hospital stay. Thus, an objective assessment of length of stay is impossible. The criterion of return to normal activity is often used in laparoscopic literature. Phillips et al (1992), Zucker et al (1994) and Van Ye et al (1994) have reported time to return to normal activity of about 1 week.

While an early return to normal activity epitomizes recuperation, the intricacies of patients' personal commitments, financial gain or loss arising from differing periods of recuperation and a host of other subjective variables elude scientific quantification, especially in small patient numbers. For instance, many patients with carcinoma are elderly and retired (Vara-Thorbeck et al 1994). Similarly, patients with inflammatory bowel disease often receive disability payments. Thus, in many series including ours, the vast majority of patients had no 'work' to which to return. A return to 'normal activity' is even more elusive and objective scientifically valid quantification of pain is impossible.

Early return of bowel function may contribute to shorter hospital stay. It is purported that laparoscopic surgery results in earlier recovery of bowel function (Table 7.3). Bohm and colleagues (1994) found that recovery from postoperative ileus is more rapid after laparoscopic than after conventional intestinal surgery by determining return of intestinal myoelectrical activity in a canine model. Jacobs, in his initial series of 20 patients (Jacobs et al 1991), noted that 18 patients 'tolerated' clear fluids on day 1 and that 14 patients were discharged within 4 days of surgery. Peters & Bartels (1993) reported that laparoscopic patients regained bowel function significantly earlier (2.7 vs 4.0 days), tolerated regular diet earlier (2.3 vs 4.6 days) and hence had a markedly shorter hospital stay (4.8 vs 8.2 days). This experience is shared by Senagore et al (1993), who compared 102 colectomies with 38 laparoscopic-assisted colectomies. They found that bowel function returned quicker (3.0 vs 4.9 days) and hospital stay was shorter (6 vs 9.9 days) in the latter group.

Scrutiny of materials and methods sections in these articles revealed dietary advancement in the

Table 7.3 Duration of Ileus

Author	Year	Number of patients	Resolution of ileus
Tucker et al	1994	114	Liquid intake 2.4 days (mean)
Wexner et al	1993	74	Flatus on day 3 (mean)
Phillips et al	1992	51	100% oral intake day 2
Senagore et al	1993	38	100% oral intake day 3
Puente et al	1994	38	74% fluids or regular diet day 2
Peters & Bartels	1993	24	Oral intake day 2–3 (mean)
Jacobs et al	1991	20	90% oral intake day 1
Vara-Thorbeck et al	1994	18	Oral intake 3.2 days (mean)

absence of objective return of bowel function, passage of flatus or stool. In fact, some of the more staunch proponents even discharged their patients from hospital prior to passage of stool. Conversely, these same surgeons waited for flatus and/or bowel motions prior to dietary advancement after laparotomy. Thus, the data become uninterpretable as the groups are not equivalent. Furthermore, Rajagopal et al (1994) have demonstrated that without the laparoscope, postcolectomy hospital stay has decreased from 9.4 days to 6.3 days over the last 10 years. Given a 6.3 day mean length of stay after standard colectomy, it is hard to expect a significantly shorter stay after laparoscopic intervention.

To ascertain if the disparity in criteria for restricting oral intake and the apparent benefit of early oral feeding in laparoscopy could be extrapolated to patients undergoing laparotomy, a prospective randomized trial testing the hypothesis that early resumption of feeding should not be confined to postlaparoscopy patients was initiated (Reissman et al 1994c). One hundred and sixty one consecutive patients who underwent elective laparotomy with colonic or bowel resection were randomized to receive postoperatively either an early oral feeding regimen (clear liquid diet on day 1 – 80 patients) or the traditional feeding regimen (feeding after clinical resolution of ileus – 81 patients). Sixty three (79%) of the early feeding group tolerated the early feeding schedule and advanced to regular diet within the next 24–48 hours. There was no significant difference between the early and regular feeding groups in vomiting (21% vs 14%), nasogastric tube reinsertion (11% vs 10%), length of ileus (3.8±0.1 vs 4.1±0.1 days), length of postoperative hospitalization (6.2±0.2 vs 6.8±0.2 days) and overall complication rate (7.5% vs 6.1%). There were no anastomotic leaks, patients who aspirated or mortality in either group. However, patients who started feeding early tolerated regular diet significantly earlier than the regular feeding group (2.6±0.1 vs 5±0.1 days). Thus early resumption of oral feeding can be tolerated safely in patients undergoing open surgery and is not unique to laparoscopic surgery. Furthermore, as seen in Table 7.1, the mean published length of hospitalization after laparoscopic or laparoscopic-assisted colectomy is 7.1 days, almost one full day longer than that achieved merely by feeding patients immediately after laparotomy. Thus, the claim by some surgeons that laparoscopy reduces the length of stay by 50% or more must be challenged. For example, Ortega et al (1994a, 1994b) cite 'multiple advantages' including a reduction in hospital stay of over 50% from 11 days to 5. However, as was shown by Binderow et al (1994), Reissman et al (1994c) and Rajagopal et al (1994), an 11-day hospitalization after standard colectomy is not generally necessary.

To address the issue of cost, Falk et al (1993) at Creighton University independently received data from four surgeons in three different institutions consisting of medical records, videos and hospital bills of 66 consecutive laparoscopic procedures (Table 7.4). Although the mean hospital stay for patients who underwent laparoscopic sigmoid or right hemicolectomies was significantly shorter, procedure and instrument costs were significantly lower in patients who underwent open surgery. The total costs were similar in both groups. Senagore et al (1993) reported that the cost was lower ($12 131 vs $14 449) for patients who underwent the laparoscopic approach. They attributed the savings not only to reduction of hospital stay, but also to the use of fewer pharmaceutical agents, intravenous infusions and intramuscular injections. The comparison made by Larach et al (1993b) concluded that despite the higher cost of operating room time and equipment, the total cost of laparoscopic-assisted colectomy was more than, although not statistically different from, open resection. When two groups of age, sex, diagnosis and operation-matched patients (40 laparoscopy and 40 open) from our institution were compared, there were no statistical differences in operating time, duration of ileus, length of hospitalization or total cost between the two groups (Reiver et al 1994).

The above discussion relates much to technical

Table 7.4 Cost

Author	Year	Open ($)	Laparoscopic ($)
Falk et al	1993	14 000	13 500
Musser et al	1994	11 207	9811
Senagore et al	1993	14 449±696	12 131±612
Reiver	1994	19 384	23 294
Pfeifer	1995	26 903	29 626

difficulties during the learning curve which may be overcome, return of bowel function, length of hospitalization and cost, none of which have long-term sequelae. By far the most important issue is the appropriateness of the laparoscopic approach to the cure of malignancy. Perhaps some of the laparoscopy institutes who currently tout their success rates should instead return in 5 years to report survival and recurrence rates. At present, surgical excision of colorectal tumours remains the primary modality for the management of colorectal carcinoma. The goal of surgery is to maximize the chance for cure through en bloc removal of the tumour and the lymphatic nodal basin with margins that are adequate to ensure removal of the entire locoregional tumour burden (Enker et al 1979, 1986, Nogueras & Jagelman 1993). In the excision of proximal lesions, vascular and lymphatic anatomy is fairly well delineated and what constitutes adequate lymphovascular resection is not controversial (Monya et al 1989). In rectosigmoid and rectal lesions, however, there exist some controversies in the literature. It is accepted that surgical technique relates closely to the rate of local recurrence. Incomplete surgical excision of the mesorectum and inadequate lateral margin clearance are both associated with locoregional recurrence and poor prognosis (Cawthorn et al 1990, Heald et al 1982). Quirke & Dixon (1986) reported a recurrence of 85% in patients in whom the tumour involved the lateral margins compared to a rate of only 5% in those patients in whom the lateral margins were free (Heald & Ryall 1986, Irene & Luk 1993). Heald et al (1982) were the first to highlight the importance of total mesorectal excision, with local recurrence rates of 3.5% and an overall survival rate of 81% after a mean 4.8 year follow-up. These rates are actually much better than the rates achieved by Krook et al (1991) using surgery and adjuvant therapy.

The wide variability of results after 'standard' colectomy is undoubtedly due to the wide disparity in techniques (Glass et al 1985). However, they make interpretation of statements by laparoscopic proponents such as 'equivalent' or 'adequate' or 'identical' meaningless. When surgeons report local recurrence rates in excess of 30% after curative resection, important basic surgical principles need to be reviewed instead of introducing new unproven techniques (Krook et al 1991). However, it was our experience as well as that of others (Guillou et al 1993) that complete excision of the mesorectum and a wide lateral clearance can be technically achieved laparoscopically in either anterior resections or abdominoperineal resections, similar to that in open surgery. When left-sided, sigmoid and rectal tumours are excised, the inferior mesenteric artery is usually ligated and divided near its origin from the aorta.

The controversy of high ligation, however, persists even in conventional techniques (Bacon & Khubchandani 1964, Moynihan 1908). Miles (1908) advocated ligation of the inferior mesenteric artery up to, but not including, the left colic artery in his description of the abdominoperineal resection. Morgan & Griffiths (1959), however, advocated a higher level of ligation to include the left colic artery at the level of its origin from the aorta. This experience was not shared with other authors who did not find any benefit of high ligation (Grinnell 1965, Surtees et al 1990). Pezim & Nichols (1984), in their study of 1370 patients, found no survival advantage between high and low ligation.

As reports of laparoscopic resections are published, the number of lymph nodes resected has been used as a denominator to compare extent and adequacy of resection. The mean number of lymph nodes excised ranges from 4.2 to 28.4 (Table 7.5) The range of individual cases, however, spans from 0 to 84. Several authors have even reported a higher lymph node yield from laparoscopic resections (Musser et al 1994, Peters & Bartels 1993, Van Ye et al 1994). It would be prudent to say that if no lymph nodes were excised, the resection would not be acceptable as a curative operation. What, if any, conclusions can be drawn from other patients in whom the number of lymph nodes excised has been deemed 'adequate'? The number of lymph nodes counted in a resected specimen is heavily dependent on not only the method of detecting the lymph nodes, but also the pathologist involved. There is great variability from institution to institution in the quantification of number of lymph nodes (Blenkinsopp et al 1981). Cawthorn et al (1986) adopted a technique of fat clearance with xylene

Table 7.5 Lymph node harvest in laparoscopic colectomy

Author	Year	No. of patients	No. of nodes mean (range)	Open colectomy mean (range)
Chindasub et al	1994	10	10 (8–18)	
Dodson	1993	3	4.2 (NS)	
Franklin	1993	24	14 (8–22)	
Guillou et al	1993	51	9 (5–21)	
Jacobs et al	1991	4 (R. hemi)	25.5 (17–35)	
		2 (L. hemi)	8 (NS)	
Larach et al	1993a	13	9.8 (0–22)	
Monson et al	1992	28	10 (5–21)	
Musser et al	1994	15	10.6 (NS)	7.9 (NS)
Peters & Bartels	1993	NS (Sig. colect)	7.3 (NS)	4.7 (NS)
		NS (R. hemi)	9 (NS)	8.5 (NS)
Phillips et al	1992	24	14 (8–22)	
Puente et al	1994	22	11 (2–28)	
Tate et al	1993	11	10 (2–14)	13 (2–18)
Van Ye et al	1994	14	10.5 (0–32)	7.6 (2–19)
Vara-Thorbeck et al	1994	17	8.5 (6–11)	
Wexner et al	1993	12	19 (3–84)	
Zucker et al	1994	23 (R. hemi)	28.4 (18–35)	
		4 (Sig. colect)	8 (6–10)	
		4 (LAR)	7.3 (5–11)	

and alcohol and identified a significantly higher number of lymph nodes (mean 23.1) in the mesorectum than did pathologists at several centres who used a different technique (mean 10.5). These differences were also reported by Scott and others (Cohen et al 1994, Scolt & Grace 1989).

Besides these differences in technique, the pathologists also have a significant role in reporting the number of lymph nodes. The pathologist who wants to help his surgeons prove the merits of laparoscopic colectomy may be more diligent than usual in his search for nodes. Bias in this respect would remain undetected in studies comparing retrospective data or historical control groups. Moreover, associating lymph node numbers with adequate cancer clearance, by itself, is also controversial. Radioimmunoguided surgery has identified occult metastases in up to 10% of patients (Arnold et al 1992, Cohen et al 1991, Doerr et al 1991, Lechner et al 1993). Shida et al (1992) evaluated the prognostic value of lymph node metastases in 357 patients who underwent curative resection for colorectal cancer. This study found no difference in the 5-year disease-free interval when the number of lymph nodes were considered. It was found that the location of lymph nodes (local(n1) vs distant(n2)) was the more important criterion in the 5-year disease-free interval (70% vs 40% respectively). There was also a 32% incidence of skip metastases (negative(n1), positive(n2)). The disease-free interval was similarly lower in the (n2) group (n1 – 57%, n2 – 35%). The number of nodes resected thus may not accurately reflect adequate clearance.

While issues such as lymph node numbers may be controversial, some current laparoscopic practices have been proven to be unacceptable. The local recurrence rate after colotomy and polypectomy is unacceptably increased (Wexner 1991). The incidence of malignant change in larger sessile polyps is significant and therefore a cancer resection should be undertaken (Haggitt et al 1985, Nivatvongs et al 1991). If a recurrence occurs after a laparoscopic colotomy and polypectomy, one should not attribute this to the type of approach but rather to the choice of procedure (Lauroy et al BJS 1995). Similarly, wedge resections are mentioned only to be condemned.

Distal resection margins are another important factor in rectal cancer surgery. It has been well accepted that adequate distal resection relates to local recurrence (Wobbes et al 1989). Although the 5 cm rule has been deemed unnecessary, the 2 cm margin is accepted (Williams et al 1983). The only study in which laparoscopic and standard anterior resection have been compared included 11 patients with tumours located a mean of 20 cm (range 7–40) from the dentate line in whom a laparoscopic anterior resection was undertaken. Fourteen patients with a mean tumour height of 15 cm (range 7–30) underwent standard anterior resection (Tate et al 1993). Despite the sigmoid location in the former group, the distal margins were as small as 5 mm whereas the smallest margins in the open group were 20 mm. Although the authors concluded that the technique was acceptable, more critical analysis should have dictated the opposite conclusion. Due to the lack of tactile sensation, proximal synchronous tumours have gone undetected during laparoscopic colectomy (Fingerhut 1995, McDermott et al 1994). These patients have all developed postoperative bowel obstructions requiring laparotomy and resection. Although improved equipment may limit this occurrence, it is difficult to fathom such a problem during 'open' colectomy.

The myriad complications relating to laparoscopy discussed above may indeed relate to inexperience. It is envisioned that with accumulated experience and sound surgical judgement, shortfalls relating to technique can be overcome. However, what remains incomprehensible is the occurrence of port site recurrence after seemingly curative resection for carcinoma. The first published report of this was by Alexander et al (1993). A 67-year-old female presented with a wound recurrence 3 months after undergoing a laparoscopic-assisted curative right hemicolectomy for a Dukes' C adenocarcinoma. O'Rourke & Heald (1993) subsequently reported another patient with port site recurrence developing 10 weeks after curative right hemicolectomy for a Dukes' B adenocarcinoma. Fusco & Paluzzi (1993) reported a recurrence 10 months after right hemicolectomy for a T3N1M0 lesion. This phenomenon was also experienced by Guillou et al (1993) and others (Gionnone 1993, Mouiel 1994, Ngoi et al 1993).

One might reasonably argue that these recurrences could be due to inadequate technique and thus the routine use of specimen bags or wound protectors should prevent tumour innoculation into the wound (Murthy & Goldschmidt 1989). Though a logical preventive measure, it still would not address reported recurrences in some patients at port sites other than that of specimen retrieval. Port site recurrences have not only been confined to advanced lesions as one would expect, but surprisingly appeared in Dukes' A and B lesions as well. Recurrences have not been limited to colorectal cancers; port site recurrences have been reported in ovarian, gastric, biliary, oesophageal and pancreatic cancers (Cava et al 1990, Clair et al 1993, Drouard et al 1991, Fung et al 1993, Gleeson et al 1993, Hsin et al 1986, Hulten 1994, Miralles et al 1989, Pezet et al 1992, Siriwardena & Samaraji 1993). A strikingly disturbing denominator in these reports is the apparent rapidity of progression of disease. O'Rourke & Heald (1993) presented a patient who underwent a laparoscopic cholecystectomy for seeming cholecystitis. The histology, unexpectedly, revealed a moderately differentiated adenocarcinoma of the gall bladder invading the serosa. She presented 3 weeks later with two port site recurrences and again 3 months later with another recurrence. A 71-year-old patient, after undergoing laparoscopic cholecystectomy, presented 6 months later with a port site adenocarcinoma. Subsequently, the patient died and necropsy revealed adenocarcinoma of the body of the pancreas (Siriwardena & Samaraji 1993). More recently, Fingerhut (1995) tabulated the results of 224 laparoscopically performed or assisted colorectal procedures in France. Fourteen of the 92 cancers resected were Dukes' B or C lesions. The overall port site recurrence rate was 3.2%, but this represented three of the 14 Dukes' B or C lesions. Nduka et al (1994), Wexner and Cohen (1995) and Guillou et al (1993) have all expressed concerns about port site recurrences.

The best evidence for port site recurrence was

Table 7.6 Resection margins for malignancy

Author	Year	Proximal margin mean (range)	Distal margin mean (range)
Guillou et al	1993	14 (5–36) cm	8 (2–24) cm
Monson et al	1992	14.2 (3–18) cm	7.1 (1.5–14) cm
Tate et al	1993	NS	2 (0.5–5) cm
Van Ye et al	1994	7.4 (1.5–20) cm	14.2 (2–30) cm

presented by Wade et al (1994). They reported a 59-year-old female who underwent laparoscopic cholecystectomy for chronic calculous cholecystitis. The pathology specimen revealed an unsuspected polypoid carcinoma. Twenty one days later, at the time of elective reexploration, several isolated 4–6 mm fibrotic inflammatory nodules were palpable in the peritoneum of the umbilical port site. Frozen section revealed a situs of metastatic gall bladder carcinoma approximately 10 cells in diameter in one of the non-palpable nodules. The authors postulated that the umbilical recurrence was a single-cell implantation at the time of initial laparoscopy. They used a doubling-time model for a sphere to confirm the 21-day growth spurt. These authors concluded that 'This demonstration of cancer recurrence in laparoscopic port sites may limit the application of laparoscopy to elective cancer resection'. Similarly Jacobi and associates (1994) reported a case in which laparoscopic cholecystectomy was converted for 'technical reasons' to a laparotomy. Two months later this patient presented with metastatic disease at two of the portsites. However the laparotomy incision was free of disease. In a recent received portsite metastasis after laparoscopic colectomy, Wexner and Cohen (1995) noted 33 cases. In six series the actual incidence was reported and ranged from 1.5% to 21% with a median of 3.5% and a mean of 6.5%.

Conversely, wound recurrences in open surgery are not often reported in the literature. Hughes et al (1983) reported abdominal wall recurrences in 16 of 1603 patients (1%) who underwent curative resection for carcinoma of the colon. However, most series do not include any wound recurrence and 1% is the *highest* published figure. The 3 to 6 fold increased incidence of this phenomenon has led to further controversy over the role of laparoscopic surgery in malignancy. The operative margins and lymphovascular margins are similar to open surgery; however, hyperbaric carbon dioxide may have a stimulatory effect on cancer growth or aid in the dissemination of cancer cells into the circulation (Fleshman 1995). In the process of laparoscopy, the pneumoperitoneum may be forcing malignant cells into the raw edges of the port sites (O'Rourke et al 1993). It has been hypothesized that attenuation of the immune response can occur as a result of blood transfusion and hence affect tumourigenesis. Though controversial (Beynon et al 1989, Blumberg et al 1988, Stephenson et al 1988, Wobbes et al 1989), extrapolation of this theory of modification of the immune response to laparoscopy and elevated intraabdominal pressure could provide an explanation. To refute this theory, investigators performing animal experiments have shown that host defences are less depressed in laparoscopy than laparotomy (Trokel et al 1994). It is even postulated that laparotomy confers a permissive effect on tumour establishment and growth in a murine model (Allendorf et al 1994). Collet et al (1994), when comparing peritoneal bacterial clearance, peritoneal and systemic monocyte class II antigen expression, peripheral blood polymorphonuclear superoxide production and peripheral blood TNFα activity in pigs undergoing either laparoscopic or open Nissen's fundoplication, found that host defence processes were less depressed by laparoscopy. Bessler et al (1994) found increased levels of epinephrine and IL-6, suggesting an exaggerated stress response in pigs undergoing laparoscopic colon resection. It remains to be seen if these experimental findings in animals can be extrapolated to humans (Skipper et al 1989).

Perhaps the advent of gasless laparoscopy and observance of meticulous techniques to prevent spillage of cancer cells would reduce the number of early recurrences. Thus, it remains that until an explanation is found, caution should be exercised in laparoscopic cancer resections (Wexner & Cohen 1995).

The future

In the immediate future, well-scrutinized, peer-reviewed, prospective, randomized controlled trials are required to address questions on the benefit of laparoscopic surgery as compared to conventional surgery (Guillou 1994). Some institutions have started these trials to establish not only differences in the immediate postoperative period relating to postoperative recovery of bowel function, pain, hospital stay, cost and return to normal activity, but also the long-term implications of the laparoscopic approach, particularly for the issue of cancer. Results of these trials in relation to immediate benefit will be available in the not too distant future, although the results of cancer resections will not be available for at least 5 years.

In the interim, it is the general consensus of most American colorectal surgeons that laparoscopic or laparoscopic-assisted colectomies for cure of malignancies be performed only within the confines of an IRB approved prospective randomized trial.

References

Alexander RJT, Jaques BC, Mitchell KG 1993 Laparoscopically-assisted colectomy and wound recurrence (letter). Lancet 341: 249–250

Allendorf JDF, Kayton ML, Libutti SK et al 1994 The effect of laparotomy versus insufflation on tumor establishment and growth (abstract). Surgical Endoscopy 8(3): 234

Altman LK 1992 Surgical injuries lead to new rule. New York Times, June 14, p 1

American Society of Colon and Rectal Surgeons 1991 Policy statement. Diseases of the Colon and Rectum 34: 35A

Arnold MN, Shneebaurs J et al 1992 Intraoperative detection of colorectal cancer with radio-immunoguided surgery qdn cc 49. A second generation monoclonal antibody. Annals of Surgery 216(6): 627–632

Bacon HE, Khubchandani IT 1964 The rationale of aortoiliopelvic lymphadenectomy and high ligation of the inferior mesenteric artery for carcinoma of the left half of the colon and rectum. Surgery, Gynecology and Obstetrics 119: 503–508

Bauer JJ, Harris MT, Gortine SR, Gelernt IM, Kreel I 1994 Laparoscopic-assisted intestinal resection for Crohn's disease (abstract). Surgical Endoscopy 8: 245

Beck DA, Wexner SD (eds) 1992 Fundamentals of anorectal surgery. New York, McGraw-Hill

Bessler M, Treat MR, Halversson A, Kayton ML, Whelan RL, Nowygrod R 1994 Laparoscopic colectomy induces a hormonal stress response (abstract). Surgical Endoscopy 8: 245

Beynon J, Davies PW, Billings PJ et al 1989 Perioperative blood transfusion increases the risk of recurrence in colorectal cancer. Diseases of the Colon and Rectum 32: 975–979

Binderow SR, Cohen SM, Wexner SD, Nogueras JJ 1994 Must early post-operative intake be limited to laparoscopy? Diseases of the Colon and Rectum 37: 584–589

Blenkinsopp WK, Stewart-Brown S, Blesovsky L et al 1981 Histopathology reporting in large bowel cancer. Journal of Clinical Pathology 34: 509–513

Blumberg N, Heal J, Chuang C et al 1988 Further evidence supporting a cause and effect relationship between blood transfusion and earlier cancer recurrence. Annals of Surgery 207: 410–415

Bohm B, Milsom JW, Fazio VW 1994 Postoperative ileus following open versus laparoscopic colectomy. Surgical Endoscopy 8(3): 234

Caushaj PF, Devereaux D, Schmitt S, Griffy S 1994 Laparoscopic-assisted colectomy: does experience improve outcome (abstract)? Disease of the Colon and Rectum 37: 21

Cava A, Roman J, Quintela AG et al 1990 Subcutaneous metastasis following 1 laparoscopy in gastric carcinoma. European Journal of Surgical Oncology 16: 63–67

Cawthorn SJ, Gibbs NM, Marks CG 1986 Clearance technique for the detection of lymph nodes in colorectal cancer. British Journal of Surgery 73: 58–60

Cawthorn SJ, Parums DV, Gibbs NM et al 1990 Extent of mesorectal spread and involvement of lateral resection margins as a prognostic factor after surgery for rectal cancer. Lancet 335: 1055–1059

Chindasub S, Charntaracharmnong C, Nimitvamit C, Akkaranurukul P, Santitarmmanon B 1994 Laparoscopic abdominoperineal resection. Journal of Laparoendoscopic Surgery 4: 17–21

Choen S, Tsunoda A, Nicholls RJ 1991 Prospective randomized trial comparing anal function after hand sewn ileoanal anastomosis vs. stapled ileoanal anastomosis without mucosectomy in restorative proctocolectomy. British Journal of Surgery 78: 430–434

Clair DG, Lautz DB, Brooks DC 1993 Rapid development of umbilical metastases after laparoscopic cholecystectomy for unsuspected gall bladder carcinoma. Surgery 113: 355–358

Cohen AM, Martin EW Jr, Lavery I et al 1991 Radio-immunoguided surgery using Iodine 125 B72.3 in patients with colorectal cancer. Archives of Surgery 126: 349–352

Cohen SM, Wexner SD, Schmitt SL, Nogueras JJ, Lucas FV 1994. Effect of xylene clearance of mesenteric fat on harvest of lymph nodes after colon resection. European Journal of Surgery 160: 693–697

Cohen SM, Wexner SD 1994 Laparoscopic colorectal surgery: are we being honest with our patients Diseases of the Colon and Rectum (in press)

Collet D, Reynolds M, Klar E, Trachtenberg MA, Vitale G 1994 Peritoneal host defenses are less improved by laparoscopic than by open operation (abstract). Surgical Endoscopy 8(3): 240

Corbitt JD 1992 Preliminary experience with laparoscopic-guided colectomy. Surgical Laparoscopy and Endoscopy 2(1): 79–81

Dodson RW, Cullado MJ, Tangen LE et al 1993 Laparoscopic assisted abdominoperineal resection. Contemporary Surgery 42: 42–44

Doerr RJ, Abdel-Nabi H, Krag D, Mitchell E 1991 Radiolabelled antibody imaging in the management of colorectal cancer. Results of a multicenter study. Annals of Surgery 214: 118–124

Drouard F, Delamarre J, Capron JP 1991 Cutaneous seeding of gall bladder cancer after laparoscopic cholecystectomy. New England Journal of Medicine 325: 1316

Dunlop MG, Farouk R, Wilson RG, Bartolo DCC 1993 Laparoscopic resection rectopexy for rectal prolapse (abstract). International Journal of Colorectal Disease 8: 230

Enker WE, Laffer UTH, Block GE 1979 Enhanced survival of patients with colon and rectal cancer is based upon wide anatomic resection. Annals of Surgery 190: 350–360

Enker WE, Heilveil ML, Hertz REL et al 1986 En bloc pelvic lymphadenectomy and sphincter preservation in the surgical management of rectal cancer. Annals of Surgery 203: 426–433

Etienne J, Jehaes C, Kartheuser A, de Neve de Roden A 1993 Laparoscopic surgery for benign colorectal disease: A multicentre prospective study (abstract). British Journal of Surgery 80: S45

Falk PM, Beart RW, Wexner SD, Thorson AG, Jagelman DG, Lavery IC, Johansen OB, Fitzgibbons RJ Jr 1993 Laparoscopic colectomy: a critical appraisal. Diseases of the Colon and Rectum 36: 28–34

Fingerhut A 1995 Laparoscopic Colectomy: The French Experience. In Wexner SD, Jager R (eds) Laparoscopic Colorectal Surgery. New York: Churchill Livingstone

Fleshman J, Fry R. Laparoscopic-assisted and mini-laparotomy approaches to colorectal diseases are similar in early outcome. Diseases of the Colon and Rectum 1995; 38: p 23 (abstract)

Franklin M 1993 Laparoscopic colectomy. Presented at the International Symposium on Advances in Laparoscopic Colectomy, Indianapolis, USA, October 29–31

Franklin ME, Ramos R, Rosenthal D, Schuessler W 1993 Laparoscopic colonic procedures. World Journal of Surgery 17: 51–56

Fung Y, Brennan MF, Turnbull A et al 1993 Gall bladder cancer discovered during laparoscopic surgery. Potential for introgenic dissemination. Archives of Surgery 128: 1054–1056

Fusco MA, Paluzzi MW 1993 Abdominal wall recurrence after laparoscopic-assisted colectomy for adenocarcinoma of the colon. Report of a case. Diseases of the Colon and Rectum 36(9): 858–861

Gionnone G 1993. Laparoscopic colectomy. Presented at the International Symposium on Advances in Laparoscopic Colectomy, Indianapolis, USA, October 29–31

Glass RE, Ritchie JK, Thompson HR et al 1985 The results of surgical treatment of cancer of the rectum by radical resection and extended abdomino-iliac lymphadenectomy. British Journal of Surgery 72: 599–601

Gleeson NC, Nicosia SV, Mark JE et al 1993 Abdominal wall metastases from ovarian cancer after laparoscopy. American Journal of Obstetrics and Gynecology 169: 522–523

Grinnell RS 1965 Results of ligation of inferior mesenteric artery at the aorta in resections of carcinoma of the descending and sigmoid colon and rectum. Surgery, Gynecology and Obstetrics 120: 1031–1036

Guillou PJ 1994 Laparoscopic surgery for diseases of the colon and rectum – quo vadis? Surgical Endoscopy 8: 669–671

Guillou PJ, Darzi A, Monson JRT 1993 Experience with laparoscopic colorectal surgery for malignant disease. Surgical Oncology 2 (suppl 1): 43–49

Haggitt RC, Glotzbach RE, Soffer EE et al 1985 Prognostic factors in colorectal carcinomas arising in adenomas: implications for lesions removed by endoscopic polypectomy. Gastroenterology 89: 328–336

Heald RJ, Ryall RD 1986 Recurrence and survival after total mesorectal excision of rectal cancer. Lancet i(8496): 1476

Heald RJ, Husband EM, Ryall RDH 1982 The mesorectum in rectal cancer surgery: the clue to pelvic recurrence? British Journal of Surgery 69: 613–616

Hoffman GC, Baker JW, Fitchett CW, Vansant JH 1994 Laparoscopic assisted colectomy: initial experience. Annals of Surgery 219(6): 732–743

Horgan PG, O'Connell PR, Shinkain LA, Kirwan WO 1989 Effect of anterior resection on anal sphincter function. British Journal of Surgery 76: 783–786

Hsin J, Given FT, Kemp GM 1986 Tumor implantation after diagnostic laparoscopic biopsy of serous ovarian tumors of low malignant potential. Obstetrics and Gynecology 68: 905–935

Hughes ES, McDermott FT, Proliglase AI, Johnson WR 1983 Tumor recurrence in abdominal wall scar after large bowel cancer surgery. Diseases of the Colon and Rectum 26: 571–572

Hulten L 1994. Pouchitis: why does it happen and how is it best treated? Presented at Colorectal Disease in 1994: An international exchange of medical and surgical concepts, Fort Lauderdale, USA, February 24–26

Irene O, Luk IS 1993 Surgical lateral clearance in resected rectal carcinomas. A multivariate analysis of clinicopathologic features. Cancer 71(6): 1972–1976

Jacobs M, Verdeja JC, Goldstein HS 1991 Minimally invasive colon resection (laparoscopic colectomy). Surgical Laparoscopy and Endoscopy 1(3): 144–150

Jacobi C, Keller HW, Said S. Implantation metastasis of unsuspected gall bladder carcinoma after laparoscopy. British Journal of Surgery 1994; 81 (suppl): 82 (abstract)

Jorge JMN, Wexner SD 1993 Etiology and management of fecal incontinence. Diseases of the Colon and Rectum 36(1): 77–97

Keighley MR 1987. Abdominal mucosectomy reduces the incidence of soiling and sphincter damage after restorative proctocolectomy and J-pouch. Diseases of the Colon and Rectum 30: 386–390

Knight CK, Griffen FD 1980 An improved technique for low anterior resection of the rectum using the EEA stapler. Surgery 88: 710–714

Krook JE, Moertel CG, Ginderson LL et al 1991 Effective surgical adjuvant therapy for high-risk rectal carcinoma. New England Journal of Medicine 324: 709–715

Larach SW, Salomon MC, Williamson PR, Goldstein E 1993a Laparoscopic-assisted colectomy: experience during the learning curve. Coloproctology (1): 38–41

Larach SW, Vayer AJ, Williamson PR, Ferrara A, Salomon MC 1993b. Cost effectiveness of laparoscopic assisted colectomy. Presented at the Tripartite Colorectal Meeting, Sydney, Australia, October 17–20

Lauroy J, Champault G, Risk N, Boutelier P. Metastatic recurrence at the cannula site: should digestive carcinomas still be managed by laparoscopy? Br J Surg 1994; 81 (suppl): 31 (abstract)

Lavery IC, Tuckson WB, Easley ICA 1989 Internal anal sphincter function after total abdominal colectomy and stapled ileal pouch–anal anastomosis without mucosal proctectomy. Diseases of the Colon and Rectum 32: 950–953

Lazorthes F, Chiotassol P 1986 Stapled colorectal anastomosis: perspective integrity of the anastomosis and risk of postoperative leakage. International Journal of Colorectal Disease 1: 96–98

Lechner P, Lind P, Binter G, Cesnik H 1993 Anti-carcinoembryonic antigen immunoscintigraphy in primary and recurrent colorectal cancer. A prospective study. Diseases of the Colon and Rectum 36: 930–935

Liljeqvist L, Lindquist K, Ljunddahl I 1988 Alterations in ileoanal pouch technique 1980 and 1987: complications and functional outcome. Diseases of the Colon and Rectum 31: 929–938

Lointier PH, Lautard M, Massoni C, Ferrier C, Dapoigny M 1993 Laparoscopically-assisted subtotal colectomy. Journal of Laparoendoscopic Surgery 3(6): 547–556

Luukkonen P, Jarvinen H 1993 Stapled vs. hand sutured ileoanal anastomosis in restorative proctocolectomy. Archives of Surgery 128: 437–440

McIntyre PB, Pemberton JH, Beart RW Jr, Devine RM,

Nivatvongs S 1994 Double-stapled vs. hand sewn ileal pouch anal anastomosis in patients with chronic ulcerative colitis. Diseases of the Colon and Rectum 37: 430–433

McDermott JP, Devereaux DA, Caushaj PF 1994 Pitfall of laparoscopic colectomy: an unrecognized synchronous cancer. Diseases of the Colon and Rectum 37(6): 602–603

Miles WE 1908 A method of performing abdominoperineal excision for carcinoma of the rectum and of the terminal portion of the pelvic colon. Lancet 2: 1812–1813

Milsom JW, Lavery IC, Bohm B, Fazio VW 1993 Laparoscopically-assisted; ileocolectomy in Crohn's disease. Surgical Laparoscopy and Endoscopy 3(2): 77–80

Miralles RM, Petit J, Gine L, Balagnero L 1989 Metastatic cancer spread at the laparoscopic puncture site. Report of a case in a patient with carcinoma of the ovary (case report). European Journal of Gynecologic Oncology 10(6): 442–444

Monson JRT, Darzi A, Carey PD, Guillou PJ 1992 Prospective evaluation of laparoscopic-assisted colectomy in an unselected group of patients. Lancet 340: 831–833

Monya Y, Hojo K, Sawada T et al 1989 Significance of lateral node dissection for advanced rectal carcinoma at or below the peritoneal reflection. Diseases of the Colon and Rectum 32: 307–315

Morgan CN, Griffiths JD 1959 High ligation of the inferior mesenteric artery during operations for carcinoma of the distal colon and rectum. Surgery, Gynecology and Obstetrics 108: 641–650

Morson BC, Bussey HJR 1985 Magnitude of risk for cancer in patients with colorectal adenomas. British Journal of Surgery 72(suppl): 523–528

Morson BC, Whiteway JE, Jones EA, Macrae FA, Williams CB 1984 Histopathology and prognosis of malignant colorectal polyps treated by endoscopic polypectomy. Gut 25: 437–444

Mouiel J 1994 Laparoscopic colectomy. Presented at the 4th World Congress of Endoscopic Surgery, Kyoto, Japan, June 16–19

Moynihan BGA 1908 The surgical treatment of cancer of the sigmoid flexure and rectum with special reference to the principles to be observed. Surgery, Gynecology and Obstetrics 6: 463–466

Murthy GM, Goldschmidt R 1989 The influence of surgical trauma on experimental metastases. Cancer 64: 2035–2044

Musser DJ, Boorse RC, Madera F, Reed JF III 1994 Laparoscopic colectomy: at what cost? Surgical Laparoscopy and Endoscopy 4(1): 1–5

Nduka CC, Monson JRT, Menzies-Gow N, Darzi A 1994 Abdominal wall metastases following laparoscopy. British Journal of Surgery 81: 648–652

Ngoi SS, Kum K, Goh PMY et al 1993 Laparoscopic colon resection: the Singapore experience. Poster presentation at the Tripartite Colorectal Surgery Meeting, Sydney, Australia, October 17–20

Nivatvongs S, Rojanasakul A, Reiman HM et al 1991 The risk of lymph node metastases in colorectal polyps with invasive adenocarcinoma. Diseases of the Colon and Rectum 34: 323–328

Nogueras JJ, Wexner SD 1992 Laparoscopic colorectal surgery. Perspectives in Colon and Rectal Surgery 579–597

Nogueras JJ, Jagelman DG 1993 Principles of surgical resection. Influence of surgical techniques on treatment outcome. Surgical Clinics of North America 73(1): 103–116

O'Donovan SC, Larach SW 1994 Postoperative herniation of small bowel through a laparoscopy port site. Coloproctology 16: 98–100

O'Rourke N, Heald RJ 1993 Laparoscopic surgery for colorectal cancer. British Journal of Surgery 80(10): 1229–1230

O'Rourke NA Priq PM, Kelly S, Sikora K 1993 Tumor inoculation during laparoscopy (letter). Lancet 342: 368

Ortega A, Beart R, Anthone G, Schlinkert R 1994a Laparoscopic bowel resection: a consecutive series (abstract). Diseases of the Colon and Rectum 37: 22

Ortega A, Beart R, Winchester D, Steele G, Green R 1994b Laparoscopic bowel surgery registry: preliminary results (abstract). Diseases of the Colon and Rectum 37: 21

Peters WR, Bartels TL 1993 Minimally invasive colectomy: are the potential benefits realized? Diseases of the Colon and Rectum 36: 751–756

Pezet D, Fondrivier E, Rothman N, Guy L, Lemesle P, Lointier P, Chipponi J 1992 Parietal seeding of carcinoma of the gall bladder after laparoscopic cholecystectomy. British Journal of Surgery 79: 230

Pezim ME, Nicholls RJ 1984 Survival after high or low ligation of the inferior mesenteric artery during curative surgery for rectal cancer. Annals of Surgery 200: 729–733

Pfeifer J, Wexner SD, Reissman P, Bernstein M, Nogueras JJ, Singh S, Weiss EG. Laparoscopic vs. open colon surgery: costs and outcome. Surg endosc (submitted)

Phillips EH, Franklin M, Carroll BJ, Fallas MJ, Ramos R, Rosenthal D 1992 Laparoscopic colectomy. Annals of Surgery 216(6): 703–707

Puente I, Sosa JL, Sleeman D, Desai U, Tranakas N, Hartmann R 1994 Laparoscopic-assisted colorectal surgery. Journal of Laparoendoscopic Surgery 4: 1–7

Quattlebaum JK Jr, Flanders HD, Usher CH 1993 Laparoscopically-assisted colectomy. Surgical Laparoscopy and Endoscopy 3(2): 81–87

Quirke P, Dixon MF 1986 Local recurrence of rectal adenocarcinoma due to inadequate surgical resection. Lancet 1: 996–998

Rajagopal AS, Thorson AG, Sentovitch SM et al 1994 Decade trends in length of postoperative stay following abdominal colectomy (abstract). Diseases of the Colon and Rectum 37(4): 26

Reissman P, Cohen SM, Weiss EG, Wexner SD 1994a Simple techniques for pelvic drain placement in laparoscopic abdomino-perineal resection. Diseases of the Colon and Rectum 37: 381–382

Reissman P, Shiloni E, Gofrit O, Rivkind A, Durst A 1994b Incarcerated hernia in a lateral trocar site: an unusual early postoperative complication of laparoscopic surgery. European Journal of Surgery 160: 191–192

Reissman P, Teoh TA, Weiss EG, Cohen SM, Nogueras JJ, Wexner SD 1994c. Is early oral feeding safe after elective colorectal surgery. Annals of surgery (in press)

Reissman P, Piccirillo MF, Ulrich A, Wexner SD, Nogueras JJ 1995a. Functional Results of the double stapled ileoanal reservoir. Journal of the American College of surgeons (in press)

Reissman P, Teoh TA, Piccirillo M, Nogueras JJ, Wexner SD 1995b. Colonoscopic assisted laparoscopic colectomy. Surgical Endoscopy 1994; 8: 1352–1353

Reiver D, Kmiot WA, Cohen SM, Weiss EG, Nogueras JJ, Wexner SD 1994 A prospective comparison of laparoscopic procedures in colorectal surgery (abstract). Diseases of the Colon and Rectum 37(4): 22

SAGES 1991 Granting of privileges for laparoscopic general

surgery. American Journal of Surgery 161:324–325

Scoggin SD, Frazee RC, Snyder SK, Hendricks JC, Roberts JV, Symmonds RE, Smith RW 1993 Laparoscopic-assisted bowel surgery. Diseases of the Colon and Rectum 36: 747–750

Scott KWN, Grace RH 1989 Detection of lymph node metastases in colorectal carcinoma before and after fat clearance. British Journal of Surgery 109–111, 1165–1167

See WA, Cooper CS, Fisher RJ 1993 Predictors of laparoscopic complications after formal training in laparoscopic surgery. Journal of the American Medical Association 73:2689–2692

Senagore AJ, Luchtefeld MA, MacKeigan JM, Mazier WP 1993 Open colectomy versus laparoscopic colectomy: are there differences? American Surgeon 59(8): 549–554

Shida H, Ban K, Matsumoto M et al 1992 Prognostic significance of location of lymph node metastases in colorectal cancer. Diseases of the Colon and Rectum 35: 1045–1050

Siriwardena A, Samaraji WN 1993 Cutaneous tumor seeding from a previous undiagnosed pancreatic carcinoma after laparoscopic cholecystectomy. Annals of the Royal College of Surgeons of England 75: 199–200

Skipper D, Jeffrey MJ, Cooper AJ, Alexander P, Taylor I 1989 Enhanced growth of tumor cells in healing colonic anastomoses and laparotomy wounds. International Journal of Colorectal Disease 4: 172–177

Sosa JL, Sleeman D, Puente I, McKenney MG, Hartmann R 1994 Laparoscopic-assisted colostomy closure after Hartmann's procedure. Diseases of the Colon and Rectum 37: 149–152

Stephenson KR, Steiberg SM, Hughes KS et al 1988 Perioperative blood transfusions are associated with decreased time to recurrence and decreased survival after resection of colorectal liver metastases. Annals of Surgery 208: 679–687

Surtees P, Ritchie JK, Phillips RKS 1990 High versus low ligation of the inferior mesenteric artery in rectal cancer. British Journal of Surgery 77: 618–621

Tate JJT, Kwok S, Dawson JW, Lau WY, Li AKC 1993 Prospective comparison of laparoscopic and conventional anterior resection. British Journal of Surgery 80: 1396–1398

Teoh TA, Reissman P, Cohen SM, Weiss EG, Wexner SD 1994 Laparoscopic loop ileostomy (letter). Diseases of the Colon and Rectum 37(5): 514

Teoh TA, Reissman P, Weiss EG, Verzaro R, Wexner SD 1995 Enhancing cosmesis in laparoscopic colon and rectal surgery. Diseases of the Colon and Rectum 1995; 38: 213–214

Trokel MJ, Allendorf JDF, Treat MR et al 1994 Inflammatory response is better preserved after laparoscopy vs laparotomy (abstract). Surgical Endoscopy 8(3): 232

Tucker JG, Ambroze WL, Orangio GR, Duncan T, Mason EM, Lucas GW 1994 Laparoscopic-assisted bowel surgery: analysis of 114 cases (abstract). Surgical Endoscopy 8: 234

Van Ye TM, Cattey RP, Henry LG 1994 Laparoscopically-assisted colon resections compare favorably with open technique. Surgical Laparoscopy and Endoscopy 4(1): 25–31

Vara-Thorbeck C, Garcia-Cabellero M, Salvi M, Gutstein D, Toscano R, Gomez A, Vara-Thorbeck R 1994 Indications and advantages of laparoscopy-assisted colon resection for carcinoma in elderly patients. Surgical Laparoscopy and Endoscopy 4(2): 110–118

Wade TP, Comitalo JB, Andrus CH, Goodwin MN Jr, Kaminski DL 1994 Laparoscopic cancer surgery: lessons from gallbladder cancer. Surgical Endoscopy 8: 698–701

Weiss EG, Wexner SD 1995a A recommended training schema for laparoscopic surgery. Surgical Oncology Clinics of North America 1994, 3(4): 759–765

Weiss EG, Wexner SD 1995b Training and preparing for laparoscopic colon surgery. Seminars in Colon and Rectal Surgery 1994, 5(4): 224–227

Wexner SD 1991 Management of the malignant polyp. Seminars in Colon and Rectal Surgery 2(1): 22–27

Wexner SD, Cohen SM 1995 Port site metastases after laparoscopic surgery for cure of malignancy: British Journal of Surgery; 1995; 82: 295–298

Wexner SD, Johansen OB 1992 Laparoscopic bowel resection advantages and limitations. Annals of Medicine 24: 105–110

Wexner SD, James KA, Jagelman DG 1991 The role of double-stapled ileal reservoir and ileoanal anastomosis. Diseases of the Colon and Rectum 34: 487–494

Wexner SD, Nogueras JJ, Jagelman DG 1992 Laparoscopic total abdominal colectomy: a prospective assessment. Diseases of the Colon and Rectum 7: 651–655

Wexner SD, Cohen SM, Johansen OB, Nogueras JJ, Jagelman DG 1993 Laparoscopic colorectal surgery: a prospective assessment and current perspective. British Journal of Surgery 80: 1602–1605

Williams NS, Dixon MF, Johnston D 1983 Reappraisal of the 5 centimeter rule of distal excision for carcinoma of the rectum: a study of distal intramural spread and of patient's survival. British Journal of Surgery 70: 150–154

Wobbes T, Jossen KHG, Kuypers JHC et al 1989 The effect of packed cells and whole blood transfusions on survival after curative resection for colorectal carcinoma. Diseases of the Colon and Rectum 32: 743–748

Zucker KA, Pitcher DE, Ford RS 1994 Laparoscopic-assisted colon resection. Surgical Endoscopy 8: 12–18

8 Obstruction and perforation

D. A. ROTHENBERGER   J. MAYORAL   K. DEEN

Introduction

Obstruction and perforation are life-threatening complications of colon carcinoma which have generally been associated with poor outcomes. In 1929, Owen H. Wangensteen observed 'Colic obstruction attended by enormous distension, limited to the colon, demands immediate surgical decompression... In most instances a diverting colostomy upon the transverse colon is performed...'. Although Dr Wangensteen's admonition to operate immediately for cases of complete colon obstruction remains good advice, the modern surgeon has numerous operative options to consider in addition to the time-honoured transverse colostomy recommended by him.

This chapter first reviews the incidence, location and prognosis of obstructing or perforated cancers. The clinical presentation and appropriate evaluation of patients with colon cancer complicated by obstruction and/or perforation are then discussed. A more detailed presentation of the preoperative management, the operative preliminaries, formulation of a suitable operative plan and a review of the many controversies surrounding the operative treatment of such patients follows.

Incidence, location and prognosis

The literature generally assumes that the definitions of obstruction and perforation secondary to colonic cancer are precise and well understood by everyone. Rarely do papers distinguish complete obstruction from partial obstruction. Similarly, the literature rarely defines whether perforations are free into the peritoneal cavity or localized and whether they occur through the cancer or through normal colon proximal to an obstructing cancer. Thus it is difficult to determine the true incidence, location and effect of these conditions on patient prognosis.

Adenocarcinoma of the colon accounts for 60–80% of large bowel obstructions in adults but only 8–30% of cancers of the colon present with clinical evidence of at least partial mechanical obstruction (Ohman 1982). If only complete obstruction (defined as total absence of flatus or faeces for at least 24 hours) is considered, the incidence drops to 2–16% (Boring et al 1992, Fearon & Vogelstein 1990, Serpell et al 1989). Most obstructing colon cancers are located in the sigmoid or splenic flexure, with the next most common site being the descending colon followed by the ascending colon (Ohman 1982, Corman 1991). Presumably right-sided colon obstruction is less common than left-sided obstruction because of its more liquid stool content, larger lumen diameter, tendency to have more polypoid cancers and lower incidence of colon cancer compared to the left colon which typically has more solid stool, smaller lumen diameter, more annular, stenosis-producing tumours and a higher incidence of colon cancer. An exception to this tendency is the annular lesion which develops at the ileocaecal valve producing right-sided colonic obstruction. The rectum is rarely the site of an obstructing cancer (Veyama et al 1991).

Perforation of the colon occurs in 6–12% of cases of colon cancer and is usually due to direct extension of the adenocarcinoma through the bowel wall (Gennaro & Tyson 1978, Ohman 1982, Rankel et al 1991). Perforation is sometimes due to a proximal (usually caecal) perforation secondary to an obstructing, left-sided colon cancer. Both obstruction and perforation occur together in only 1% of all colon cancers but in those with an obstructing cancer, approximately 12–19% will have a perforation (Runkel et al 1991, Umpleby et al 1984). Iatrogenic perforation can occur either during diagnostic tests or during an operation for cancer and will not be discussed here.

Controversy exists about the impact of obstruction on patient prognosis. Several studies suggest that obstruction is an independent variable predictive of a poorer prognosis than similar staged non-obstructing cancers (Chapuis et al 1985, Crucitti et al 1991, Griffin et al 1987, Serpell et al 1989, Steinberg et al 1986, Wolmark et al 1983). Conversely, other studies suggest that the only effect of obstruction on prognosis is by adversely affecting the stage of disease – i.e. there are more advanced tumours in patients presenting with obstructing cancers than in patients without obstruction (Garcia-Valdescasas et al 1991, Korenaga et al 1991, Ueyama et al 1991). These studies suggest that patients with obstruction have the same prognosis as those without obstruction if compared stage for stage.

If both obstruction and perforation are present, the prognosis is worse, perhaps because of increased local recurrences or because of the increased need for emergency surgery which correlates in elderly patients with an increased morbidity and mortality (Fielding et al 1989, Griffin et al 1987, Willet et al 1985).

Clinical presentation and examination

Obstruction

The onset of symptoms is usually insidious with the patient experiencing progressive constipation. Patients often begin using laxatives, first rarely and then more regularly. Weeks or months later, they present for medical evaluation because of abdominal pain and distension, obstipation and sometimes nausea and vomiting. The patient with a carcinoma may have had previous symptoms of tenesmus and alternating constipation and diarrhoea. If the neoplasm has disseminated, there may be weight loss and symptoms related to the metastases. In a small number of cases the acute obstruction is more sudden, particularly with neoplasms at the ileocaecal valve. Such a patient presents with sudden onset of colicky, abdominal pain accompanied by profuse vomiting.

On examination, the distended abdomen often precludes palpation of an obstructing mass. When present, a non-tender or mobile mass is more likely to be due to carcinoma than to diverticular disease. Localized tenderness and peritoneal signs may be present at the site of the obstructing or locally perforated cancer. Localized tenderness or peritoneal signs in the right lower quadrant in the setting of a left-sided obstructing cancer implies acute caecal distension and impending perforation dictating urgent intervention.

If the carcinoma has metastasized, there may be hepatomegaly or other features of dissemination. Occasionally, a rectal carcinoma causing obstruction may be palpable on digital rectal examination or a sigmoid carcinoma may be palpated through the anterior rectal wall if it lies in the rectal vesicle or rectovaginal pouch of Douglas.

Perforation

For the 12–19% of patients with obstruction who develop a concomitant perforation, the major presenting symptoms may be due to the perforation and secondary peritonitis (Runkel et al 1991, Umpleby et al 1984). Runkel et al reported that half of the perforations were free into the abdominal cavity resulting in diffuse peritonitis and sepsis. Half of the patients perforated locally. Presumably because of its gradual development, the peritoneal defence mechanisms wall off and localize the site of perforation, often resulting in a localized abscess or phlegmon. Not surprisingly, diverticulitis, appendicitis or Crohn's disease is often considered in the differential diagnosis. As noted above, localized peritonitis in the right lower quadrant is an ominous sign of impending or partial caecal perforation.

Ancillary diagnostic evaluation

Plain abdominal radiography, apart from indicating that an obstruction is present, is usually not helpful in establishing its cause. The exact pattern of gas distribution and extent of associated small bowel distension depend on the location of the cancer, the status of the ileocaecal valve and the time course of the development of the obstruction. Free air or retroperitoneal air should be excluded. A contrast enema can, in certain circumstances, demonstrate the radiologic signs of a carcinoma and may reveal a perforation or fistula. More often, however, there is merely a cut-off of contrast material at the point of obstruction without diagnostic features of a cancer (Fig. 8.1). An annular carcinoma of the left colon which products acute, complete obstruction will rapidly produce massive colonic distension but no significant small bowel gas if the ileocaecal valve is competent. The identical lesion in a patient with an incompetent ileocaecal valve will more slowly result in diffuse distension of both small and large bowel.

The primary goals of the contrast enema are to confirm the presence, site and degree of colon obstruction and to exclude other pathologies such as a volvulus. A water-soluble contrast such as gastrografin eliminates the risk of barium peritonitis in cases with associated perforation. Additionally, the gastrografin acts as a cathartic to cleanse the colon distal to the obstructing lesion and occasionally it converts a completely obstructing tumour to a partially obstructing tumour, perhaps by diminishing associated bowel wall oedema through its hydrostatic properties.

A CT scan may provide useful information especially if there is a large, palpable mass which might be fixed to other organs. Such information would be useful in anticipating a particular area of difficult dissection such as an obstructing cancer invading into the splenic hilum. It may also prepare the surgeon for the possibility of ureteral displacement or compression from an obstructing or perforating carcinoma. In the latter instance, one should place ureteral stents at the time of laparotomy to minimize risk of ureteral injury. A CT scan can also help define the aetiology of the colon obstruction and is

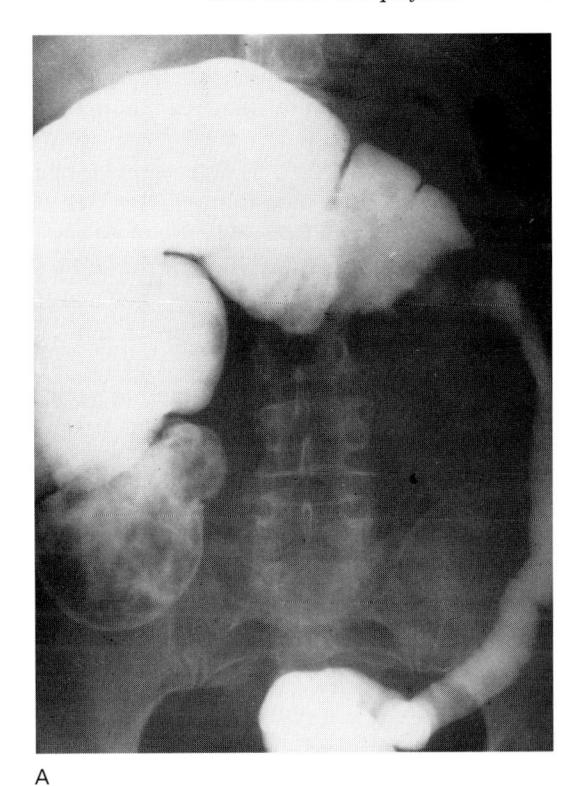

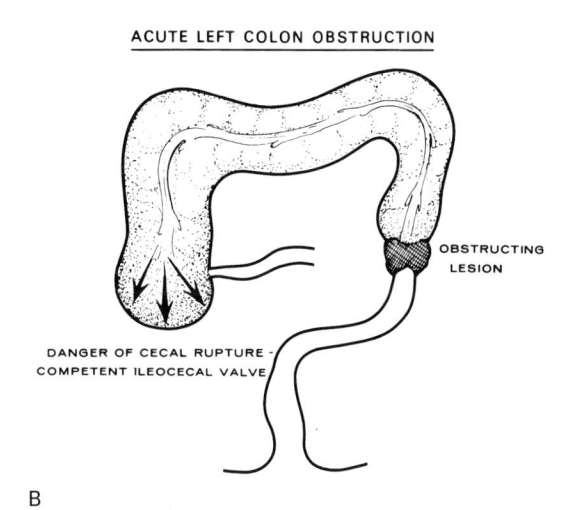

Fig. 8.1 (A) A gastrografin enema demonstrating complete obstruction to retrograde flow with proximal colonic dilation. (B) The artist's drawing emphasizes the potential danger of proximal perforation from an obstructing colonic cancer.

especially useful in the diagnosis of diverticulitis which can present with colon obstruction. The clinician must be aware that carcinoma and diverticulitis can coexist.

The role of proctoscopy, flexible sigmoidoscopy or colonoscopy in evaluating patients with a colon obstruction or possible perforation is controversial because of the risk of insufflating air which might increase the risk of perforation. Digital rectal examination and proctosigmoidoscopy without insufflation of air can be done safely to assess the anal sphincters and to exclude rectal pathology. No patient should undergo laparotomy for a colon obstruction without first undergoing a proctosigmoidoscopy.

Preoperative management

Obstruction or perforation due to colorectal cancer demand that the clinician determines whether this is a true emergency or an urgent situation which can be converted to a more elective operation. If the patient has evidence of diffuse peritonitis or if vital signs are unstable, fluid resuscitation and institution of antibiotics with immediate laparotomy are essential. Preoperative management with invasive monitoring is sometimes necessary in the critically ill patient.

If the patient's vital signs are stable and there is no evidence of diffuse peritonitis, one can take the time to better control the degree of bowel obstruction by placing a nasogastric tube to decompress the upper tract and by doing a gastrografin enema as described earlier. At a minimum, this will purge the bowel distal to the obstruction or perforation and in some instances, it helps avoid emergency surgery so a more elective operation can be performed after the patient has been fully resuscitated and has completed a full bowel preparation. This can sometimes make the difference between a one-stage resection and anastomosis versus a multiple-stage procedure with the use of a temporary stoma. An alternative advocated by some surgeons is endoscopic decompression using a laser or cautery to 'core out' a lumen within an obstructing cancer (Bright et al 1992, Eckhauser & Mansour 1992). This allows a complete bowel preparation to be performed before a definitive laparotomy is undertaken.

If after placement of a nasogastric tube, fluid resuscitation and gastrografin enema, the patient still has localized peritoneal signs either at the site of the cancer or overlying the caecum, early intervention is necessary to avoid catastrophic perforation. Conversely, if the patient becomes more comfortable, less distended and begins to pass some gas and stool, one can use a modified bowel preparation routine and prepare for surgery in 24–48 hours. A modified bowel preparation consists of tap water enemas and low doses of mild oral laxatives or polyethylene glycol solution. If the patient develops increased abdominal distension or signs of complete obstruction, the modified bowel preparation is stopped and an urgent operation is undertaken.

Other preoperative preparation includes education of the patient as to the problem confronted and the possible operative alternatives including the likelihood of the need for a colostomy or ileostomy, either temporary or permanent. Ideally, the patient should be seen by an enterostomal therapy nurse and either the surgeon or enterostomal therapy nurse should mark the patient's abdomen for a temporary or permanent stoma site.

Operative preliminaries

Positioning

Once in the operating room, the patient should be positioned in a modified lithotomy position so that the surgeon has access to the anorectum and rectosigmoid. This also allows easy positioning for the second assistant who can stand between the legs which are elevated in stirrups but only positioned such that they do not interfere with the abdominal exploration. This position also facilitates cystoscopy and ureteral stent placement, intraoperative colonoscopy, intraoperative bowel preparation by rectal irrigations or proximal lavage and per anal placement of surgical staplers.

Exploration

Thorough exploration through a midline incision is essential to determine:

1. the extent and location of the primary cancer;
2. the presence of direct spread to adjacent structures or of abdominal metastases;
3. the degree of peritoneal contamination or intraabdominal abscess;
4. the condition of the bowel proximal and distal to the cancer;
5. other pathology.

When undertaking a laparotomy for colonic obstruction, one must be extremely careful not to create an inadvertent colotomy which would result in disastrous spillage of faecal contents. Often marked colonic distension prevents accurate assessment of the abdomen until decompression is performed.

Decompression

If the colon is found to be markedly distended and about to perforate, it is essential to decompress the colon before handling it. This can be done in one of the following ways. If the colon is grossly distended by a large volume of air, a 16 gauge intravenous catheter needle is used to penetrate the colon wall. The needle is removed leaving the sheath from the catheter in the lumen of the colon and the gas is easily aspirated by suction to decompress the colon. Since the puncture site of the intravenous needle is tiny, it is readily closed with a previously placed purse string suture.

This technique will not work to remove stool and if the patient has a large volume of liquid or solid stool proximal to an obstructing cancer, an alternative decompression technique described by Khoo et al (1988) is useful and can be done very safely through the terminal ileum. A large bore soft chest tube with multiple holes in the distal 5–7 cm is connected proximally via a Y adapter with one limb of non-collapsible tubing connected to a suction device and the other limb of tubing connected to an irrigation syringe. The chest tube is inserted via an ileotomy surrounded by a purse string suture 8–10 cm from the competent ileocaecal valve. As the chest tube reaches the caecum, the purse string is tightened to prevent spillage of faeces from the ileotomy and the bowel is decompressed as stool is suctioned from the colon. If tubing gets plugged with solid stool, irrigation via the other limb of the Y adapter will facilitate complete emptying of the colon. Once the colon is decompressed, it can be more safely handled and assessed as can the rest of the abdominal viscera.

Operative plan

The surgeon must next formulate a treatment plan based on the ability to do a resection, either for palliation or cure, and the safety of performing an anastomosis. Can resection be safely performed? If so, will it be potentially curative or will there be residual cancer? Should an anastomosis be performed? Should a temporary stoma be constructed? It is difficult to answer these questions categorically.

If the surgeon is uncertain whether he possesses the expertise or experience to meet the technical demands that may be required by an obstructing or perforated carcinoma or if appropriate support (anaesthesia, operating room assistant, nurses, intensive care unit, blood bank, etc.) is unavailable, the patient is best served by a proximal diversion to decompress the colon without resection of the lesion and prompt referral to a tertiary care centre which can offer the full range of care needed to manage such cases successfully.

Assessment of resectability

Almost all obstructive or perforated carcinomas can be resected either for palliation or cure and as a general rule, resection is indicated. Only rarely is a lesion so fixed to secondary structures that resection is highly dangerous and thus contraindicated. An example is an obstructing colon carcinoma directly invading the duodenum and encasing the vena cava. Spread to adjacent organs or other structures is not, in and of itself, a contraindication to resection and often does not preclude a curative resection. The presence of multiple, retroperitoneal, peritoneal, liver or other abdominal metastases dictates a palliative approach but usually does not preclude resection of the primary obstructing lesion.

It may occasionally be unwise to attempt a primary resection of an obstructing carcinoma of the colon. An unstable patient whose general condition is poor in whom there is a combination of a fixed growth and considerable colonic distension is one who may be best served by a proximal diversion as an initial stage.

Intent of treatment

Many obstructing and even perforated cancers can be resected with curative intent. En bloc resection of the colon and adjacent tissues or organs directly invaded by the cancer without cutting across tumour produces cure rates comparable to those achieved after resection of non-obstructed cancers of the same pathological stage (Bright et al 1992, Osteen et al 1980, Spears et al 1988, Turnbull et al 1989). If the patient has no distant spread, aggressive local resection including presumed inflammatory attachments to loops of bowel or other viscera is indicated even if this requires multiple anastomoses. One cannot separate attached loops of bowel or other organs adherent to the primary tumour without potentially compromising curability.

Palliation may be necessary because of an extensively fixed, non-resectable primary lesion (as described above) or because resection cannot eliminate distant metastases or carcinomatosis. Palliative treatment can nonetheless minimize pain and provide the patient with a reasonable quality of life for a limited time. Principles useful for providing palliative care are:

1. Resect the primary lesion if technically safe to do so.
2. Preserve gastrointestinal continuity if safe to do so, i.e. after resection, perform a primary anastomosis or if resection is not feasible, construct an internal bypass.
3. Avoid staged procedures for palliation, i.e. the operative plan should not contemplate a later, elective return to the operating room to perform a second or third stage procedure on a patient with a very limited lifespan. Instead, the operative plan should provide the best function possible while relieving as many of the patient's symptoms as possible. Thus, if resection and anastomosis or internal bypass are not viable options, one should opt for a resection of the primary obstructing cancer and a permanent end stoma generally placed as distally as feasible in the gastrointestinal tract, thus minimizing the stoma output and maximizing ease of care of the stoma. The distal end of bowel can be closed as a long Hartmann pouch or a separate mucus fistula can be constructed. If resection of the primary is not feasible, a proximal loop colostomy or ileostomy is advised since this will vent in both directions.

Consideration of staged procedures

Traditionally, a three-stage procedure was used for obstructed cancers. An ostomy was constructed at the first stage to overcome the immediate problems posed by the obstruction. A subsequent radical cancer operation was done as the second stage, followed by a third operation to restore bowel continuity. In recent decades, in an effort to decrease morbidity of multiple laparotomies, surgeons more commonly used a two-stage approach combining stages one and two or two and three of the original, classic three-stage procedure (Barillari et al 1992, Dutton et al 1976, Irvin & Greaney 1977, Jarvinen et al 1988, Korenaga et al 1991, Welch & Donaldson 1974). Perforated cancers generally require resection to remove the septic focus since drainage and proximal diversion without resection leaves a column of stool between the stoma and the perforation. In addition, desquamated cells from the tumour itself may continue to seed the abdomen and further worsen the already grim prognosis.

Today, there is increasing use of a one-stage approach especially for obstructing right-sided colonic cancers. Surgeons learned that obstructing carcinoma of the proximal colon, even when a closed loop obstruction produced marked caecal distension, could be treated safely by decompression, resection and anastomosis (Ota 1995). This approach had many advantages over the formerly used first stage procedures of an ileotransverse colostomy for bypass or a defunctioning ileostomy. Not only were subsequent operations avoided but the risk of caecal perforation from continued caecal distension if the ileocaecal valve remained competent was also obviated.

The principle of immediate resection for left-sided colonic obstruction was introduced by Wangensteen in 1949. Numerous authors since argued that with appropriate attention to detail, an immediate excision followed by a primary colocolic anastomosis would be the simplest and best way to treat obstructing cancers of the left colon. Despite the obvious advantages of removing the cancer immediately and avoiding the need for additional surgery, morbidity and mortality were high (Umpleby et al 1984). Thus, it soon became surgical dogma that left-sided colon obstruction should be treated with a two-stage approach. Currently, this policy is questioned and as noted below, subtotal colectomy and on-table bowel preparation enhance the safety of using a one-stage operation even for left-sided obstructing cancers.

In general, it is advisable to avoid staged procedures for palliation since most patients will not live long enough to justify the morbidity associated with reoperation. However, if the patient is likely to live for a year or more or when cure is possible, a staged approach may be indicated. It is often unsafe to perform a primary anastomosis after resection of an obstructed or perforated carcinoma. Malnutrition, faecal or purulent peritonitis, and other systemic conditions such as shock, may make a staged approach mandatory. Questionable viability of the cut edges of bowel, bowel wall oedema or other secondary effects of obstruction or perforation and sepsis may dictate use of a temporary stoma.

Operative options – technique

The surgeon synthesizes all of the information gathered from the patient's preoperative assessment and the findings at laparotomy to decide which of the many operative options best fits a particular patient (Buechter et al 1988, Crooms & Kovalcik 1984, Waldron & Donovan 1986). Special aspects and technical tips of the available options are discussed below.

Immediate resection

In a general sense, resection of an obstructing or perforated carcinoma of the colon is performed in the same way as any elective colectomy for cancer. Oncologic principles must be followed. However, the acute setting of obstruction or perforation creates some special technical problems for the surgeon. Despite decompression, the bowel wall remains stretched and oedematous and there may be areas of near full-thickness necrosis which are easily disrupted during mobilization, resulting in faecal contamination and potential tumour spillage. The mesentery is often thickened and oedematous and thus prone to tearing or bleeding. Suture ligation of vascular pedicles and mesenteric edges can overcome this problem. As noted above, direct extension to other organs or attached limbs of bowel must be resected en bloc if the intent of resection is curative. At times, this can require partial removal of the liver, abdominal wall or other viscera, thus complicating the resection.

The extent of colonic resection is primarily dictated by the location of the obstructing or perforated primary cancer. For caecal and ascending colon cancers, a standard right hemicolectomy is performed with ligation of the ileocolic and right colic vessels. For lesions of the hepatic flexure and right transverse colon, an extended right hemicolectomy with additional ligation of the middle colic vessels is indicated. If the lesion is in the left transverse colon, the splenic flexure or the descending colon, oncologic principles would be satisfied by a left hemicolectomy but this has the significant disadvantage of leaving the non-prepared, dilated right colon for an anastomosis or for a right transverse colostomy which is a 'wet' stoma and often difficult to care for. A preferred alternative is to extend the resection to a subtotal colectomy which has significant

Table 8.1 Potential advantages of total or subtotal colectomy and primary ileocolic or ileorectal anastomosis for obstructing cancer of the colon

1. Pathology fully defined
2. Synchronous lesions resected
3. Single hospitalization and single operation
4. Minimal morbidity/mortality*
5. No special bowel preparation necessary
6. No intraoperative contamination
7. No size discrepancy**
8. Good functional result***

* Assumes conditions favourable for primary anastomosis – see text
** Assumes ileocaecal valve is competent – see text
*** Assumes competent anal sphincter and normal small bowel and rectum – see text

advantages, as noted in Table 8.1. An obstructing or perforated sigmoid cancer is often best treated by a sigmoid colectomy. Alternatively, a total colectomy to achieve the advantages noted above may be performed. This is especially useful if the patient has partial thickness tears in the right colon from proximal distension. If an ileorectal anastomosis would probably result in significant diarrhoea, an alternative is to resect the sigmoid, decompress and oversew the right colon tears and construct a proximal ileostomy.

Primary anastomosis after resection

The decision to perform a primary anastomosis after resection of an obstructing or perforated colon cancer requires mature judgement. The surgeon must consider not only the patient's overall status (nutrition, shock, etc.), the degree of peritoneal contamination and the technical demands of constructing a well-vascularized, accurate anastomosis without tension but also the condition of the two limbs of bowel to be anastomosed and the likely functional result to be expected. If the ileocaecal valve is competent, the distal small bowel is generally well suited for an anastomosis. The colon distal to the obstruction can be irrigated and cleansed either preoperatively via enemas or intraoperatively via rectal irrigations or antegrade lavage irrigations. A clamp can be placed distal to the obstructing cancer and a large bore catheter inserted into the colon just distal to the clamp. A lavage solution of saline is instilled via the catheter after an assistant inserts a proctoscope into the rectum to suction the returns until the distal colon is clean. The site of the catheter placement is resected with the colectomy specimen. Next an ileocolic anastomosis is performed either by handsewn or stapled technique. This assumes the patient's anal sphincter is functional and that the extent of colonic resection will not result in diarrhoea. For most patients, regardless of age, an ileosigmoid anastomosis will provide reasonable function without diarrhoea providing the rectosigmoid is not diseased. Thus for most obstructing or perforated cancers of the colon proximal to the left colic artery, a subtotal colectomy with ileosigmoid anastomosis is the preferred operation.

If the sigmoid is the site of the obstruction or perforation or if the sigmoid is unsuited for anastomosis because of the disease (diverticular, etc.), one can consider the alternative of segmental colectomy, distal rectal washout, proximal on-table bowel preparation and colorectal anastomosis. The on-table lavage introduced by Dudley et al (1980) is performed by mobilizing both the hepatic and splenic flexures, placing two clamps proximal to the tumour: one at the point of the proposed anastomosis and the other approximately 8–10 cm distally. The colon cancer distal to this second clamp is then excised in the usual way. A large bore anaesthetic tubing is fed into the proximal colon at its cut edge and secured to the bowel. The other end of the tubing is passed off the operative field to a closed container to collect the effluent. Proximal instillation of saline via a catheter placed into the caecum through the appendix stump is begun until the colon is clean. The 8–10 cm segment of colon at the site of the tubing placement is resected. After irrigating the distal rectum and colon, a primary anastomosis is performed. Extensive intraperitoneal lavage is used with appropriate antibiotic or saline solutions (Stewart et al 1993).

Diversion after resection and anastomosis

Occasionally, after resection of a perforated or obstructed cancer, one or more primary anastomoses is performed under less than ideal circumstances, thus increasing the risk of an anastomotic leak. A proximal loop or end stoma to divert faeces may minimize the consequences of a leaked anastomosis. This is an unusual circumstance and a proximal stoma is not an excuse to perform a less than adequate anastomosis.

Diversion without resection

On occasion, the best option is a simple diversion proximal to the obstructing or perforated cancer. Tube caecostomy was commonly used in the early 1900s but its role today is questioned. It does not totally divert the faecal stream, does not drain adequately even if irrigated daily and is often very difficult to manage postoperatively because of its flush construction and relatively liquid output. Advocates point out that it can be done expeditiously if necessary under local anaesthesia through a small incision in the right lower abdomen and that it has the advantage of exteriorizing the most dilated and often partially disrupted portion of the intestine (Hoffmann & Jensen 1984). The disadvantages are so significant, however, that caecostomy is not recommended.

Another area of controversy relates to the use of a so-called 'blind stoma'. A 'blind stoma' implies that a limb of bowel presumed proximal to the obstruction is mobilized, opened and matured as a diverting stoma. This technique carries a small but definite risk of a wrong diagnosis, incorrect anatomic location for the stoma or the failure to detect a complication such as an impending perforation. Its use should be confined to patients with known malignant obstruction without clinical signs of bowel infarction, peritonitis or localized sepsis. A small incision is made in the abdomen to gain access to the dilated bowel proximal to the obstructing cancer. Bowel viability and peritoneal contamination are assessed. A 'blind' loop of dilated bowel is gently delivered through the wound and decompressed. An immediate mucocutaneous suture is used to mature the stoma. The surgeon must be prepared to proceed with laparotomy if this technique is unsuccessful. This procedure is rarely performed.

Controversy exists regarding the relative advantages of a loop vs end stoma and colostomy vs ileostomy. For permanent stomas, an end stoma is generally preferred over a loop stoma as it is easier to care for and a left-sided colostomy is preferred over a proximal stoma since the stool is more solid and faecal volume is less. However, a Brooke ileostomy is often easier to manage than a right transverse colostomy. If an ileostomy is used and there is concern that the ileocaecal valve is competent and the caecum is distended, a large Foley catheter should be passed through the distal limb of the ileostomy, the balloon inflated and the catheter pulled back against the ileocaecal valve and connected to low suction to act as a vent.

Personal series

In a recent survey of patients with left colon obstruction at the University of Minnesota Hospitals, 74 were due to carcinoma. Most patients were elderly – median age 74 years (range 34–100 years). Forty eight of these patients were women.

The site distribution of obstruction was:

- splenic flexure – 15%
- descending colon – 12%
- sigmoid colon – 46%
- rectosigmoid – 27%

Four patients (5%) were found to harbour synchronous cancers at operation. Two were in the caecum, one at the hepatic flexure and one was in the transverse colon. Furthermore, sigmoid diverticular disease was found to coexist with malignancy in four (5%) patients. Modified Astler–Coller staging of index cancers were: Dukes' A – 3, Dukes' B1 – 2, Dukes' B2 – 26, Dukes' C – 23 and Dukes' D – 20. Thus, extracolonic spread of cancer was present in 55% of patients.

At operation, no free perforations were present although several patients had serosal tears of the caecum. Two patients had localized perforations through tumour resulting in abscess formation. Colonic lavage was performed in 18 patients. Primary resection of the disease segment and restoration of bowel continuity was achieved without an accompanying stoma in 61 (82%) patients. A diverting stoma was performed following anastomosis in one patient and a Hartmann procedure in four. Hence, resection of primary disease was possible in 89% of patients. Only one patient developed a clinical anastomotic dehiscence which required reoperation.

Conclusion

The surgeon plays a critical role in the care of patients with an obstructed or perforated carcinoma of the colon. The surgeon must recognize the clinical presentation and quickly make an accurate diagnosis of the problem so immediate non-operative treatment can be instituted in the hopes of reversing or at least controlling sequelae of the obstruction or perforation. Attention to details during the initial phase of surgery can avoid disastrous faecal or tumour spillage into the abdomen and allow accurate assessment of the patient's status. This information is used to create a rational operative plan individualized to the patient's needs (Fig. 8.2).

All operative options should be part of the surgeon's armamentarium. Although the trend increasingly is to perform a primary resection and anastomosis, there are still occasions when resection and diversion or diversion alone are indicated. Mature judgement is necessary to make this distinction properly.

Fig. 8.2 Colonic cancer: obstruction and perforation

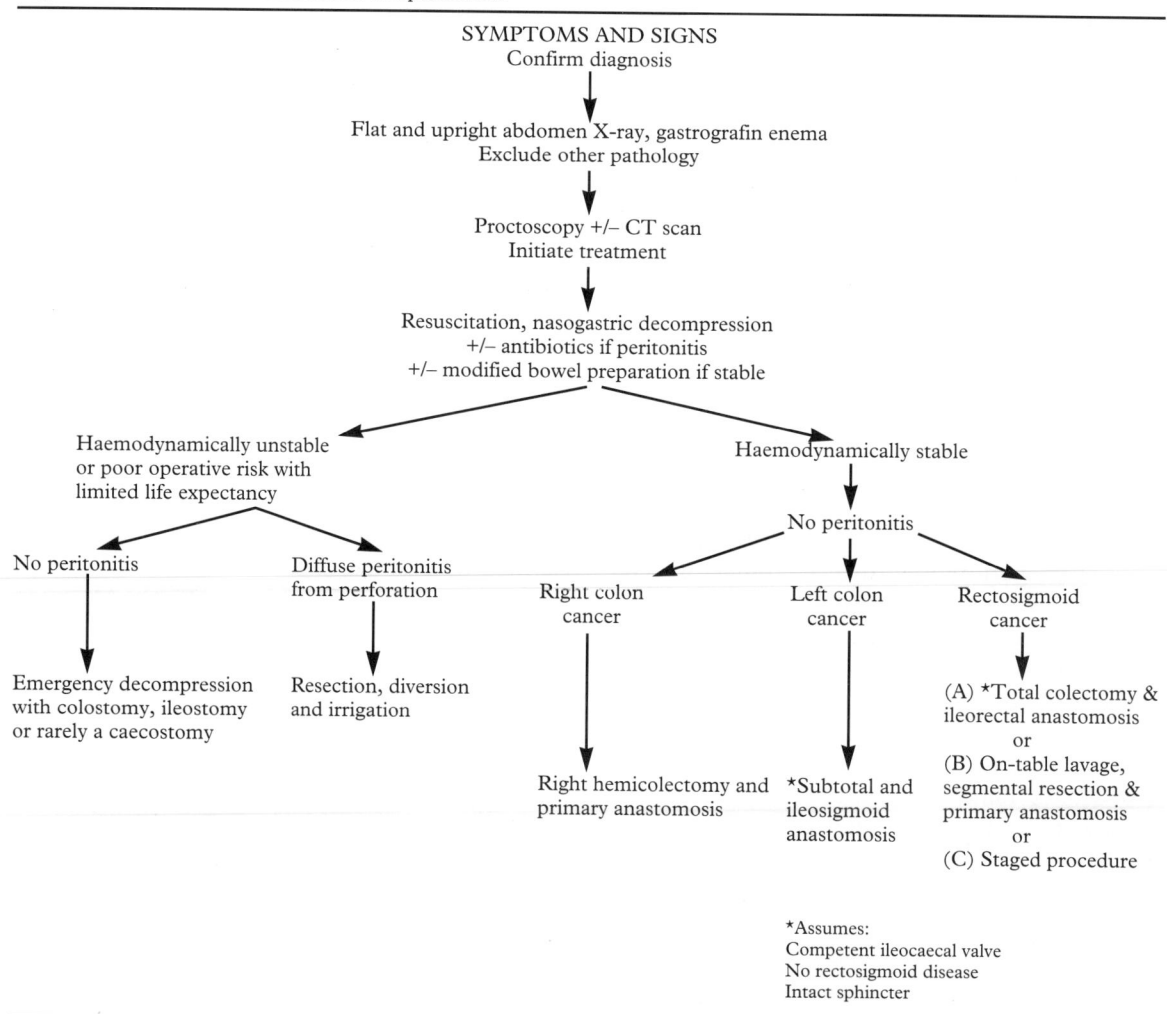

```
                    SYMPTOMS AND SIGNS
                     Confirm diagnosis
                            ↓
        Flat and upright abdomen X-ray, gastrografin enema
                    Exclude other pathology
                            ↓
                   Proctoscopy +/− CT scan
                      Initiate treatment
                            ↓
              Resuscitation, nasogastric decompression
                    +/− antibiotics if peritonitis
                +/− modified bowel preparation if stable
```

Haemodynamically unstable or poor operative risk with limited life expectancy

Haemodynamically stable
↓
No peritonitis

- No peritonitis → Emergency decompression with colostomy, ileostomy or rarely a caecostomy
- Diffuse peritonitis from perforation → Resection, diversion and irrigation
- Right colon cancer → Right hemicolectomy and primary anastomosis
- Left colon cancer → *Subtotal and ileosigmoid anastomosis
- Rectosigmoid cancer →
  (A) *Total colectomy & ileorectal anastomosis
  or
  (B) On-table lavage, segmental resection & primary anastomosis
  or
  (C) Staged procedure

*Assumes:
Competent ileocaecal valve
No rectosigmoid disease
Intact sphincter

References

Barillari P, Aurello P, DeAngelis R et al 1992 Management and survival of patients affected with obstructive colorectal cancer. International Surgeon 77: 251–255

Boring CC, Squires TS, Heath CW Jr 1992 Cancer statistics for African Americans. Cancer 42: 7–17

Buechter KJ, Bousany C, Caillouette R, Cohn Jr I 1988 Surgical management of the acutely obstructed colon. American Journal of Surgery 156: 163–168

Bright N, Hale P, Mason R 1992 Poor palliation of colorectal malignancy with the neodymium yttrium-aluminium-garnet laser. British Journal of Surgery 79: 308–309

Chapuis PH, Dent OF, Fisher R et al 1985 A multivariate analysis of clinical and pathological variables in prognosis after resection of large bowel cancer. British Journal of Surgery 72: 698–702

Corman ML 1991 Principles of surgical technique in the treatment of carcinoma of the large bowel. World Journal of Surgery 15: 592–596

Crooms JW, Kovalcik PJ 1984 Obstructing left-sided colon carcinoma. Appraisal of surgical options. Annals of Surgery 50: 15–19

Crucitti F, Sofo L, Doglietto GB et al 1991 Prognostic factors in colorectal cancer: Current status and new trends. Journal of Surgical Oncology 2 (suppl): 76–82

Dutton JW, Hreno A, Hampson LG 1976 Mortality and prognosis of obstructing carcinoma of the large bowel. American Journal of Surgery 131: 36–41

Dudley HAF, Radcliffe AG, McGeehan D 1980 Intraoperative irrigation of the colon to permit primary anastomosis. British Journal of Surgery 67: 80–81

Eckhauser ML, Mansour EG 1992 Endoscopic laser therapy for obstructing and/or bleeding colorectal carcinoma. American Surgeon 58(6): 358–363

Fearon ER, Vogelstein B 1990 A genetic model for colorectal tumorigenesis. Cell 61: 759–767

Fielding LP, Phillips RKS, Hittinger R 1989 Factors influencing mortality after curative resection for large bowel cancer in elderly patients. Lancet i: 595–597

Garcia-Valdescasas JC, Lovera JM, deLacy AM et al 1991 Obstructing colorectal carcinomas: prospective study. Diseases of the Colon and Rectum 34: 759–762

Gennaro AR, Tyson RR 1978 Obstructive colonic cancer. Diseases of the Colon and Rectum 21(5): 346–351

Griffin MR, Bergstralh EJ, Coffey RJ et al 1987 Predictors of survival after curative resection of carcinoma of the colon and rectum. Cancer 60: 2318–2324

Hoffmann J, Jensen HE 1984 Tube cecostomy and staged resection for obstructing carcinoma of the left colon. Diseases of the Colon and Rectum 27: 24–32

Irvin TT, Greaney MG 1977 The treatment of colonic cancer presenting with intestinal obstruction. British Journal of Surgery 64: 741–744

Jarvinen HJ, Ovaska J, Mecklin JP 1988 Improvements in the treatment and prognosis of colorectal carcinoma. British Journal of Surgery 75: 25–27

Khoo RE, Rothenberger DA, Wong WD, Buls JG, Najarian JS 1988 Tube decompression of the dilated colon. American Journal of Surgery 156: 214–216

Korenaga D, Ueo H, Mochida K et al 1991 Prognostic factors in Japanese patients with colorectal cancer: the significance of large bowel obstruction – univariate and multivariate analyses. Journal of Surgical Oncology 47: 188–192

Ohman U 1982 Prognosis in patients with obstructing colorectal carcinoma. American Journal of Surgery 143: 742–747

Osteen RT, Guyton S, Steele G, Wilson RE 1980 Malignant intestinal obstruction. Surgery 87: 611–615

Ota DM 1995 Surgical considerations. In Cohen AM, Winawer SJ, Friedman MA, Gunderson LL (eds) Cancer of the colon, rectum, and anus. McGraw-Hill, New York, pp 431–435

Runkel NS, Schlag P, Schwarz V et al 1991 Outcome after emergency surgery for cancer of the large intestine. British Journal of Surgery 78: 183–188

Serpell JW, McDermott FT, Katrivessis H et al 1989 Obstructing carcinomas of the colon. British Journal of Surgery 76: 965–969

Spears H, Petrelli NJ, Herrera L, Mittelman A 1988 Treatment of bowel obstruction after operation for colorectal carcinoma. American Journal of Surgery 155: 383–386

Steinberg SM, Barkin JS, Kaplan RS et al 1986 Prognostic indicators of colon tumors: the Gastrointestinal Tumor Group experience. Cancer 57: 1866–1870

Stewart J, Diament RH, Brennan TG 1993 Management of obstructing lesions of the left colon by resection, on-table lavage, and primary anastomosis. Surgery 114(3): 502–505

Turnbull ADM, Guerra J, Starnes HF 1989 Results of surgery for obstructing carcinomatosis of gastrointestinal, pancreatic, or biliary origin. Journal of Clinical Oncology 7(3): 381–386

Ueyama T, Yao T, Nakamura K et al 1991 Obstructing carcinomas of the colon and rectum: clinicopathologic analysis of 40 cases. Japanese Journal of Clinical Oncology 21: 100–109

Umpleby HC, Williamson RCN, Chir M 1984 Survival in acute obstructing colorectal carcinoma. Diseases of the Colon and Rectum 27: 299–304

Wangensteen OH, Wangensteen SD (eds) 1978 The rise of surgery from empiric craft to scientific discipline. University of Minnesota Press, Minneapolis, MN, p 128

Wangensteen OH. Evolution of surgery for large intestinal obstruction. Diseases of the Colon and Rectum 21: 135–139

Waldron RP, Donovan IA 1986 Mortality in patients with obstructing colorectal cancer. Annals of the Royal College of Surgeons of England 68: 219–221

Welch JP, Donaldson GA 1974 Management of severe obstruction of the large bowel due to malignant disease. American Journal of Surgery 127: 492–499

Willett C, Tepper JE, Cohen A et al 1985 Obstructive and perforative colonic carcinoma: patterns of failure. Journal of Clinical Oncology 3: 379–384

Wolmark N, Wieand HS, Rockette HE et al 1983 The prognostic significance of tumor and location and bowel obstruction in Dukes B and C colorectal cancer: findings from the NSABP clinical trials. Annals of Surgery 198: 743–752

9 Adjuvant radiotherapy

R. D. JAMES

Introduction

Referrals of patients with colorectal cancer for non-surgical (adjuvant) treatment have increased markedly in the last decade (Table 9.1). Policies for adjuvant treatment have followed those for breast cancer a decade ago. Most notable is the increased use of postoperative adjuvant cytotoxic chemotherapy, dealt with in Chapter 10. Radiotherapy (XRT) has also been used increasingly for patients with rectal cancer, often in combination with chemotherapy.

The aim of this chapter is to introduce the concept of treatment quality or cost-effectiveness, to define how it can be measured and how it is modified by various combinations of surgery, XRT and chemotherapy. There is no attempt to quantify cost-effectiveness, merely to indicate in which direction improvements are most likely to emerge.

Cost-effectiveness seeks to define 'the intervention that results in the lowest cost for achieving a given outcome' (Brown et al 1994). Improvements in effectiveness (efficacy) of treatment frequently involve an increase in the cost of treatment.

The most reliable data on relative cost-effectiveness are from prospective, randomized clinical trials which contain a surgery–only arm. Most of them measure effectiveness in terms of survival. Fewer report local recurrence or the preservation of the anal sphincter or sexual function (Table 9.2). Only a few measure and report costs (Tables 9.3 and 9.4). Even rarer is any attempt to measure the multitude of variables which might influence cost-effectiveness and confound conclusions drawn from the data. These include the extent of spread of the cancer (stage), its grade and radio sensitivity (Table 9.5). Although these can be measured to a greater or lesser extent, their

Table 9.1 Colorectal cancer, non-surgical treatment. New registrations, by year, at the Christie Hospital, Manchester, United Kingdom

1984	304
1985	323
1986	285
1987	330
1988	324
1989	333
1990	339
1991	517
1992	563
1993	603

Table 9.2 Measures of effectiveness of adjuvant XRT

Survival
Local recurrence
Sphincter preservation
Sexual potency

Table 9.3 Measures of direct costs of adjuvant XRT

Proportion of patients experiencing:
Toxic death
Anastomotic leaks
Extended (more than 1 week) XRT schedule
Non-compliance with XRT schedule
Diarrhoea, weight loss
Laparotomies for XRT enteritis

Table 9.4 Measures of indirect costs of adjuvant XRT

Proportion of patients experiencing:
Needless irradiation
Needless delay in surgical intervention
Unreliable pathologic staging
Hospitalization
Loss of earnings
Adverse quality of life

Table 9.5 Non-controllable factors modifying cost-effectiveness of XRT

Stage
Grade
Radiosensitivity

Table 9.6 Controllable factors modifying cost-effectiveness of XRT

XRT dose, field size and shape
Timing of chemotherapy and surgery

control is beyond the scope of current XRT practice.

A further series of variables can not only be measured, but may be controlled by the radiotherapist (Table 9.6). These include XRT dose and field size and the timing of chemotherapy or surgery relative to XRT. Comparisons of the cost-effectiveness of certain schedules used in published trials are unreliable if no attempt is made to control confounding variables. If, for example, postoperative XRT + chemotherapy is thought to be more effective than postoperative XRT alone, the only reliable way to ascertain this is to compare the two directly in a clinical trial.

If XRT and chemotherapy are given before rather than after surgery, the traditional staging system (Dukes' or Astler–Coller) and grading system (Broders), which rely on a complete removal of the surgical specimen, may no longer be reliable. The issue of non-surgical staging, dealt with in Chapter 4, is therefore particularly relevant to adjuvant XRT and is mentioned briefly at the end of this chapter.

Measurements of cost-effectiveness

Measures of cost

Any therapeutic advantage to rectal cancer patients from XRT may be paralleled by a concomitant increase in side-effects which are not quantified by overviews and are much more difficult to measure than deaths. These include hospitalization costs, loss of earnings, inconvenience and psychological upset. The time schedule of XRT is the most important single factor influencing XRT cost: published trials have used schedules varying from one day to 60 days. The longer, more expensive schedules are not necessarily the most effective.

Some costs directly attributable to adjuvant treatment may threaten the life of the patient. One large European trial reported an excess of non-cancer deaths in patients over 75 years treated with a preoperative XRT arm compared with age-matched patients in the control arm (Stockholm Rectal Cancer Study Group 1990). Most deaths were cardiovascular and were due to some as yet unexplained effect of the combination of large XRT fractions with large field sizes. This toxic effect was abolished in subsequent trials by a reduction in XRT field size (Swedish Rectal Cancer Trial 1993).

A less serious, but occasionally fatal cost of XRT is radiation bowel disease (XRT enteritis). This has deterred many surgeons from referring patients for adjuvant XRT. The incidence of XRT enteritis varies with uncontrollable factors like hypertension, diabetes, vascular disease, diverticular disease, pelvic inflammatory disease, previous bowel surgery, physique and age.

XRT enteritis may be acute or late. When the gut is irradiated, an acute reaction, due to epithelial stem cell death, appears approximately 2 weeks after XRT is started and continues 2–3 weeks after its end. The epithelial lining of the gastrointestinal tract is depopulated by XRT because it sterilizes the self-renewal stem cells at the base of the intestinal crypts. Macroscopically, the villi shorten and shrink, giving rise to a syndrome similar to malabsorption. Acute XRT enteritis occurs during or shortly after treatment and is measured by diarrhoea, fatigue, weight loss and nausea. Following preoperative XRT, further complications of acute XRT enteritis may include anastomotic dehiscence and thus its frequency may be a useful measure of any deleterious effect. Since the timing and dose of XRT is so critical, a measure of the compliance of patients with the planned schedule is as important as the incidence of side-effects.

The chronic or late XRT reaction appears months or years after the acute reaction has settled and is due to progressive endothelial changes. The serosal surface is thickened and several bowel loops may be matted together. Segments may show dilatation, variable lengths of stenosis and irregular defects of various sizes in the wall. Stenotic segments suggest features of late Crohn's or ischaemic bowel disease, with a cobblestone appearance to the mucosa. Microscopically, the lamina is fibrous and contains ectatic, thinwalled vessels, many of which are thrombosed. Capillaries exhibit intimal thickening and contain fibrin platelet thrombi associated with damaged endothelial cells (Carr et al 1984). Changes in small arterioles include medial necrosis due to ischaemia and medial hypertrophy, presumed to be secondary to the increased resistance to blood flow in the microvascular bed.

Measurements of late XRT enteritis may require years of follow-up. Common symptoms include bowel disturbance and food intolerance. More serious are obstruction, bleeding and fistula formation. The most accurate measure is the frequency of late surgical interventions required for non-cancer causes.

Measures of effectiveness (efficacy)

The two measures of efficacy most used in rectal cancer are reductions in local recurrence and metastases. Whether this is achieved is only discovered by a careful record of patterns of recurrence following adjuvant therapy. Therapeutic strategies for improvement should take into account patterns of recurrence. One trial of preoperative XRT maintained a permanent record of the XRT treatment field for each patient as defined by CT scanning (Marsh et al 1994a). Of 16 patients with suspected local pelvic recurrence recalled for scanning, 10 had recurrence within and six outside the XRT field. An increase in effectiveness would therefore imply not only an increase in field size, but also in dose.

If deaths from distant metastases are reduced by chemotherapy, more patients may live long enough to develop local recurrence. Conversely, if deaths from local recurrence are reduced by XRT or more extensive surgery, more patients may live long enough to develop metastases. Any treatment that improves survival may produce an increase in the number of individuals susceptible to late treatment-induced effects like XRT enteritis, which may be fatal. This sort of bias in clinical results is difficult to detect in overviews of surgical trials which concentrate on survival rates.

Local recurrence

Local recurrence rates, like survival rates, may be altered according to a definition of surgical procedure (Marsh et al 1994b). Many series report local recurrence rates only after resections with curative intent. Patients with tumours which are unresectable at laparotomy may be considered recurrent from the first postoperative day or alternatively excluded from analysis. Other series record local recurrences only if they occur with no evidence of distant metastases.

Like surgery, XRT is a local form of treatment. The size of the XRT field or portal is analogous to the extent of surgical resection margins. When XRT is combined with surgery, the aim is to reduce local recurrence. In breast carcinoma, XRT has enabled surgeons to perform less mutilating operations with no increase in local recurrence. Although such a trend towards conservative surgery may be possible for mobile cancers in the lower rectum further clinical trials are required before this policy can be recommended. Nevertheless, most prospective adjuvant trials which include a surgery-only arm have shown an improvement in local recurrence in favour of XRT (Table 9.7).

In rectal cancer, the aim of adjuvant chemotherapy is to reduce metastases, mainly in the liver. However, a related but different aim of combining chemotherapy with surgery is to enhance the local effectiveness of the resection: for many years cytotoxic agents have been instilled in the pelvis during laparotomy with the aim of reducing local recurrence. The corresponding use of chemotherapy with XRT, therefore, would be equivalent to an increase in XRT dose.

Survival

Most rectal cancer deaths are due to liver metastases. A few patients die as a direct result of local recurrence. The effect of combining

138 Colorectal cancer

Table 9.7 Reported local recurrence rates in randomized trials of adjuvant radiotherapy for operable rectal cancer

Trial (reference)	Dose	No. patients randomized	Local recurrences Radiotherapy	Control	p-value[†]	Endpoint
Preoperative radiotherapy						
MRC 1	5 or 20 Gy	824	235/549	112/275	NS	Local
EORTC 2	34.5 Gy	466	6/152	21/166	**	Local only
			17/152	42/166	**	Local + distant
VASOG 2	31.5 Gy	361	37/180	40/181	NS	Residual or recurrent disease
Stockholm	25 Gy	694	23/271	54/274	***	Pelvic recurrence
MRC 2	40 Gy	261	41/129	50/132	NS	'Local recurrence'
ICRF	25 Gy	478	'Significant difference'		*	'Local recurrence'
North-west	25 Gy	284	26/143	58/141	***	'Local recurrence'
Postoperative radiotherapy						
GITSG	40 Gy	202	15/96	27/106	NS	Local as the first sign of recurrence
Denmark	50 Gy	494	18/244	20/250	NS	Local only
			38/244	44/250	NS	Local + distant
NSABP	46.5 Gy	368	30/184	45/184	NS	Local ± distant
MRC 3	40 Gy	369	14/180	42/189	***	'Local recurrence'

[†]NS=not conventionally significant: *=p<0.05, **=p<0.01, ***=p<0.001

Table 9.8 Mortality in trials comparing adjuvant radiotherapy with no radiotherapy (including trials with identical chemotherapy for both treatment and control groups)

Trial**		Deaths/no. entered Radiotherapy	Control	O-E	Variance	Odds ratio* comparing treatment with control mortality rates (and c.i.)
Preoperative radiotherapy						
VASOG-20	20 Gy	225/347	251/353	−11.0	38.1	
Yale	40 Gy	9/15	11/16	−0.7	1.8	
Toronto	5 Gy	46/60	52/65	−1.0	5.3	
MRC 1	5/20 Gy	318/549	166/275	−4.5	44.5	
EORTC-40761	34.5 Gy	55/201	61/209	−1.9	20.8	
VASOG-28	31.5 Gy	121/180	114/181	3.8	20.6	
Stockholm	25 Gy	147/351	140/343	1.8	42.1	
North-west	25 Gy	83/143	84/141	−1.1	17.3	
MRC 2	40 Gy	60/129	73/132	−5.7	16.4	
■ Total preoperative		1064/1975	952/1715	−20.2	206.9	9% ± 7
Postoperative Radiotherapy						
Denmark	50 Gy	105/244	104/250	1.8	30.2	
GITSG-7175	40 Gy	49/101	63/110	−4.6	13.2	
NSABP R-01	46.5 Gy	113/184	116/184	−1.5	21.7	
MRC 3	40 Gy	23/180	39/189	−7.2	12.9	
■ Total postoperative		290/709	322/733	−11.6	78.0	14% ± 11
■ TOTAL: All trials		1354/2684	1274/2448	−31.8	284.9	11% ± 6

0.0   0.5   1.0   1.5   2.0
Treatment better | Treatment worse

Treatment effect 2P<0.06

* For each trial the observed odds reduction in the figures is represented by a black square, with its 99% confidence interval as a horizontal line. A diamond shape represents the odds reduction and 95% confidence interval for the overview of the individual trials (see EBCTCG 1988, 1990 for details of statistical calculations)
** Data derived from Buyse et al 1988 except for MRC 1, 2 and 3 (MRC Working Party 1984), Stockholm (Stockholm Rectal Cancer Study Group 1990), North-west (James et al 1991) and NSABF R-01 (Fisher et al 1988)

chemotherapy with local treatments like XRT and surgery is analogous to increasing the volume of a conventional surgical resection to include a liver resection. The analogy for the radiotherapist is to increase XRT field size to include the liver.

Large overviews of the use of XRT in breast carcinoma have shown no survival advantage. In contrast, a recent overview of the use of adjuvant XRT in resected rectal cancer suggested a slight survival advantage (Table 9.8). This might be because more patients may die as a direct result of local recurrence in rectal cancer than in breast cancer. Alternatively, non-cancer deaths may be increased in irradiated breast cancer patients compared with unirradiated controls and this may offset any survival benefit.

Sphincter preservation, sexual potency

The proportion of patients who are treated by conservative surgery for early cancer of the lower rectum might in the future be a reasonable measure of the effectiveness of XRT. However, at the moment, this type of project can only be recommended in centres with access to specialized XRT machines and surgeons with a particular interest in colorectal surgery. Radical pelvic dissection is associated with sexual and urinary problems. If the need for radical dissection is reduced by XRT, the incidence of these complications might also be used as a measure of the effect of XRT.

Factors modifying cost-effectiveness

Stage, grade and radiosensitivity

Clinical trials containing small numbers of patients are less likely to reveal statistically significant treatment effects than those containing large numbers. For the same reason, any effect of adjuvant treatment on deaths from cancer is likely to be more noticeable in a group of patients where deaths are frequent than in a group where deaths are rare. Provided selection bias is avoided, clinical trials which include patients with high-grade or advanced stage rectal cancer are therefore more likely to show a statistically significant treatment effect than those with low-grade, early tumours.

Two Medical Research Council (MRC) trials were launched simultaneously in order to test the relative effectiveness of pre- and postoperative pelvic XRT in rectal cancer. XRT field sizes and doses were identical. However, comparisons of efficacy between the two trials are compounded by a non-controlled variable, namely disease stage (MRC personal communication). The postoperative trial (MRC III) included only patients with completely resected Dukes' B and C rectal cancer, who were fit to receive XRT. In contrast, the preoperative trial (MRC II) included only patients with much more advanced tumours (partially or completely 'fixed' on pelvic examination). Not surprisingly, the survival figures for patients allocated surgery alone in MRC II are significantly lower than the comparable arm in MRC III (23% vs 43%).

The effect of stage is illustrated by attempts to compare XRT alone with XRT combined with conservative surgery as an alternative to abdominoperineal excision for mobile, well-differentiated tumours in the lower rectum. A cure rate of 80% has been reported by most series for XRT alone for tumours of less than 5 cm in diameter (Basrur and Knight 1983, Kovalic 1988, Lavery et al 1987, Papillon 1975, Parturier Albot & Albot 1981, Sischy et al 1988). However, in one series (Roth et al 1989), efficacy, measured by local control, varied according to size and fixity from 97% (for superficial, exophytic tumours less than 3 cm diameter) to 60% (for tethered tumours 3–5 cm diameter). In contrast, the efficacy of XRT for large, fixed, inoperable rectal cancer is much reduced. In one series of 29 such patients subjected to laparotomy 2 months after radical pelvic XRT, resection was impossible in 11. Of the 18 tumours resected, only three showed complete clinical remission following XRT (James and Schofield 1985). Efficacy (local control) is approximately 15% for recurrent tumours, which often exceed 10 cm (James et al 1983).

A great deal of laboratory-based research has been dedicated to identifying tumour-tissue variables which may predict radiosensitivity and chemosensitivity preoperatively, so that more patients can be selected before surgery for adjuvant therapy. Laboratory definitions of radiosensitivity include a number of variables like cellular kinetics and intrinsic radiosensitivity. The latter has been studied most in the laboratory and is related to the efficiency of DNA repair. Much is now known about the genetic basis for such repair for both proliferative and stromal elements.

XRT dose, field size and shape

The relationship between XRT dose and volume of tissue irradiated is complex. Large tumours clearly require larger XRT fields and higher XRT doses for cure than small tumours. However, this inevitably means that larger volumes of normal tissue are irradiated to higher doses. A margin is always included in the planning of an XRT field around a tumour for a number of reasons. First, histological studies show that malignant infiltration can extend many millimetres beyond the visible margin of a tumour. Second, most organs and tumours in the abdomen move with respiration or peristalsis. Third, there is often uncertainty over the exact location of a tumour in relation to skin marks used to direct radiotherapy beams.

XRT dose

COST OF TREATMENT AS A FUNCTION OF XRT DOSE Because more normal tissue is irradiated with large tumours, there is an increased probability of serious XRT enteritis. Single fraction total abdominal XRT in doses as low as 7 Gy can be fatal. Small bowel obstruction due to late XRT enteritis varies from 30% for extended abdominal fields to 9% for shaped pelvic fields (Mak et al 1994). For large tumours, most radiotherapists order a reduction rather than an elevation in XRT dose and accept that the probability of cure is also reduced. This tendency is reflected in the schedules of published clinical trials. Two studies conducted by the MRC, designed to irradiate the true pelvis, specified a dose of 40 Gy. Two conducted by the European Organization for Research on Treatment of Cancer (EORTC) using extended abdominal fields, specified 34.5 Gy.

EFFECTIVENESS OF TREATMENT AS A FUNCTION OF XRT DOSE Many of the disappointing results in early XRT trials were due to inadequate overall XRT dose. In one trial, for example, local recurrence was recorded in 48 of 97 patients offered a postoperative XRT dose of 25 Gy in 2 weeks and the authors concluded this was inadequate (Feigen et al 1989). Tables 9.9 and 9.10 illustrate the effect of XRT dose on local recurrence in published randomized trials with a surgery-only arm. The nominal standard dose (NSD) (Orton and Ellis 1973) is one method of estimating the biological effectiveness of XRT by taking into account radiation repair between separate daily fractions. It was not designed to compare tumour doses, but it gives an approximation of the cumulative effects of XRT on subcutaneous tissues. There is a trend in these tables towards more effective local tumour control with higher XRT dose as measured by NSD. This trend is more notable if data from non-randomized trials are included.

The planned XRT dose is often determined by the presence or absence of small bowel in the XRT field. This allows an ethically acceptable but indirect retrospective analysis of the efficacy of postoperative XRT as a function of dose. In one study of 206 patients with completely resected Dukes' stage B rectal cancer, a statistically significant ($p=0.017$) trend for improved tumour control was noted with increased XRT dose (Aleman et al 1992). However, the relationship between dose and tumour volume is complex. In one series, a positive correlation between post-

Table 9.9 Local recurrence as a function of postoperative XRT nominal standard dose (NSD) – prospective randomized trials with surgery-only arm

NSD	Significant difference	Centre	No. of patients	Follow-up (months)
1510	Yes	NSABP	368	36
1501	Yes/No	Denmark	494	24
1415	No	GITSG	202	94
1362	Yes	MRC III	247	13

Table 9.10 Local recurrence as a function of preoperative XRT nominal standard dose (NSD) – prospective randomized trials with surgery-only arm

NSD	Significant difference	Centre	No. of patients	Follow-up (months)
1423*	Yes	Stockholm	545	34
1362	No	MRC II	204	35
1303	Yes	EORTC II	410	60
1231*	Yes	NW	280	14
1010*	Yes	ICRF	478	24
1021	No	VASAG II	361	60
876	Yes	VASAG I	700	60
876	No	MRC I	'824'	60
500*	No	MRC I	'824'	60
500*	Yes	Toronto	250	60

*Immediate surgery.

operative XRT dose and effectiveness (local control) was found for patients with microscopic residual disease but not for those with macroscopic, unresectable disease (Allee et al 1989).

XRT field size and shape

COST OF TREATMENT AS A FUNCTION OF XRT FIELD SIZE AND SHAPE Normal tissue damage can be separated from tumour damage spatially. The spatial shaping of XRT fields is important in excluding normal bowel from radiation effects. The simplest shaping technique uses fields directed entirely from the posterior pelvis rather than parallel opposed fields which include the bladder and anterior abdominal wall. Modern imaging technology has helped in field-shaping, particularly if the tumour itself can be imaged, as is the case for preoperative XRT. In a retrospective series, the Houston group showed that mechanical devices which exclude small bowel from XRT fields can reduce late XRT enteritis from 9% to 3% (Mak et al 1994).

A carefully conducted series of Swedish trials has done much to clarify the relationship between preoperative XRT dose, field size and postoperative mortality. In the Stockholm–Malmo Trial (Stockholm Rectal Cancer Group 1990), a subgroup analysis showed that postoperative non-cancer deaths were significantly higher in the XRT than the control arm (7% vs 2%: p<0.01). Suggestions that this excess was due to an accelerated XRT dose schedule were discounted by a comparison with the Uppsala Trial (Pahlman et al 1985), which used a biologically higher dose (25 Gy vs 25.5 Gy) and recorded no increase in mortality. However, the XRT field size was much larger in the Stockholm than in the Uppsala trial (lower pelvis to L1–L2 interface, two-field vs. lower pelvis to L3–L4 interface, three-fields). This cost of preoperative XRT has not been seen in a subsequent Swedish national study (Swedish Rectal Cancer Group 1993) using the Stockholm dose but the Uppsala fields size (postoperative mortality: XRT: 4%, control: 3%).

EFFECTIVENESS OF TREATMENT AS A FUNCTION OF XRT FIELD SIZE AND SHAPE One of the reasons why XRT dose was inadequate in early adjuvant trials was because XRT field size was inappropriately large and doses were reduced to avoid XRT enteritis. It is now generally accepted that local recurrence is due to posterior or lateral spread of carcinoma into adjacent, unresected organs or the pelvic side wall. Computerized tomography (CT) of locally recurrent tumours confirms that the vast majority occur in the posterior pelvis (Zheng et al 1984). An appropriate XRT field encompasses the tumour bed within a margin of approximately 10 cm (Figs. 9.1 and 9.2).

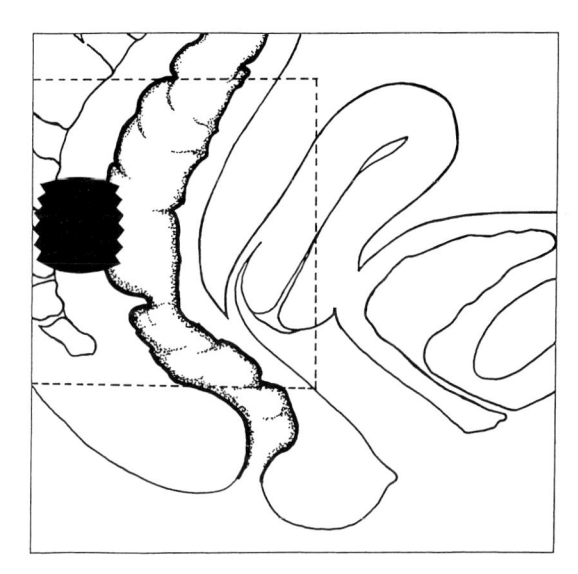

Fig. 9.1 Preoperative radiotherapy includes the tumour within a field in the posterior pelvis, but no small bowel.

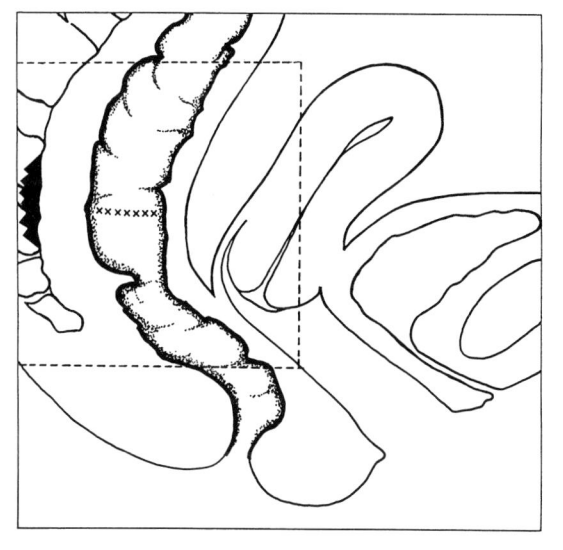

Fig. 9.2 Postoperative radiotherapy following anterior resection. The pelvis usually contains small bowel and the tumour bed may be difficult to identify. For handsewn anastomoses, sites of suspected residual tumour should be marked by clips.

Timing of chemotherapy and surgery

Timing of chemotherapy

In order for chemotherapy to improve the effectiveness of XRT, it must be present in the tumour at the time XRT-inflicted DNA damage is being repaired. A similar argument applies to an increase in cost (XRT enteritis) due to chemotherapy. The biological half-life of 5-fluorouracil (5-Fu) is of the order of 20 minutes. For concomitant therapy to work, chemotherapy must obviously be given whilst the patient is on the XRT treatment machine. This mode of administration of chemotherapy with XRT is called concomitant therapy. Modern techniques of giving cytotoxics by continuous ambulatory infusion have made this more feasible. A North Central Cancer Treatment Group Trial (NCCTG 86-47-51) is comparing the enhancement of postoperative XRT by concomitant 5-Fu delivered by either bolus injection or continuous infusion. A planned interim analysis (Gunderson 1994) showed a significant advantage to infusion in terms of 3-year survival (76% vs 68%, p=0.02), local recurrence (8% vs 11%, p=0.04) and distant metastases (33% vs 41%, p=0.04).

Concomitant infusion of chemotherapy during XRT may be most effective in terms of local tumour control, but may also be most toxic in terms of XRT enteritis. One method of overcoming this is by a spatial separation of XRT and chemotherapy, such as portal vein infusion of 5-Fu. This is less likely to increase XRT-induced enteritis from pelvic XRT than systemic infusion. An unreported, ongoing British trial of adjuvant X-ray infusion (AXIS) is seeking to evaluate this combination.

If chemotherapy is not intended as a specific radiosensitizer, it may be given at another time. This technique is called sequential therapy. It is less likely to alter the cost-effectiveness of local XRT but may influence survival by changing the pattern and timing of liver metastases. Many centres, for example, now deliver XRT preoperatively and chemotherapy postoperatively.

Effectiveness of chemotherapy

Adjuvant chemotherapy seems more important than adjuvant XRT in terms of survival: a three-armed trial conducted by the National Surgical Adjuvant Breast and Bowel Program (NSABP R-01) showed a survival advantage for adjuvant chemotherapy but not for adjuvant XRT in a direct comparison with surgery (Fisher et al 1988). A more important question is whether concomitant chemotherapy is more effective than sequential, since it may be more costly in terms of XRT enteritis. A direct comparison of preoperative XRT and concomitant chemotherapy versus preoperative XRT alone in resectable rectal cancer (EORTC 40741) showed no survival advantage (Boulis-Wassif et al 1984). However, a similar, non-randomized study of concomitant chemotherapy and preoperative XRT in patients with primary unresectable cancer showed an improved resectability rate compared with historical controls (Frykholm et al 1989).

There has been no equivalent trial for postoperative XRT, but the question has been answered indirectly by two trials (GI-7175 and NCCTG 79-47-51). Both showed a survival advantage for postoperative XRT plus chemotherapy over, respectively, surgery alone and postoperative XRT (Gastrointestinal Tumor Study Group 1992, Krook et al 1991). However, both used a combination of concomitant and sequential techniques. In contrast, an Eastern Cooperative Oncology Group (ECOG) trial, which showed no survival advantage for post-operative XRT plus chemotherapy, used a sequential technique (Mansour et al 1991).

In the light of these reports, a recent National Cancer Institute (NCI) Clinical Announcement advocated the use of adjuvant combined XRT and chemotherapy (concomitant plus sequential), rather than adjuvant XRT alone for patients with stage III rectal cancer not included in clinical trials (National Cancer Institute 1989).

Cost of chemotherapy

In the postoperative XRT trials analysed by the NCI for effectiveness, there was a clear indication of increased cost for the combined arms over XRT alone. In the Gastrointestinal Study Group (GTSG 7175) Trial, severe non-haematological toxicity was reported in 35% of those receiving combined modality XRT–chemotherapy, compared with 16% of those receiving XRT alone, whilst two cancer-free patients in the combined arm died of their complications (Gastrointestinal Tumor Study Group 1992). In the Mayo/North Central Cancer Treatment Group (NCCTG) trial, the comparable figures were 20% versus 5% (Krook et al 1991).

A trial which randomized patients with more advanced disease to either postoperative XRT alone or XRT combined with chemotherapy (concomitant + sequential) reported severe late XRT enteritis (necrosis, stenosis and fistulae) more commonly in the combined group (20% vs 14%). Ten patients developed life-threatening complications (Rominger & Gelber 1985). A further, non-randomized pilot study of concomitant 5-Fu with postoperative XRT reported severe late XRT enteritis in 35% of patients (Danjoux and Catton, 1979).

An indirect comparison of toxicity due to preoperative XRT and concomitant chemotherapy versus that due to preoperative XRT alone is available from two trials conducted by the European Organisation for Research on Treatment of Cancer (EORTC 40741 and 40761). Both trials used the same XRT schedule (dose, fractionation, field size) and aimed to recruit patients with similar stage disease. Both randomized between treatment and surgery only. However, EORTC 40741 added concomitant chemotherapy to the preoperative XRT. This resulted in an increase, compared with surgical controls, in both postoperative (30 day) mortality (8.9% vs 5%) and in overall non-cancer intercurrent mortality (16% vs 5%), as well as a doubling of postoperative pulmonary complications (16% vs 8%). More patients experienced more severe acute XRT toxicity before surgery in the combined arm than in the XRT-only arm. This was particularly striking for weakness and pain (16% vs 5%, p=0.004) and for severe diarrhoea (9% vs 1%, p=0.006). Life-threatening XRT-related complications were not seen in the XRT-only arm, but occurred in 6% of patients in the combined arm (Gerard et al 1980). In contrast, in trial 40761, in which the same schedule of preoperative XRT was delivered without concomitant chemotherapy, XRT was completed with no discernible toxicity in 162 of 166 patients and there was no reported increase in postoperative mortality compared with unirradiated controls (Gerard et al 1988).

Timing of surgery

The incidence of XRT enteritis rises as more collagenous material forms around dissection lines. In this way, the ability of normal bowel mucosa to repair a surgical incision is likely to be compromised by previous XRT. Conversely, a mechanical insult like surgery can be thought of as converting a radio-resistant normal tissue into a radiosensitive tissue if XRT is given in the immediate postoperative period. Most clinical trials therefore recommend that postoperative XRT starts within one month of surgery.

Surgery alters the cellular kinetics of tumours and normal tissues by initiating tissue repair mechanisms. The inflammatory reaction following a surgical incision is an acute phenomenon. It includes an increase in cellular division of tissues which might otherwise contain a majority of intermitotic or resting cells. It is now known that this alteration in cellular kinetics is under the control of a series of growth factors, some of which have been cloned and are available as recombinant products.

A number of DNA repair mechanisms have been identified which determine the extent of XRT-mediated endothelial cell death. If dividing cells have been damaged by preoperative XRT, a surgical insult might precipitate the expression of XRT damage which would otherwise be repaired. Some angiogenic growth factors have been cloned and their effects on DNA repair determined in experimental systems, but it is not known if these are amplified as a result of surgical trauma. If some of the resistance of tumours to XRT is determined by stromal cellular kinetics, growth factors released by surgery might alter such kinetics.

In this way, irradiated tumours or normal tissues might be made more sensitive by surgical trauma. The duration and mechanism of this interaction between tissue repair and DNA repair is poorly understood, but there may be potential for an improvement in cost-effectiveness. Certain XRT schedules are followed by immediate resection of the irradiated tumour whilst others impose a delay of weeks or months. In rectal cancer, the former appear to be more effective and less toxic than the latter.

For the interaction of XRT with surgery, timing may be critical in determining cost-effectiveness: efficacy in terms of tumour control falls as the tumour regrows. Preoperative XRT takes this logical sequence to further extremes: efficacy is maximized if surgery is performed within 24 hours of the final XRT fraction. At long intervals following surgery, tumour cells are more likely to be poorly oxygenated and out of cell cycle, both factors which are known to influence radiosensitivity.

Cost of surgery

Prolonged preoperative XRT schedules impose delays on surgery and are less likely to be acceptable to surgeons and patients than short, sharp XRT schedules which allow immediate surgery and are equally effective. This may have been one of the reasons why the preoperative British trial (MRC II) was less popular with surgeons than the postoperative trial (MRC III) launched at the same time. Accrual was 279 patients in 7 years for MRC II compared with 516 patients in 5 years for MRC III.

XRT enteritis is minimized during preoperative XRT in comparison with postoperative since, before surgery, there is no small bowel in the pelvis to be irradiated. The most dangerous time to operate on irradiated tissue is months or years following XRT. In contrast, leak rates following bowel anastomosis are not significantly increased in reported trials of preoperative XRT followed by immediate surgery.

Although XRT enteritis is comparatively rare, surgeons may need to take these pathological changes into account when scheduling surgery for malignant bowel cancers following XRT. If radical surgery is scheduled within 3 weeks of the start of XRT, the acute reaction is unlikely to render the patient unfit for anaesthetic. However, when late XRT enteritis is established, there is serious danger of anastomotic breakdown if the full extent of affected bowel is not resected. It is fairly common for experienced surgeons to resect over 50 cm of small bowel to ensure that they are dealing with well-vascularized mucosa (Schofield 1989).

In the Uppsala trial, in which patients were randomized to receive either preoperative or postoperative XRT, there was a marked difference in cost between the two schedules (Frykholm et al 1993, Påhlman et al 1985, Påhlman and Glimelius 1990). First, the preoperative schedule was planned for 1 week, whilst the postoperative schedule was planned for 8 weeks. Second, in terms of compliance with planned treatment, postoperative XRT was significantly less likely to be delivered according to schedule. Fewer than 50% of the patients allocated postoperative XRT were able to start XRT as planned (within 6 weeks of surgery), whilst only 60% completed XRT as planned (within 8 weeks). Third, more direct measures of toxicity seemed to favour preoperative XRT: all patients allocated this arm experienced nil or minimal XRT-related morbidity and there was no measurable excess of postoperative mortality or anastomotic dehiscence, although significantly more patients in this arm experienced perineal wound sepsis.

In contrast, amongst those allocated postoperative XRT, over 90% experienced XRT-related complications: 52% moderate or severe diarrhoea (5% requiring parenteral nutrition), 21% fatigue, 18% urinary disorders and 18% skin reactions. Furthermore, late small bowel obstruction due to XRT enteritis (defined radiologically or at laparotomy) was twice as likely in the postoperative as in the preoperative arm (11% vs 5%). Patients who live longer are clearly more at risk for developing late XRT enteritis than those who die early as a result of cancer recurrence, but this potential bias is not present in the Uppsala trial, since survival rates were identical.

The MRC trials II and III confirm the impression that measures of cost, such as treatment compliance, favour preoperative over postoperative XRT. In MRC II, 90% of patients allocated preoperative XRT received it in the scheduled period. The corresponding figure for MRC III was 75%. Early XRT morbidity was also more common during postoperative than preoperative XRT: twice as many patients experienced nausea, abdominal pain and urinary symptoms. There was an excess of diarrhoea (46% vs 33%) and of obstruction and colovesical fistula (MRC personal communication).

A non-randomized comparison of relative cost, but not effectiveness, is available from the Adjuvant X-ray Infusion Study (AXIS), an ongoing British trial (MRC personal communication). Patients randomized to receive XRT are treated according to the preference of each local centre: some prefer preoperative, others postoperative XRT. Data are available on 69 patients allocated preoperative XRT and on a further 124 allocated postoperative XRT over the same period. No serious morbidity was reported for any patient allocated preoperative XRT: one patient refused and another was not treated in error. In contrast, amongst 124 postoperative patients, two suffered severe diarrhoea, requiring hospitalization and two suffered severe skin reactions requiring a break in treatment, whilst delayed starts were recorded in 16 patients (MRC personal communication).

Effectiveness of surgery

In the Uppsala trial (Påhlman and Glimelius 1990), 471 patients were randomly assigned to receive either pre- or postoperative XRT through identical pelvic portals. The XRT doses were made as comparable as possible using the cumulative radiation effect (CRE) formula (preoperative CRE=15.4; postoperative CRE=17.0). Efficacy measured by survival was identical in the two arms. However, efficacy measured by local recurrence rates was significantly superior in the preoperative arm (13% vs 22%: p=0.02).

The Stockholm–Malmo trial is probably the most impressive example of the efficacy of preoperative XRT in the literature (Stockholm Rectal Cancer Study Group 1990). The authors report a significant reduction in local recurrence (25% vs 11%: p<0.05) in favour of the preoperative XRT arm and an identical overall 5-year survival for the two trial arms (XRT – 55%, control – 50%).

Measures of efficacy in the two British trials, MRC II and MRC III, launched simultaneously, are particularly interesting in view of the fact that the preoperative trial contained patients with more advanced disease than the postoperative trial (MRC personal communication). In MRC II (preoperative) there was a reduction in favour of the preoperative XRT arm compared to control of the following parameters: overall deaths (p=0.09), cause-specific deaths (p=0.03) and metastases (p=0.02). The corresponding figures for MRC III (postoperative) were less impressive (p=0.1, p=0.04 and 0.18, respectively). In contrast, although both trials showed a significant reduction in local recurrence in favour of XRT, the result was more impressive in the postoperative than the preoperative trial (p=0.0007 vs p=0.04).

Recommendations

XRT technique and dose (Table 9.11, Figs. 9.3 and 9.4)

The optimal XRT technique is applied to patients treated either pre- or postoperatively. Treatment should be carried out with the patient prone on a linear accelerator, using three or four portals resulting in a 'brick' or 'box' of dimensions between 8×8×8 cm and 12×12×12 cm. The commonest volume is 10×10×10 cm. Since the rectum lies in the curve of the sacrum, the distance of this 'brick' from the skin of the natal cleft will vary, being most superficial in the midrectum and deepest in the upper or lower rectum. In the last case, the perineal skin should be included in the volume, using appropriate tissue-equivalent 'bolus', but this is not required for more proximal tumours. The position of the centre of the 'brick' should be determined from CT scanning or surgical information but in the midrectum is usually between 7 and 9 cm below the skin surface (Fig. 9.3).

The prescribed XRT dose for 'tethered' tumours (Dukes' B or C) should be approximately equivalent to 60 Gy in 30 fractions over 6 weeks. Dose reductions should be applied if CT scanning suggests considerable small bowel tethering in the treatment volume. These is anecdotal evidence that surgical as opposed to XRT techniques may reduce XRT enteritis. The commonest of these is the insertion of a mesh to exclude small bowel from the pelvis at the time of surgery. For postoperative XRT, a 4–6 week fractionation is probably best. For preoperative XRT, since the rectum is extraperitoneal preoperatively and is rarely

Table 9.11 Recommended radiotherapy technique

Patient prone
Posterior pelvic 'brick'
Four orthogonal portals
10 × 10 × 10 cm

146 Colorectal cancer

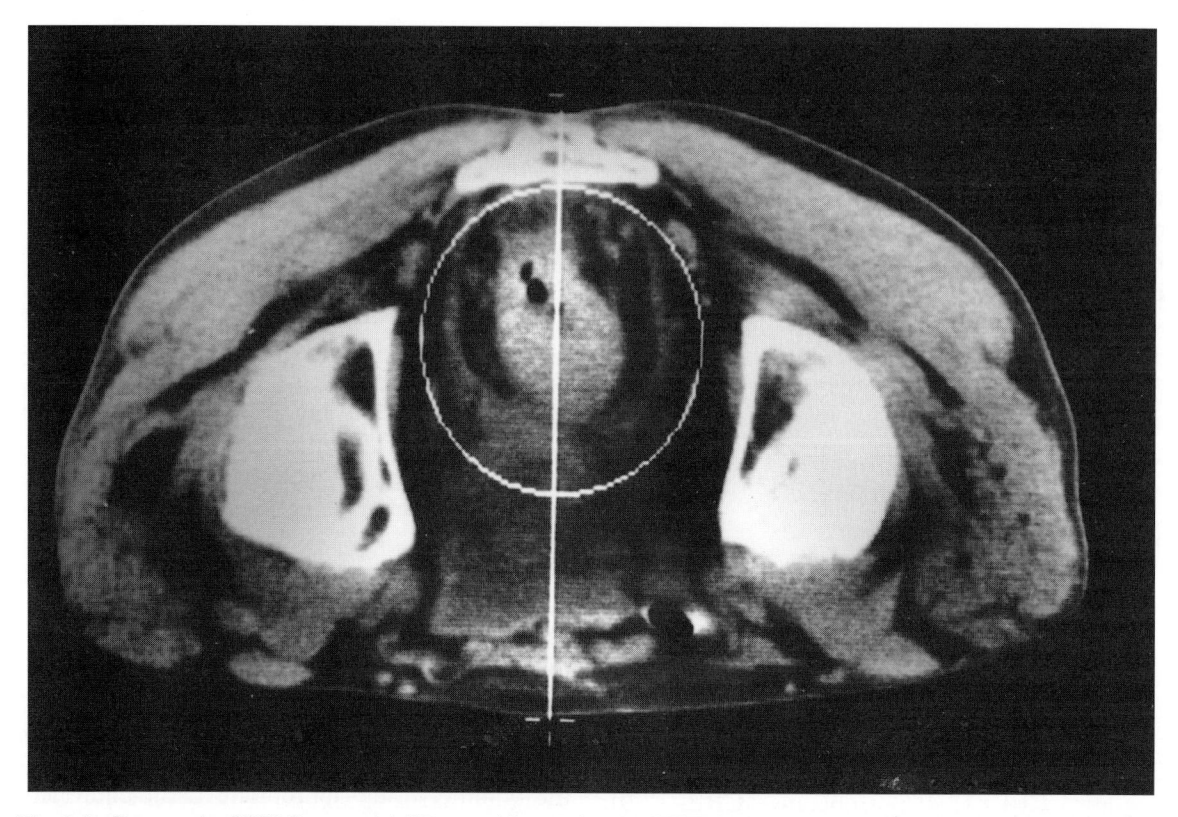

Fig. 9.3 Preoperative XRT. Prone, axial CT scan with superimposed XRT field centred 8 cm from the skin of the natal cleft.

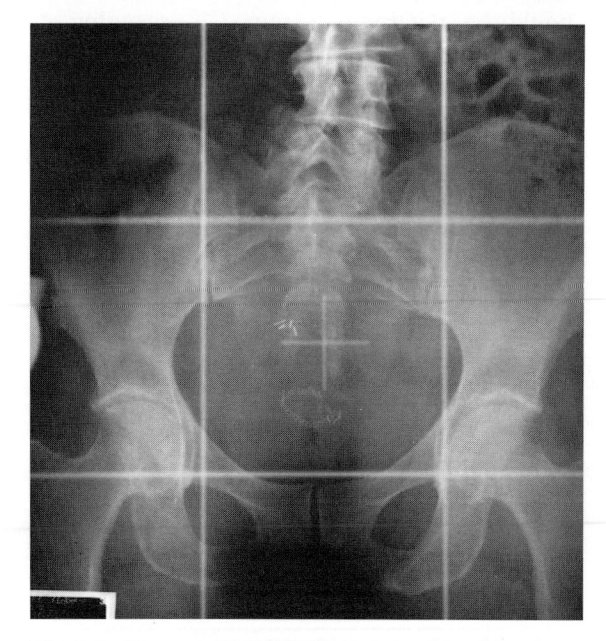

Fig. 9.4 Postoperative XRT. Prone anteroposterior radiograph in a patient following staple resection, with site of residual tumour marked by clips.

surrounded by small bowel, a more accelerated fractionation schedule can be employed safely, followed by immediate surgery ('short, sharp XRT').

The dose for 'fixed, inoperable' rectal cancer is less critical, since a proportion of patients will become unfit for surgery due to distant metastases or local pain during the 6–8 week delay for tumour volume reduction. In the author's institute a dose of between 30 Gy (over 2 weeks) and 45 Gy (over 3 weeks) is associated with a resection rate of 44%, similar to centres using much higher doses (Dosoretz et al 1983, Emami et al 1982, Frykholm et al 1989, Glimelius et al 1982, James & Schofield 1985).

Chemotherapy

Until the results of current clinical trials are available, it is difficult to determine the most effective chemotherapy schedule to be used in conjunction with XRT. 5-Fluorouracil will be an essential part of most schedules, probably modified by high or low dose folinic acid. In terms of costs, intrahepatic, perioperative schedules are cheaper and less toxic than intravenous schedules and concomitant schedules are cheaper than sequential schedules. The most effective regime, however, may well prove to be a combination of intrahepatic, concomitant and sequential schedules (Ch. 10).

Clinical staging

'Downstaging' by preoperative XRT

If preoperative XRT is more cost-effective than postoperative, there may have to be a change in the philosophy of the surgeon towards clinical assessment of the patient. For many years the selection of patients with rectal cancer for adjuvant treatment has been based on Dukes' (Astler–Coller) staging and Broders grading. However, preoperative XRT may alter the reliability of staging based on lymph node invasion. This is less likely with XRT schedules given over a week followed by immediate surgery than with those taking over 4 weeks, with a gap before surgery. In one series, 93% of tumours were resected within 2 weeks of the start of XRT and showed no detectable differences in tumour volume or Dukes' staging compared with unirradiated controls (James et al 1991). In contrast, a similar biological dose but at an interval extended to 6 weeks resulted in a significant downstaging compared with controls in both lymph node invasion (18.4% vs 27.5%, $p<0.05$) and tumour size ($p<0.05$), as well as complete tumour regression in 4.4% of patients (Horn et al 1990).

Digital assessment

One possible cost of preoperative XRT is that patients with early (Dukes' A) tumours may be offered XRT when it may not be necessary. However, a number of these patients are currently offered radical surgery when it may not be necessary. Both of these costs are less likely with a reliable clinical staging system. A related measure of effectiveness, therefore, is the degree to which preoperative XRT may encourage more surgeons to perform sphincter-preserving surgery for selected tumours of the lower rectum (Billingham 1992).

Modern radiology, including computerized tomography, magnetic resonance and endoluminal ultrasound (Ch. 4), has done much to improve clinical assessment. However, the most useful measure of tumour spread remains the digital assessment by the surgeon of tumour fixity under anaesthetic. York Mason (1976) first documented the usefulness of digital examination; experienced surgeons can probably achieve an accuracy of over 80% (Nicholls 1982).

In the first MRC trial of preoperative XRT (MRC I), surgeons were asked to record the degree of fixity before XRT was commenced. Patients with any degree of fixity had a probability of death from cancer twice that of those with mobile lesions and a statistically significant reduction in the probability of having a 'curative' resection (MRC Working Party 1984). This sort of diagnostic accuracy by experienced surgeons suggests that a group of patients assessed preoperatively and offered preoperative XRT is unlikely to include many with Dukes' A lesions. As a result, radiotherapists and surgeons are able to plan a treatment policy for individual patients and audit the results of this policy (Buhre et al 1994, Fleshman et al 1985).

Recommended staging system

A simplified version of the staging used at the author's institute is shown in Table 9.12. Patients are divided into three groups on the basis of digital assessment under anaesthetic.

Table 9.12 Preoperative staging and radiotherapy in rectal adenocarcinoma. Based on examination under anaesthetic

Examination	Frequency	XRT	Surgical delay*
Fully mobile	30%	None	None
Tethered	60%	Short (20–25 Gy/1 wk)	None
Fully fixed	10%	Long (40–60 Gy/ 4–6 wks)	6 weeks

*Surgical delay following completion of XRT.

Fully mobile

In general, these patients should be offered no adjuvant XRT or chemotherapy and should proceed to immediate surgery. However, there may be a place for considering alternatives to abdominoperineal resection in selected patients with small tumours in the lower rectum. Conservative surgery is generally recommended only for well-differentiated tumours less than 3 cm in diameter, but centres with access to specialized XRT machines and dedicated colorectal surgeons have reported promising results for larger tumours. Of 34 patients with mobile or tethered tumours up to 6 cm treated by preoperative XRT followed 6–8 weeks later by a variety of conservative procedures (transanal, transsacral, anterior or local excision), 80% were alive at 2 years with only two colostomies (Marks et al 1985). Two similar series of 17 and 16 patients respectively reported local failure in only one patient each (Ramming et al 1986, Rich et al 1985).

Tethered

These tumours are likely to be advanced Dukes' B or C tumours and are known to require extensive posterior dissection in order to reduce the risk of local recurrence (Heald et al 1982). Less careful dissection can be associated with permanent sexual or urinary problems (Enker 1992, Williams & Johnston 1983). Surgeons who feel that adjuvant XRT is required are advised to refer patients for preoperative XRT followed by immediate surgery (within 1 week of completion of XRT). Less cost-effective schedules are delivered postoperatively.

Fixed

A number of published series document the advantage of a combined approach for this type of tumour, with a trial dissection at laparotomy 6–8 weeks after the completion of radical pelvic XRT (Dosoretz et al 1983, Emami et al 1982, Glimelius et al 1982, James & Schofield 1985).

Conclusions

Tethered/fixed tumours

The most cost-effective adjuvant treatment for patients with advanced (tethered/fixed, Dukes' B/C) is a combination of radical pelvic XRT with chemotherapy. Preoperative XRT is more cost-effective than postoperative, but should be combined with a clinical staging system based on digital examination under anaesthetic. Short, sharp preoperative XRT is less likely to alter Dukes' staging than prolonged preoperative XRT.

The most cost-effective adjuvant chemotherapy schedule (intrahepatic vs intravenous, concomitant or sequential, preoperative vs postoperative) remains unclear and may prove to be a combination of different schedules. At the moment, continuous infusion of 5-Fu looks particularly attractive. However, wherever possible, patients should be included in ongoing clinical trials.

Mobile tumours

In the upper rectum, low anterior resection is the most cost-effective treatment. In the lower rectum, an alternative to abdominoperineal resection might be conservative, sphincter-preserving surgery with adjuvant XRT. However, such a policy is only recommended in the confines of a clinical trial, conducted by specialist centres.

Acknowledgement
Tables 9.7 and 9.8 are reprinted, with permission, from the AXIS trial protocol.

References

Aleman BMP, Lebesque JV, Hart 1992 Postoperative radiotherapy for rectal and rectosigmoid cancer: the impact of total dose on local control. Radiotherapy and Oncology 25: 203–206

Allee PE, Tepper JE, Gunderson LL et al 1989 Postoperative radiation therapy for incompletely resected colorectal carcinoma. International Journal of Radiation, Oncology and Biological Physics 17: 1171–1176

Basrur VR, Knight PR 1983 "intracavitary" radiation for rectal cancer. Journal of the Canadian Association of Radiologists 34: 42–46

Billingham RP 1992 Conservative treatment of rectal cancer. Cancer 70 (suppl): 1355–1363

Boulis-Wassif S, Gerard A, Loygue J et al 1984 Final results of a randomised trial on the treatment of rectal cancer with preoperative radiotherapy alone or in combination with 5-fluouracil, followed by radical surgery. Cancer 53: 1181–1818

Brown ML, Nayfield SG, Shibley LM 1994 Adjuvant therapy for stage III colon cancer: economics returns to research and cost-effectiveness of treatment. Journal of the National Cancer Institute 86: 424–430

Buhre LMD, Mulder NH, Oldhoff J et al 1994 The clinical staging of rectal cancer in patients treated by preoperative radiotherapy. Clinical Oncology 6: 157–161

Buyse M, Zeleninch-Jacquotte A, Chalmers TC 1988 Adjuvant therapy of colorectal cancer: why we still don't know. Journal of the American Medical Association 259: 3571–3578

Carr ND, Pullen BR, Hasleton P et al 1984 Microvascular studies in radiation bowel disease. Gut 25: 448–453

Danjoux CE, Catton GE 1979 Delayed complications in colorectal carcinoma treated by combination radiotherapy and 5-fluouracil – Eastern Cooperative Oncology Group (E.C.O.G.) Pilot Study. International Journal of Radiation, Oncology and Biological Physics 5: 311–315

Dosoretz DE, Gunderson LL, Hedberg S et al 1983 Preoperative irradiation for unresectable rectal and rectosigmoid carcinomas. Cancer 52: 814–818

Early Breast Cancer Trials Collaborative Group 1988 Effects of adjuvant tamoxifen and of cytotoxic therapy on mortality in early breast cancer. New England Journal of Medicine 319: 1681–1692

Early Breast Cancer Trials Collaborative Group 1990 Treatment of early breast cancer. Vol I Worldwide evidence 1985–1990. Oxford University Press, Oxford

Emami B, Pilepich M, Willett C et al 1982 Effect of preoperative irradiation on resectability of colorectal carcinomas. International Journal of Radiation, Oncology and Biological Physics 8: 1295–1299

Enker WE 1992 Potency, cure and local control in the operative treatment of rectal cancer. Archives of Surgery 127: 1396–1402

Feigen M, Cummings B, Hawkins N et al 1989 Low dose postoperative adjuvant radiation therapy is ineffective. Radiotherapy and Oncology 13: 181–186

Fisher B, Wolmark N, Rockette H et al 1988 Postoperative adjuvant chemotherapy or radiation therapy for rectal cancer: results from NSABP protocol R-01. Journal of the National Cancer Institute 80: 21–29

Fleshman JW, Kodner LJ et al 1985 Adenocarcinoma of the rectum. Diseases of the Colon and Rectum 11: 810–816

Frykholm GJ, Glimelius B, Pahlman L 1989 Preoperative irradiation with and without chemotherapy (MFL) in the treatment of primarily non-resectable adenocarcinoma of the rectum. European Journal of Cancer and Clinical Oncology 25: 1535–1541

Frykholm GJ, Glimelius B, Pahlman L 1993 Preoperative or postoperative irradiation in adenocarcinoma of the rectum: final treatment results of a randomized trial and an evaluation of secondary effects. Diseases of the Colon and Rectum 36: 564–572

Gastrointestinal Tumor Study Group 1992 Radiation and fluorouracil with or without semustine for the treatment of patients with surgcal adjuvant adenocarcinoma of the rectum. Journal of Clinical Oncology 10: 549–557

Gerard A, Loygue J, Liegois P et al 1980 Controlled clinical trial for the treatment of rectal cancer using surgery, radiotherapy and chemotherapy – post-operative and delayed complications. In: Gerard A (Ed) Progress and perspectives in the treatment of gastrointestinal tumours. Pergamon Press, Oxford, p 76

Gerard A, Buyse M, Nordlinger B et al 1988 Preoperative radiotherapy as adjuvant treatment in rectal cancer. Annals of Surgery 208: 606–614

Glimelius B, Grafman S, Pahlman L et al 1982 Preoperative irradiation with high dose fractionation in adenocarcinoma of the rectum and rectosigmoid. Acta Radiologica: Oncology 21: 373–379

Gunderson LL 1994 Adjuvant therapy for rectal cancer. In: ASCO education book. American Society of Clinical Oncology, p 164

Heald RJ, Husband EM, Ryall RDH 1982 The mesorectum in rectal cancer surgery – the clue to pelvic recurrence. British Journal of Surgery 69: 613–616

Horn A, Morild I, Dahl O 1990 Tumour shrinkage and down staging after preoperative radiation of rectal adenocarcinomas. Radiotherapy and Oncology 18: 19–28

James RD, Schofield PF 1985 Resection of 'inoperable' rectal cancer following radiotherapy. British Journal of Surgery 72: 279–281

James RD, Johnson RJ, Eddleston B et al 1983 Prognostic factors in locally recurrent rectal carcinoma treated by radiotherapy. British Journal of Surgery 70: 469–472

James RD, Haboubi N, Schofield PF et al 1991 Prognostic factors in colorectal carcinoma treated by preoperative radiotherapy and immediate surgery. Diseases of the Colon and Rectum 34: 546–551

Kovalic JJ 1988 Endocavitary irradiation for rectal cancer. International Journal of Radiation, Oncology and Biological Physics 14: 261–264

Krook JE, Moertel CG, Gunderson LL et al 1991 Effective surgical adjuvant therapy for high risk rectal carcinoma. New England Journal of Medicine 324: 709–715

Lavery IC, Jones IT, Weakley FL et al 1987 Definitive management of rectal cancer by contact (intracavitary) irradiation. Diseases of the Colon and Rectum 30: 835–838

Mak AC, Rich TA, Schultheiss TE et al 1994 Late complications of postoperative radiation therapy for cancer of the rectum and rectosigmoid. International Journal of Radiation, Oncology and Biological Physics 28: 597–603

Mansour EG, Letkopoulou M, Johnson R et al 1991 A comparison of postoperative adjuvant chemotherapy, radiotherapy or combination therapy in potentially curable resectable rectal carcinoma (abstract). Proceedings of the American Society of Clinical Oncology 10: 154

Marks G, Mohiuddin M, Borenstein RD 1985 Preoperative

radiation therapy and sphincter preservation by the combined abdominosacral technique for selected cancers. Diseases of the Colon and Rectum. 28: 565–571

Marsh PJ, James RD, Schofield PF 1994a Adjuvant preoperative radiotherapy for locally advanced rectal carcinoma: results of a prospective, randomised trial. Diseases of the Colon and Rectum 37: 1205–1214

Marsh PJ, James RD, Schofield PF 1994b What is local recurrence after surgery for rectal carcinoma? British Journal of Surgery (in press)

MRC Working Party 1984 Second report. The evaluation of low dose preoperative X-ray therapy in the management of operable rectal cancer: results of a randomly controlled trial. British Journal of Surgery 71: 21–25

National Cancer Institute 1989 Clinical Announcement. NCI, Bethesda, Md

Nichols RJ 1982 The staging of rectal cancer. British Journal of Surgery 69: 404–409

Orton CG, Ellis F 1973 A simplification of the use of the NSD concept in practical radiotherapy. British Journal of Radiology 46: 529–537

Pahlman L, Glimelius B, Graffman S 1985 Pre- versus postoperative radiotherapy in rectal carcinoma: an interim report from a randomized multicentre trial. British Journal of Surgery 72: 961–966

Pahlman L, Glimelius B 1990 Pre- or postoperative radiotherapy in rectal and rectosigmoid carcinoma. Annals of Surgery 211: 187–189

Papillon J 1975 Intracavitary irradiation of early rectal cancer for cure. Cancer 36: 696–701

Parturier Albot M, Albot G 1981 Deux mille quarante cinq cas de cancer du rectum traites par radiotherapie de contact endocavitaire seule, ou preoperatoire, ou palliative. Annals de Gastroenterologie et de Hepatologie 17: 313–320

Ramming KP, Juillard G, Parker R et al 1986 Management of carcinoma of the rectum and anus without abdominoperineal excision. American Journal of Surgery 152: 16–20

Rich TA, Weiss DR, Mies C et al 1985 Sphincter preservation in patients treated with radiation therapy with or without local excision or fulguration. Radiology 156: 527–531

Rominger JC, Gelber RD 1985 Radiation therapy alone or in combination with chemotherapy in the treatment of residual or inoperable carcinoma of the rectum and rectosigmoid or pelvic recurrence following colorectal surgery. Radiation Therapy Oncology Group study (76–16). American Journal of Clinical Oncology 8: 118–127

Roth SL, Horiot JC, Calais G et al 1989 Prognostic factors in limited rectal cancer treated with intracavitary irradiation. International Journal of Radiation, Oncology and Biological Physics 16: 1445–1451

Schofield PF 1989 Treatment of radiation pelvic disease. In: Schofield PF, Lupton EW (eds) Causation and management of pelvic radiation disease. Springer, London

Sischy B, Hinson EJ, Wilkinson DR 1988 Definitive radiation therapy for selected cancers of the rectum. British Journal of Surgery 75: 901–903

Stockholm Rectal Cancer Study Group 1990 Preoperative short term radiation therapy in operable rectal carcinoma. Cancer 66: 49–56

Swedish Rectal Cancer Trial 1993 Initial report from a Swedish multicentre study examining the role of preoperative irradiation in the treatment of patients with resectable rectal carcinoma. British Journal of Surgery 80: 1333–1336

Williams NS, Johnston D 1983 The quality of life after rectal excision for low rectal cancer. British Journal of Surgery 70: 460–462

York Mason A 1976 Rectal cancer: the spectrum of selective surgery. Proceedings of the Royal Society of Medicine 69: 30–36

Zheng G, Eddleston B, Schofield PF et al 1984 Computed tomographic scanning in rectal carcinoma. Journal of the Royal Society of Medicine 77: 915–920

10 Adjuvant chemotherapy and immunotherapy for colorectal cancer

D. J. KERR

There is increasing awareness of the role of the specialist surgeon in the management of colorectal cancer and, in parallel with this, the emerging concept that multidisciplinary clinical teams (comprising surgeon, radiotherapist and medical oncologist) have the combined potential to offer optimal therapy. The requirement for an interdisciplinary approach reflects the natural history and biology of colorectal cancer; although 70–90% of patients are considered suitable for surgical intervention – the main treatment option – only approximately one-third of those patients survive to 5 years.

Clearly there are several stage-related prognostic factors which will determine the likelihood of long term survival for a given individual (Ch. 4), but the clinical implication is that microscopic metastases have occurred at some time prior to surgical intervention and have, therefore, rendered that patient potentially incurable. The aim of 'adjuvant' treatment (derived from the Latin verb *adjuvare* meaning 'to help') is to deliver additional anticancer therapy, either regionally (Ch. 9) to prevent local recurrence or systemically to prevent the emergence of distant metastases and perhaps prolong disease-free and overall survival.

There is a compelling biological rationale for the use of adjuvant therapies, either conventional cytotoxics or immunomodulatory agents, following surgical debulking of the primary tumour:

1. *The cancer burden is minimally low*. The received wisdom in delivering cytotoxic drugs and immunotherapies is that the smaller the tumour volume, the greater the likelihood of tumour eradication. Small tumour nodules are likely to be better vascularized, less necrotic and, therefore, have an improved capacity for homogeneous drug delivery than, say, a cancer nodule several centimetres in diameter which will have hypoxic compartments, compressed or obliterated vasculature and much larger distances, in molecular terms, for drugs or immune effector cells to diffuse from the vascular compartment to their site of action.

2. *Fewer mutations will have occurred*. The basis of tumour heterogeneity is of increased mutation rates within an expanding uncoordinated cancer cell population. Mutations occur at random, but with a higher frequency in cancer cells relative to normal host, proliferative, cellular compartments (e.g. bone marrow, mucosal crypt cell, hair follicle cells, etc.). This intrinsic genetic instability means that there is a greater likelihood of spontaneous, random mutations occurring which could confer resistance to the anticancer therapy. For example, a mutation which leads to greatly amplified levels of the target enzyme for the antineoplastic drug, within the cancer cells, would greatly reduce the likelihood of that cell being killed by the appropriate drug. This mechanism is important in the development of cellular resistance to methotrexate and 5-fluorouracil (5-Fu), both of which have been used in the treatment of colorectal cancer. Goldie & Coldman have described a formal, statistical model relating the likelihood of mutation to the development of drug resistance and, not surprisingly, the take-home message is that the greater the tumour volume at the time of treatment, the greater the chance that a resistant colony of cancer cells will have grown out (Tannock 1978).

3. *Favourable cell cycle kinetics*. The majority of cytotoxic drugs are DNA synthesis inhibitors and, therefore, are more active against tumours which have a higher proportion of their cells in the S phase (DNA synthetic phase) of the cell cycle. There have been many studies of the prognostic importance of aneuploidy and the proportion of cells in S-phase in colorectal cancer but there is additional information to suggest that when the primary tumour is resected, the growth fraction of residual micrometastases increases. This phenomenon may be mediated by a humoral factor secreted by the primary cancer, although it remains to be fully characterized.

Selection of patients for adjuvant therapy

In any clinical undertaking which is potentially toxic, like adjuvant chemotherapy or immunotherapy, consideration must be given to the benefits relative to the likely cost. An important factor in refining cost-benefit analysis is the definition of subgroups based on some aspect of the natural history of the disease and then allotting treatment appropriately. There is no doubt that access to pathological expertise is an essential part of the multidisciplinary team involved in making therapeutic decisions. We are dependent upon staging systems (e.g. TNM) that define the extent of tumour invasion and metastasis, conversant with the relative importance of histopathological features like tumour grade, the degree of aneuploidy and the proportion of cells actively synthesizing DNA (% S-phase cells) but it is clear that we must be openminded and considerate of the stream of information which is coming from biologists who are defining the molecular lesions which determine the malignant phenotype. The next decade should see a great increase in our capacity to further refine prognostic markers which may control subsequent therapeutic choice. The majority of prognostic work lionizing novel molecular or immunocytochemical markers is retrospective and, although the statistics are usually well done by multivariate analysis, this must be considered a means of generating prognostic hypotheses which can be prospectively tested in randomized clinical trials rather than a fait accompli which can be instantly plugged into a clinical formula to help choose treatments for individual patients.

Regardless of the complexity of the model derived to help inform choice of adjuvant therapy, and this could range from Dukes' staging (which must surely be considered a mandatory minimum) to a sophisticated battery of additional information including tumour grade, ploidy, immunocytochemical staining for proteases such as the cathepsins and molecular hybridization techniques to assess the presence or absence of key tumour repressor genes (Ch 1), we must compress this information into lay terms when explaining the need for adjuvant therapy or eliciting informed consent for a clinical trial from a patient.

In our clinic, we explain that:

> Surgery has gone well, but even with the best will in the world, it is possible that seeds of the cancer have escaped and have the capacity to reform other cancer nodules. We have a drug treatment which can cut down the chance of the cancer coming back and now is the best opportunity to administer the drugs while you are fit and the cancer (if there) is invisibly small. Better treatment now, rather than be faced with the possibility of having to treat an established cancer nodule years hence. There are no guarantees that the drug therapy will be 100% successful, but it is the best that we can offer at the moment.

This framework allows the attending surgeon or physician to bolt on as much specific information as is deemed appropriate, for example, a 50:50 chance of the cancer recurring within 5 years or the possibility of the drug treatment reducing the odds of dying of colorectal cancer by a third, etc. It also leads one naturally to discuss the chemotherapy schedule and all that it involves in terms of social impact and side-effects. One must remember that the patient will retain little information from this first conversation, therefore reiteration and plain speaking are important and a variety of methods can be used to reinforce the content of the consultation such as taped interview, simple consent form-type documents, subsequent interview by nurse specialists who will be involved with therapy.

Which chemotherapy works for colorectal cancer?

Many anticancer drugs have been tested in advanced colorectal cancer but the therapeutic mainstay has been, and still is, 5-Fu. 5-Fu is a prodrug which, when activated, is an antimetabolite, i.e. it is mistaken by the enzymes involved in the cell's own housekeeping functions as an essential metabolite, is then falsely incorporated into a number of vital, biochemical processes and ultimately sabotages them, because it simply cannot fulfil the complete role of the normal cell metabolite which it has mimicked (Kerr 1989). An analogy could be the recruitment of a new star to a tug-of-war team. Unbeknown to his colleagues, the newcomer resembles them only because his wife made a bizarre padded suit which makes him look like Charles Atlas (or his modern equivalent). The tug-of-war team looks sturdy but on the first pull they do their best, stand their ground for a while, but even they cannot compensate for the weedy imposter and eventually are pulled across the losing line.

5-Fu is metabolised to 5-FdUMP (5-fluoro deoxyuridine monophosphate) (Fig. 10.1) and can inhibit the enzyme thymidylate synthetase (TS) and hence the production of thymidine which is an essential building block for DNA synthesis. 5-Fu can be further metabolized and incorporated falsely into DNA and RNA. 5-Fu has been used clinically for 30 years (Brackner & Matward 1991) and, therefore, there is a plethora of different doses, routes and schedules of administration. In general, and in the absence of specific, powerful clinical trials to direct choice, there are a few observations which can be made about single agent 5-Fu:

- Oral 5-Fu should not be used, given its wide interindividual variation in bioavailability and hence toxicity.
- Intermittent, weekly or fortnightly bolus administration of 5-Fu is probably inferior to the more toxic, dose-intensive, five times daily schedules which are administered once a month.
- Recent advances in pump technology and in pharmaceutical support services make prolonged infusion of 5-Fu an attractive therapeutic option for those centres with sufficient community resource. Prolonged infusional schedules make sense of two pharmacokinetic principles:

1. that prolonged exposure to antimetabolites which are active in the S-phase of the cell cycle makes cell kinetic sense;
2. that 5-Fu has non-linear or saturable kinetics, therefore, there is likely to be a greater capacity for tumour cell drug uptake if it is given by a slow, steady trickle.

How active is 5-Fu?

Single agent response rates (the percentage of patients who show >50% diminution in tumour volume) in colorectal cancer hover around 10–20% (Brackner & Matward 1991). In a recent randomized study comparing weekly intravenous bolus 5-Fu (600 mg/m^2) versus prolonged infusional 5-Fu (300 mg/m^2 daily for 12 weeks) the respective response rates were 7% and 30% although there was no significant survival benefit from infusion (Lokich et al 1989). This is consistent with the pharmacokinetic hypothesis suggested above.

What side-effects are associated with 5-Fu?

Toxicity is schedule-dependent and includes nausea, vomiting, myelosuppression, mucositis,

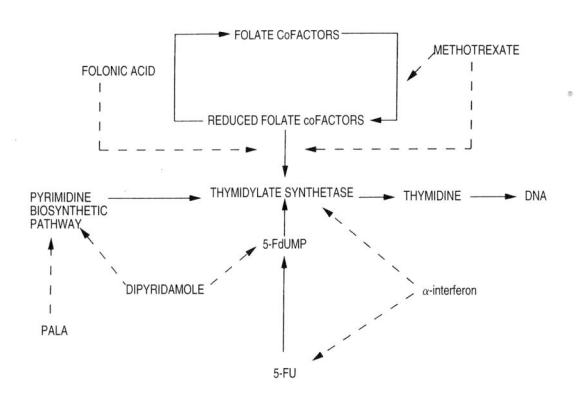

Fig. 10.1 Biochemical modulation of 5-Fu.

diarrhoea and, more rarely, a desquamative hand–foot syndrome with prolonged infusions, cardiac and neurological toxicities.

Recent advances in the use of 5-Fu

Perhaps the most exciting advance in the clinical use of 5-Fu has come from its combination with folinic acid (FA) (Kerr 1989). FA modulates the activity of 5-Fu by stabilizing the ternary complex of 5-FdUMP with TS, thereby increasing the degree of inhibition of the enzyme and enhancing the likelihood of cell death following thymidine depletion (see Fig. 10.1). So, a pharmocological observation has led to a rational drug development programme combining 5-Fu and FA. Over 2000 patients have been entered into clinical trials in advanced colorectal cancer comparing a number of different 5-Fu and 5-Fu/FA schedules. Metaanalysis of the results of these studies indicates that the response rate for the 5-Fu/FA combination is 23% compared with 9% for single agent 5-Fu and there is a trend towards improved overall survival in the 5-Fu/FA groups (Journal of Clinical Oncology 1992). The keystone of any drive to establish an adjuvant therapy is access to a treatment with proven efficacy in advanced disease and it would appear that the 5-Fu/FA combination is a likely contender.

Immunotherapy of colorectal cancer

This is a complex therapeutic area to review and has suffered, to an extent, scientifically in that much of the immunological work performed in the 1960s and 1970s was not hypothesis driven, poorly constructed and tended to give the field a rather negative reputation. Given enormous advances in molecular biology, however, and the technological capacity to produce large quantities of genetically engineered pure proteins, there has been a major resurgence of interest in immunotherapy. This can be considered under the following headings.

Cytokines

Interferon

The interferons have a complex anticancer effect which comprises both a direct antiproliferative action and an immunomodulatory role to up-regulate tumour cell surface expression of MHC and stimulate production of helper and cytotoxic T lymphocytes. Neither γ-interferon nor α-interferon is clinically active in the therapy of advanced colorectal cancer and they do not have a convincing role to play in adjuvant therapy. There was a flurry of interest over the potential synergy between 5-Fu and α-interferon (Wadler et al 1989), but a recent large randomized study performed by the MRC has shown that α-interferon adds to the toxicity of 5-Fu/FA combinations but adds nothing to tumour response rate and survival.

Interleukin 2 (IL-2)

IL-2 is a 15.5 kD glycoprotein which plays a central role in immune responses. Activation of lymphocytes by specific antigen results in increased expression of IL-2 receptors and subsequent binding of the ligand will lead to lymphocyte proliferation and immune response. IL-2 has been used in a number of dose schedules in the treatment of advanced colorectal cancer. There is significant toxicity (malaise, nausea and vomiting, hypotension, fluid retention and organ dysfunction) but the tumour response rate is neither high nor durable. There have been combinations of IL-2 interferon and tumour necrosis factor, but this approach worsens toxicity without conferring appreciable therapeutic benefit.

Small molecular weight immunomodulators

Levamisole

Levamisole has been used, empirically, to treat a wide number of diseases ranging from helminthic infestations to autoimmune disorders. Although the drug is widely held to have immunostimulating properties, the scientific evidence culled from the literature is conflicting with both positive and negative data reported. There have been three small randomized studies in which levamisole was used to treat patients with advanced cancer (Stevenson et al 1991) and no effects on response rate or survival were documented.

Cimetidine

There is some evidence to suggest that the H_2-receptor antagonists have immunomodulatory properties and can alter the ratio of helper:suppressor T cells. A Danish group (Torresen et al 1988) investigated the effect of cimetidine on survival of a group of 180 gastric cancer patients. Immediately after operation or the decision not to operate, the patients were randomized to placebo or cimetidine. Survival in the cimetidine group was significantly longer than the placebo group. There are parallel adjuvant studies in colorectal cancer, the results of which are awaited with interest.

Monoclonal antibody therapy

There have been many phase II trials of a number of murine, chimaeric and humanized monoclonal antibodies raised against a variety of tumour antigens. The antibodies have been coupled to cell toxins such as ricin, radiopharmaceuticals, cytotoxic drugs and enzymes capable of activating prodrugs. The trials are labour-intense and a number of intellectual problems remain to be overcome such as antihuman mouse antibody responses, poor tumour delivery and penetration of the therapeutic antibody, variation in antigen expression, crossreaction with normal tissues and expense. It is doubtful whether the complexity of the treatment justifies the rather meagre clinical gains associated with currently available antibody directed therapy.

Active specific immunotherapy

Although there was a vogue for IL-2-induced ex vivo expansion of lymphokine activated killer (LAK) cells and their reinfusion into autologous donors and a similar approach to expand tumour infiltrating lymphocytes, neither of these approaches has been useful in colorectal cancer (Rosenberg et al 1989). There have been studies of adjuvant active specific immunotherapy in colorectal cancer, where the tumours were disaggregated postsurgically into single cell suspension and cryopreserved. Subsequently treated patients received one intradermal vaccination per week for 2 weeks consisting of 10^7 viable, irradiated, autologous tumour cells and 10^7 viable bacillus Calmette-Guérin (BCG) organisms. Ninety eight patients were randomized into the study and, with a median follow-up of 6.5 years, there was a significant but slight improvement in survival seen for the colon cancer patients as distinct from patients with rectal cancer who had no benefit.

Adjuvant chemotherapy for colorectal cancer

There is a large but scattered literature on the use of adjuvant chemotherapy in colorectal cancer, predominantly based on administration of the antimetabolite 5-Fu. Metaanalysis of published data from these studies suggests that the more dose-intense chemotherapy schedules providing at least 6 months treatment with 5-Fu may reduce the risk of death by 10–15% although this difference is of borderline statistical significance (Gray et al 1991).

The trial with the most striking result was the American intergroup study comparing one year of 5-Fu and levamisole with levamisole alone and an untreated control group. This trial reported a one-third reduction in the death rate in a subgroup of high-risk (Dukes' stage C) colon cancer patients who received combination therapy (Moertel et al 1990). However, the contribution of levamisole to the strikingly improved outcome can be questioned. The 5-Fu levamisole combination appears no more effective than 5-Fu alone in advanced disease and a clear understanding of the biological mechanism of the hypothesized synergy between these drugs has proved elusive. The large survival benefit seen in this study may, therefore, not be due to synergy between 5-Fu and levamisole but simply a 'random high', i.e. a 5-Fu effect that, by chance, turned out larger in the stage C patients in this study than in previous studies of 5-Fu on its own.

A second smaller study by the American NCCTG group has also reported a large reduction in mortality, this time achieved by adding systemic 5-Fu to radiotherapy in rectal cancer (Krook et al 1991). Again, radiotherapy alone has, at best, a moderate influence on survival and so it is unclear whether the benefit seen in this study was inflated by chance or was due to synergy between 5-Fu and radiotherapy.

Three recent studies which recruited almost 3000 patients comparing a no-treatment control versus 6 months treatment with adjuvant 5-Fu coupled with its biomodulator folinic acid (Fu/FA) provide more convincing evidence of a worthwhile survival benefit for adjuvant chemotherapy. First, an overview of three randomized studies from Italy, France and Canada that had tested 6 months of 5-Fu with high doses ($250 \, mg/m^2$) of FA has reported a significant benefit of this combination in terms of recurrence-free survival (RFS) but not, to date, in survival (Zaniboni et al 1993). Second, an American intergroup study of 5-Fu with much lower doses ($20 \, mg/m^2$) of folinic acid has reported a significant reduction in RFS but, again, not in survival (O'Connell et al 1993). Finally, an NSABP study comparing 5-Fu and very high dose ($500 \, mg/m^2$) FA with chemotherapy methyl CCNU + vincristine + 5-Fu (MOF) chemotherapy has shown a significant improvement in RFS and also a survival benefit for the 5-Fu/FA combination (Wolmark et al 1993). These apparent benefits from adjuvant 5-Fu/FA are made more plausible by an understanding of the pharmacological rationale for this 5-Fu potentiation (Kerr 1989), coupled with definite evidence that folinic acid enhances the activity of 5-Fu in advanced disease.

These encouraging results are likely to lead to much wider use of 5-Fu/FA based chemotherapy for colorectal cancer. However, there is still real doubt about the size of the survival benefit relative to toxicity, quality of life and health service resource usage and there is, as yet, no convincing evidence which allows a rational selection of competing adjuvant chemotherapy regimens. A recent survey by the UKCCCR suggested that less than 50% of clinicians polled in the United Kingdom offer adjuvant chemotherapy; nevertheless, there is an increasing patient-led demand for action and our purchasing colleagues need advice. What practical answer could there be that would assuage the needs of these different communities? By a timely quirk of academic fate QUASAR, a UKCCCR study of adjuvant therapy for colorectal cancer, has just been launched.

Patients without metastases or apparent residual disease for whom there is *substantial uncertainty* over whether or not they should receive chemotherapy in addition to surgery for colorectal cancer are randomized equally between chemotherapy and control groups. Patients with a *clear indication* for chemotherapy but for whom there is substantial uncertainty which regimen to use are randomized between chemotherapy options. The chemotherapy tested is a practicable outpatient regimen involving intravenous 5-Fu combined with either low-dose or high-dose L-folinic acid and either levamisole or placebo.

QUASAR aims to randomize 8000 patients over the next 3 years and will provide an opportunity for the surgical and oncological communities in the UK to address this emergent clinical practice.

Portal venous infusional adjuvant chemotherapy

It is worthwhile considering postoperative portal venous infusion (PVI) of 5-Fu as a special case. Administration of 1 g of 5-Fu daily by PVI for 7 days has been compared against control in six studies, comprising approximately 1500 patients. The treatment is well tolerated and a recent metaanalysis suggests that it can confer a significant reduction in the odds of dying of colorectal cancer by approximately 30%. This therapy is rational and is based on the capacity of the liver to extract significant quantities (up to 60%) of 5-Fu from the portal venous circulation, generating very high intrahepatic 5-Fu concentrations, and the fact that the portal vein drains effluent blood from the bowel and is, therefore, a prominent 'highway' for metastasizing colorectal cancer cells. There is debate about the importance of local control in terms of reduction in the incidence of hepatic metastases and, through this, contributing to improved overall survival but this would seem the likeliest mechanism of action as PVI of 5-Fu is pharmacologically unlikely to contribute to control of systemic metastases.

Adjuvant immunotherapy for colorectal cancer

This is a rapidly evolving field, but to date there have been no major randomized studies which have indicated that adjuvant immunotherapy, other than for the 5-Fu/levamisole combination, has any significant effect on disease-free or overall survival following apparently curative resection of colorectal cancers.

There has been a chequered history for adjuvant immunomodulatory trials, but it is possible that recent advances in understanding the nature of the process of antigen recognition and cloning of several of the molecules involved could lead to genetic manipulation of autologous cancer cells ex vivo before they are vaccinated back into the patient with a far greater potential for exciting the sorts of immune responses which are required to activate the organism's host defence mechanisms and reject residual tumour cells.

Future prospects

As always, time, tide and therapeutic concepts move on and evolve and it is worth a little space to speculate on the innovative treatment modalities which may be subject to clinical trials over the next decade.

There are several potent thymidylate synthetase inhibitors in phase II and phase III clinical trials in advanced disease which one might expect to have a better therapeutic ratio than 5-Fu/FA. Novel molecular targets have been identified in the therapy of colorectal cancer: topoisomerase I, an enzyme involved in 'untwisting' DNA during replication; isoforms of protein kinase C and certain tyrosine kinases involved in growth factor–receptor–signal transduction pathways. It will be interesting to see if small molecular weight inhibitors of these proteins can be developed and brought forward to clinical trial (Kerr & Workman 1994).

Perhaps most innovative will be the application of gene therapy, first in an advanced setting and, if successful, introduced into the adjuvant area. There is one strategy which has been developed by Dr Brian Huber which would seem particularly applicable to the adjuvant therapy of colorectal cancer.

Huber and colleagues (1993) have synthesized DNA vectors which contain the carcinoembryonic antigen (CEA) promoter linked to the bacterial enzyme cytosine deaminase (CD), packaged into retroviruses and adenoviruses which have the capacity to infect human cells (Kerr & Workman 1994). The 'tumour-specific' CEA promoter ensures that the bacterial CD will only be 'switched on' and synthesized in cells which are CEA-positive, therefore imparting a tumour targeting effect. Tumour cells (Fig. 10.2) which express CD exposed to the inactive, non-toxic prodrug 5-flucytosine will convert it to 5-Fu and will be killed along with a significant proportion of surrounding cells (the 'bystander' effect, brought

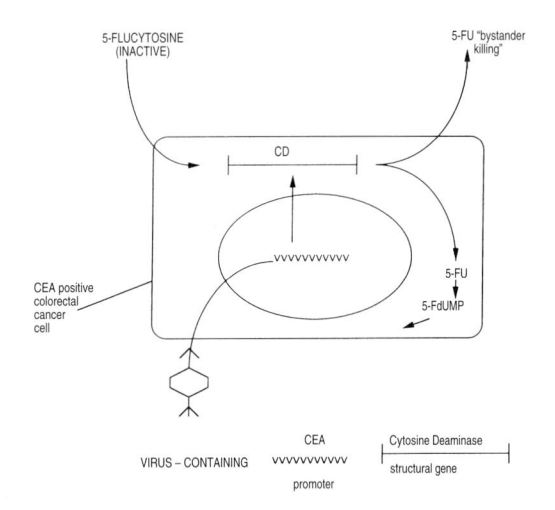

Fig. 10.2 Schematic representation of virally directed enzyme prodrug therapy.

about by 5-Fu secretion from the CD-expressing tumour cells). In vivo studies in mice with hepatic metastatic colorectal cancer nodules, established by subcapsular injection of mixtures of colorectal cancer cells (some of which have been transfected with the CD gene), have shown that <10% of the total tumour cell population needs to express the CD gene for some of the tumours to be cured by intrahepatic arterial infusion of 5-flucytosine. We plan to perform a phase I study of hepatic arterial infusion of the viruses containing the CD gene followed by the prodrug 5-flucytosine and, if safety permits and efficacy dictates, one could imagine the same system being administered via the portal vein.

The future is bright and a dialectical synchretism between scientists and clinicians beckons.

Acknowledgements
The author wishes to thank Lisa McCorrie and Suzanne Witcomb for typing the manuscript and acknowledges grant support from the Cancer Research Campaign and the Medical Research Council.

References
Brackner HW, Matward BT 1991 Chemotherapy of advanced cancer of colon and rectum. Seminars in Oncology 18: 443–461

Gray R, James R, Mossman J, Stenning S 1991 AXIS – a suitable case for treatment. British Journal of Cancer 63: 841–845

Huber BC, Austin EA, Good SS et al 1993 In vivo antitumour activity of 5-flucytosine on human colorectal cancer cells genetically modified to express cytosine deaminase. Cancer Research 53: 4619–4626

Journal of Clinical Oncology 1992 Advanced colorectal cancer meta-analysis project. Modulation of fluorouracil by leucovorin in patients with advanced colorectal cancer; evidence in terms of response rate. Journal of Clinical Oncology 10: 896–903

Kerr DJ 1989 5-fluorouracil and folinic acid; interesting biochemistry or effective treatment (editorial)? British Journal of Cancer 60: 807–808

Kerr DJ, Workman P 1994 New molecular targets for cancer chemotherapy. Cancer Research Campaign Press, Philadelphia

Krook JE, Moertel CG, Gunderson LL et al 1991 Effective surgical adjuvant therapy for high-risk rectal carcinoma. New England Journal of Medicine 324: 709–715

Lokich JJ, Aldgren JD, Gullo JJ et al 1989 A prospective randomised comparison of continuous infusion 5-fluorouracil with a conventional bolus schedule in metastatic colorectal cancer. Journal of Clinical Oncology 7: 425–432

Moertel CG, Fleming TR, MacDonald JS et al 1990 Levamisole and fluorouracil as adjuvant therapy of resected colon carcinoma. New England Journal of Medicine 322: 352–358

O'Connell M, Mailliard J, MacDonald J et al 1993 An intergroup trial of intensive course 5-FU and low-dose leucovorin as surgical adjuvant therapy for high-risk colon cancer (abstract). Proceedings of the American Society of Clinical Oncology 12(190): 552

Rosenberg SA, Lotze MT, Yang JC et al 1989 Experience with the use of high-dose interleukin 2 in the treatment of 652 cancer patients. Annals of Surgery 210: 474–485

Stevenson HC, Green I, Hamilton JM et al 1991 Levamisole: known effects on the immune system, clinical results and future applications to the treatment of cancer. Journal of Clinical Oncology 9: 2052–2066

Tannock I 1978 Cells, kinetics and chemotherapy; a critical review. Cancer Treatment Reviews 62: 1117

Torresen H, Bulow S, Fischerman K et al 1988 Effect of cimetidine on survival after gastric cancer. Lancet (8618)ii: 990–991

Wadler S, Schwartz EL, Goldman M et al 1989 Fluorouracil and recombinant alpha-2 interferon: an active regimen against advanced colorectal carcinoma. Journal of Clinical Oncology 7: 1769–1775

Wolmark N, Rockette H, Fisher B et al 1993 The benefit of leucovorin modulated fluorouracil as postoperative adjuvant therapy for primary colon cancer. (Results from National Surgical Adjuvant Breast and Bowel Project protocol C-03). Journal of Clinical Oncology 1: 1879–1887

Zaniboni A, Ehrlichman C, Seitz JF et al 1993 FU/FA increased disease-free survival in resected B2C colon cancer: results of a prospective pooled analysis of 3 randomised trials (abstract). Proceedings of the American Society of Clinical Oncology 12(191): 555

11 Surveillance and recurrence

L. PÅHLMAN

Surveillance

Follow-up programmes for patients operated upon for colorectal cancer cover a huge volume of visits to the outpatient clinic at a surgical department. The rationale for a surveillance regimen is mainly based on three factors.

The most important is to detect recurrences or metachronous tumours. Theoretically the advantage of this is prolonged survival if a recurrence is diagnosed early when no symptoms have occurred, compared with treatment of symptomatic recurrences. Also, palliative treatment might be more effective if early recurrence is detected.

The second reason is that patients feel more secure if they are under surveillance. Both the examination and repeated check-ups and the fact that the patient has contact with a doctor can be seen as security. A third argument for routine follow-up consultations is the collection of data for research and quality assurance. Such a systematic data collection to study effects and side-effects of treatment is important so that the natural history of the disease can be better understood.

A fourth important reason is to evaluate quality of life. Patients operated upon for a colorectal cancer need to discuss functional problems with the surgeon. Information about the surgical procedure as well as the outcome must repeatedly be explained and discussed. This is of special importance for those having a stoma. Regular visits to a stoma therapist are necessary to assist the patient. The aim is to educate and give psychosocial support enabling patients to cope with a stoma. This part of the follow-up programme is obvious and will not be discussed further in this chapter.

Several surveillance programmes have been used and also reported in the literature (Böhm et al 1993, Safi et al 1993, Schiessel et al 1986, Törnqvist et al 1982, Vernava III et al 1994). However, all those studies have compared the results with historical controls. Therefore the value of surveillance after surgery for colorectal cancer is not established. No randomized controlled trials have been reported, but two trials are ongoing (see below).

Who shall we follow?

Initially it is important to decide which group of patients we should place in a surveillance programme. Patients not operated upon for cure, in whom disease-related symptoms are to be expected in the near future, must be followed to detect those symptoms as soon as possible, with the aim of starting palliative treatment before the patients have suffered too much.

In most series with specific follow-up regimens, criteria for curative treatment are not addressed. 'Curative' surgery indicates no sign of distant metastases present at surgery and a curatively resected primary tumour, i.e. no signs of tumour left at surgery and confirmed by a detailed histopathological report. It is important to take biopsies if the intraabdominal exploration indicates suspicious metastatic tumour outside the resected area. This includes paraaortic lymph nodes, liver metastases and peritoneal seedings. Also elimination of synchronous distant metastases is important if a patient is to be recommended for regular follow-up. A perioperative chest X-ray has to be performed to disclose synchronous lung metastases and perioperative evaluation of the liver is recommended. Different techniques for scanning the liver are available including computed tomography (CT), magnetic resonance imaging (MRI) and pre- or peroperative ultrasonography. A preoperative abnormal liver function test may indicate the necessity of performing perioperative scanning of the liver. This topic, as well as the surgical treatment of secondaries in the liver, is discussed in Chapter 12.

A pre- or postoperative colonoscopy is important to evaluate synchronous adenomas and cancers. If this investigation is performed preoperatively it may have an impact on the surgical strategy regarding the length of the resected specimen (Langevin & Nivatvongs 1984, Pagana et al 1984), since peroperative examination of the bowel by the surgeon is not a reliable method (Heald & Bussey 1975). However, it is debatable whether preoperative colonoscopy is advisable since there is the risk of tumour cell spread to other areas of the colon via the colonoscope (Umpleby et al 1984). Moreover, a total examination of the colon is not possible in one-third of the patients due to an obstructing tumour (Kronborg et al 1983). For these reasons, an early postoperative colonoscopy is advisable.

The value of a preoperative screening programme for synchronous distant metastases and synchronous colonic lesions is debatable. The rationale for such a screening procedure is to detect a lesion before it has became symptomatic. Whether such an approach will have an impact on survival is not known, since no randomized trial has evaluated this specific question. However, before a patient is recommended for a follow-up programme, the absence or presence of distant metastases, as well as a 'clean' colon, i.e. no synchronous adenomas or cancer, should be established.

When the patient is considered to have been curatively treated according to the guidelines above it is important to identify the risk groups. Prediction of prognosis as a guide to selecting patients at risk can be of value (see below). Another important judgement is to evaluate whether a patient, due to age or concomitant disease, will survive another major surgical procedure for recurrence or not. If not, there is no reason to follow such a patient extensively.

Follow-up programme

No prospective randomized trial comparing an intensive follow-up schedule with no regular follow-up at all has been performed, although two studies are ongoing (see below) (Kronborg et al 1988, Northover & Slack 1984). Several studies have been reported from institutions with special follow-up regimens. In most of the surveillance programmes a clinical examination, including laboratory examination and selective tumour markers, has been carried out every third to fourth month up to 24 months after surgery and thereafter twice per year for 5 years postoperatively. Chest X-ray, barium enema or colonoscopy and different imaging procedures (ultrasonography, CT scan or MRI scan) have been used annually or every second year (Böhm et al 1993, Enker & Kramer 1982, Safi et al 1993, Schiessel et al 1986, Törnqvist et al 1982).

The results of these studies are disappointing with a very low benefit for the treatment. The number of patients available for a second operation for cure is very low (3–6%) and the survival after such a procedure is approximately 75% after 12 months, 50% after 24 months and <25% after 5 years. Only very few patients can be cured in such a follow-up programme and the question raised is of course whether those patients could be cured anyway if they were admitted some months later when they had developed symptoms from their recurrence. In a prospective population-based Swedish trial, patients were followed twice per year. Most recurrences were diagnosed in between visits because they were symptomatic. As a result of these findings a second trial was conducted with four regular follow-ups per year within the first 2 years and then twice yearly for 5 years postoperatively. Most recurrences were found at the clinical visit when the patient was asymptomatic. However, the number of cured patients was similar, indicating that it might not be important to find a recurrence before symptoms are present (Törnqvist et al 1982).

Tumour markers

A number of tumour markers such as CEA (carcinoembryonic antigen), TPA (tissue polypeptide antigen), TPS (tissue polypeptide specific antigen) and different monoclonal antibodies (CA 19–9, CA 50 and CA 242) have been used in predicting outcome as well as in a follow-up programme (Begent & Rustin 1989, Lindmark 1992, Moertel et al 1986, Moore et al 1989, Ståhle et al 1988b, 1989). Patients with an elevated CEA preoperatively have a high risk of developing a recurrence despite 'curative' surgery. This is also true for several other tumour markers like CA 19–9, CA 50 and TPA (Lindmark et al 1994, Ståhle et al 1988b). However, no prospective randomized trial has evaluated the benefit of these tumour markers. The value of using serum markers in a follow-up programme if a preoperative serum level is normal has been contemplated. The problem is that recurrence may occur even in the presence of a normal serum CEA level (Zeng et al 1993).

The main point in using serum markers in a follow-up programme is to find patients with an asymptomatic recurrence and to offer them a 'second look' operation with a curative potential. The initial trials within this field used CEA measurements every 4–8 weeks during the first 2 years and then every 3 months to 5 years postoperatively. If the CEA level was increased irrespective of any symptoms indicating a recurrence, a 'second look' laparotomy was performed. Approximately 10% of the patients were operated upon due to an elevated CEA level and one-third of this group had a resectable recurrence (Attiyeh & Stearns 1981, Martin et al 1985). By measuring plasma CEA levels a relationship has been established to distant metastases but not to local recurrence (Lunde & Havig 1982, Moertel et al 1978, Staab et al 1978).

Only one prospective randomized trial within this field has been conducted, an ongoing multicentre trial in the UK sponsored by the National Institutes of Health and the Cancer Research Campaign (Northover & Slack 1984). In this trial patients are followed intensively with repeated CEA examinations and are randomly allocated to two groups. In one group the responsible surgeon will be contacted if an elevated CEA level has been detected. The surgeon is then given the opportunity to investigate the patient for a recurrence or to perform a 'second look' operation. In the other group the responsible surgeon is not informed about the increased CEA level. The aim of this study is to evaluate whether early intervention due to an elevated CEA level postoperatively will increase the number of asymptomatic recurrences amenable to a second, curative operation with the possibility of improving survival. This trial is now completed but not yet officially reported but early indications are that the 'second look' procedure has had no major impact on survival or improved the effective surgical treatment of the recurrence (Northover, personal communication). Similar studies with other tumour markers have not been done.

Colonoscopic surveillance

The rationale for colonoscopic surveillance is to find metachronous adenomas or cancers. It is well known that the risk of having a metachronous tumour is 3–5% (Agrez et al 1982, Bussey et al 1967, Cunliffe et al 1984, Heald & Lockhart-Mummery 1972, Kronborg et al 1983). The risk of developing a metachronous adenoma or cancer is probably increased with the length of follow-up, indicating that the younger the patient the higher is the risk of having a metachronous lesion (Cali et al 1993, Luchtefeld et al 1987). Support for such an aggressive follow-up policy also comes from the results achieved after repeated sigmoidoscopy and subsequent polypectomy in an unselected group of patients (Gilbertson & Nelms 1978). After a mean of 4 years of follow-up, 13 rectal cancers occurred among the 21 000 subjects who underwent a 'clearing' proctosigmoidoscopy and subsequent annual endoscopy with removal of all lesions compared to the calculated estimate of 90 rectal cancers which might have been expected to occur in this group. Two case control studies have shown that patients who had undergone a rigid proctosigmoidoscopy had a 70–85% reduction in risk of developing a rectal cancer compared with controls who were not offered the examination (Atkin et al 1992, Selby et al 1992).

Another technique which has been used in screening programmes is a simple faecal occult blood test. In a study to evaluate the efficacy of Haemoccult-II in a surveillance programme after curative surgery for colorectal cancer or polypectomies, it was found that the faecal blood test was positive in three of nine patients with local recurrence, in two of 13 patients with metachronous cancer and in 31 of 186 with adenomas. The test was positive more often if the lesion was large. It was concluded that a faecal occult blood test should not be used in a surveillance programme. If the remaining colon is to be screened, colonoscopy is mandatory (Jahn et al 1992).

One ongoing trial in Funen, Denmark, is intended specifically to study the value of postoperative follow-up in patients with colorectal cancer operated upon for cure. Within 3 months postoperatively all patients are subjected to a colonoscopy so that the remaining colon can be examined. After this 'cleaning' procedure patients are randomly alloted either to have repeated colonoscopy and follow-ups or no regular follow-up at all (Kronborg et al 1988). This important trial is still running and the results are eagerly available.

Other techniques

In all reported follow-up programmes the clinical investigations, including laboratory tests, have been combined with different imaging techniques, such as chest X-ray, ultrasonography, CT (Fig. 11.1) and MRI, although the latter have been carried out less frequently than clinical examination (Böhm et al 1993, Safi et al 1993, Schiessel et al 1986, Törnqvist et al 1982). In patients with symptoms these techniques are of value and the local tradition at each hospital is often the reason to use a specific technique. However, none of the above methods has been critically evaluated in a surveillance programme.

Prediction of prognosis

Before starting a mass screening programme for recurrent or metachronous disease after radical

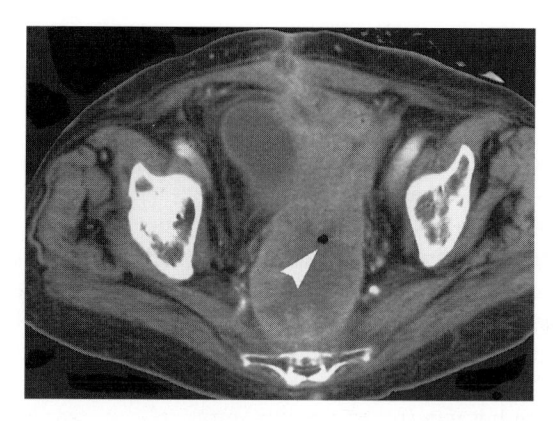

Fig. 11.1 A huge recurrence from a sigmoid cancer with a fistula to the abdominal wall and to the bowel. Air within the recurrence (arrow).

surgery for colorectal cancer, it might be of value to determine the risk groups. Dukes' classification, first applied to rectal cancer, is still the best prognostic indicator available (Dukes & Bussey 1958). Several modifications of the Dukes' staging system have been described, none of which has shown any further prognostic predictive capability (Nathanson et al 1986). The cell morphology and the growth pattern of the tumour are also important. A poor differentiation pattern has constantly been demonstrated to be a predictor of shorter survival (Chapuis et al 1985, Halvorsen & Seim 1988, Jass et al 1986, Ståhle et al 1988a). DNA disturbances are another observation in colorectal cancers and aneuploidy has been considered as a marker of poor outcome after curative surgery (Armitage et al 1985, Quirke et al 1987) although contradictory findings have been reported (Enblad et al 1985, Lindmark et al 1991). However, the heterogeneity in ploidy and S-phase fraction limits the use of DNA measurements (Lindmark et al 1991).

More sophisticated analysis of the tumour morphology has been used to further improve the prediction of prognosis. The morphology of the basement membrane has been suggested to be of importance (Levy et al 1991, Lindmark et al 1993, Offerhaus et al 1991). Also the tumour stroma with several growth factors and neoangiogenesis have been studied in order to find prognostic markers (Anzano et al 1989, Weidner et al 1991). The value of a more sophisticated analysis of the tumour is still questionable (Lindmark

1992). The lack of expression of the tumour suppressor gene p53 may predict an adverse outcome in colorectal cancer (Nathanson et al 1994).

Conclusions

No firm data support a meticulous follow-up programme for patients operated upon for cure and the value of surveillance after colorectal cancer surgery has been discussed (Ballantyne & Modlin 1988, Kronborg 1986). Better tumour markers to predict prognosis and identify those at high risk of developing new adenomas or recurrences are likely to be found in the future but until the results of prospective randomized trials are available, each surgeon must decide on their own follow-up programme. If a patient is excluded from a surveillance regimen, it is important to inform them about symptoms which could indicate recurrence and allow them immediate access to the physician.

As mentioned above, it is important to 'clean' the colon once by colonoscopy and preferably early in the postoperative period. Patients should also be seen soon after surgery to discuss surgery-related problems. It is the author's opinion that patients should be seen regularly during the first 5 years postoperatively. An increased level in a serum CEA test will indicate a recurrent tumour with high specificity (Northover 1986). Therefore if the CEA level is increasing, a thorough investigation dependent upon symptoms should be undertaken by the best techniques available. Furthermore, young patients and those with multiple adenomas at surgery should have a colonoscopy every third or fourth year.

Recurrent colorectal cancer

A recurrence after curative surgery for colorectal cancer is either distant or local or a combination thereof. The most frequent sites of recurrent tumour after 'curative' surgery are the liver, the local tumour site and the lung (Gilbert et al 1984, Gunderson & Sosin 1974, Gunderson et al 1985). Hepatic metastases are more common if the primary tumour is situated in the colon, whereas rectal cancers relatively more commonly spread to the lungs (Lavin et al 1980). A local recurrence refers to a recurrent tumour within the area where the primary tumour was situated and is more common after rectal cancer surgery, i.e. in the pelvis.

Diagnosis of recurrence

The patient may present with a specific symptom indicating a recurrence. Patients with lung secondaries often have dyspnoea or cough and if liver metastases are present pain or tenderness in the right hypochondrium is common. Jaundice can also be a sign of hepatic metastases. Other typical signs of recurrent disease can be distension of the abdomen indicating ascites or abdominal pain with signs of bowel obstruction. Pain in the back or pathological fractures can be a sign of spread to the bone. Although rare, brain metastases have their own symptomatology with loss of specific functions and sometimes epilepsy. Other obvious but rare signs of disseminated disease are subcutaneous nodes.

A local recurrence after rectal cancer surgery can have many different clinical features. The most common symptom is perineal or sacral pain. Also symptoms from the urogenital organs like vaginal bleeding or bladder dysfunction may indicate a recurrence. Ureteral obstruction may also be the result of a local recurrence as well as leg oedema or thrombosis indicating a recurrence in inguinal lymph nodes. If a sphincter-saving procedure has been performed the first sign of a recurrence can be peranal bleeding or changing bowel habit.

When a specific symptom is present it is often rather easy to confirm the recurrence. By the use of modern imaging techniques like ultrasound, CT or MRI scan, the liver and the paraaortic lymph nodes can easily be investigated. A plain chest X-ray may often disclose pulmonary metastases, although a CT scan of the lungs often gives more information. If recurrence is suspected an elevated serum CEA strongly supports the diagnosis. When symptoms of bone metatsases are present plain radiography over the suspicious area is often enough. Sometimes the use of a scintigraphic method is necessary to confirm the diagnosis.

The diagnostic procedure for a pelvic recurrence is sometimes difficult. In those having a sphincter-saving operation endoscopy combined with a rectal examination and a biopsy will often disclose the diagnosis. Vaginal examination is also important. Endoluminal ultrasonography via rectum or vagina is often helpful to confirm the clinical findings and is also a help for needle biopsies (Benyon 1989, Waizer et al 1991).

However, if patients just have perineal pain, and especially in those operated upon by abdominoperineal excision, the diagnosis can be difficult. The use of CT or MRI scan can in those cases be of value (Fig. 11.2), although most patients have postoperative fibrosis which can be difficult to distinguish from a recurrence (Adalsteinsson et al 1987). MRI scan is probably better able to distinguish recurrent tumour from fibrosis (Gromberg et al 1986, Waizer et al 1991). However, a CT-guided biopsy is often necessary. The use of a PET scan (positron emission tomography) has been claimed to be better than both CT and MRI scan, but this technique has to be investigated further before it can be recommended as a standard investigation (Schlag et al 1989).

The local recurrence rate after 'curative' surgery for rectal cancer differs enormously in the literature from <5% to >50% (Gunderson & Sosin 1974, Kranjia et al 1990, Morson et al 1963, Påhlman & Glimelius 1984, Phillips et al 1984). This difference can be explained by selection bias and how intensively patients have been followed.

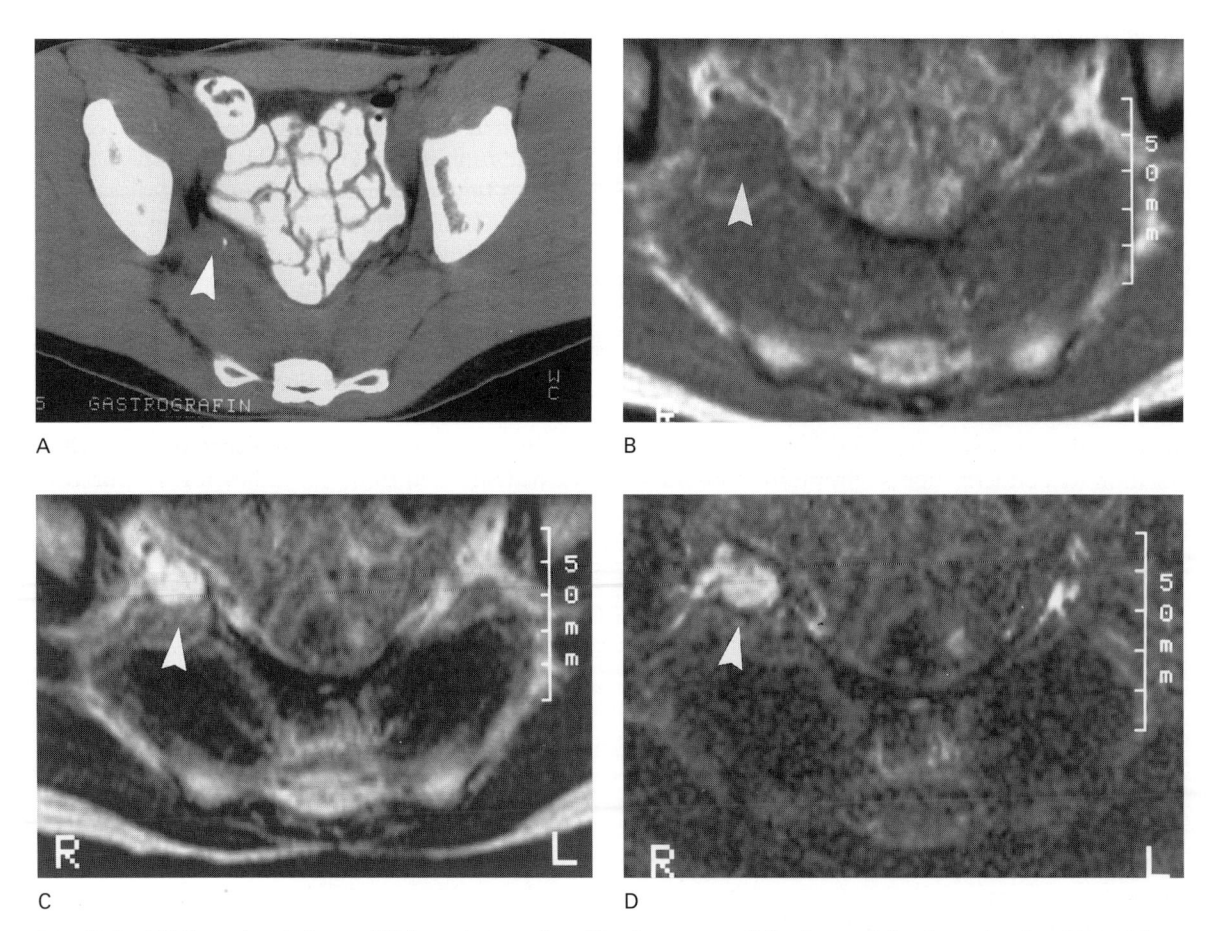

Fig. 11.2 (A) Suspicious lesion on CT (arrow) suggestive of local recurrence following an abdominoperineal excision of the rectum for rectal cancer. MRI improved the definition of this area and virtually confined it to be a recurrence. (B) T_1 weighted image. (C) T_2 weighted image. (D) Inversion recovery image.

However, the skill and experience of the surgeon is probably of the utmost importance. The best figures are presented from institutions with a special interest in colorectal surgery indicating that surgical skill is paramount.

It is difficult to interpret the data within this field. Several randomized trials evaluating perioperative radiotherapy as an adjuvant treatment have been carried out during the last two decades and interestingly no trial has demonstrated a local recurrence rate below 20% in the surgery-alone arm, indicating that local recurrence after 'curative' surgery for rectal cancer is an enormous problem (Påhlman & Glimelius 1992). Local recurrence following 'curative' surgery for colon cancer is not so well established but some studies indicate that the recurrence rate is of the same magnitude as for rectal cancer, i.e. approximately 20% (Gunderson et al 1985, Willett et al 1984).

Surgical treatment of recurrent cancer

The only possibility of curing patients with recurrent disease is a surgical resection of the recurrence. Liver resection for colorectal metastases is a well-documented therapy with a 5-year survival rate of approximately 30% and with almost no postoperative mortality today (see Ch. 12).

Most patients with pulmonary metastases are inoperable because of simultaneous disseminated recurrent disease to other organs. Approximately 10% of all patients with colorectal cancer will develop pulmonary metastases and in 10% of those patients, the metastatic disease is confined to the lung only (McCormack & Attiyeh 1979) and in this group thoracotomy and segmental resection of the lung will improve survival with a five-year survival rate varying from 20–40% (Brister et al 1988, Goya et al 1989, McCormack & Attiyeh 1979, Mansel et al 1986, Sauter et al 1990). The postoperative mortality after segmental or wedge resection is almost nil and in the future a thoracoscopic wedge resection for metastases is possible. The outcome is worse if multiple metastases are present, i.e. a similar result as after liver resection for colorectal cancer metastases.

The surgical management of non-hepatic intra-abdominal recurrences is often a challenge. The most common situation is to perform a laparotomy for bowel obstruction or an acute abdomen. It is often known that the patient has disseminated disease and a laparotomy should be avoided if at all possible due to the short life expectancy. However, conservative treatment is often unsuccessful and in quite a few patients surgical intervention is necessary for symptom relief or because of alarming symptomatology. Morbidity and mortality are high since patients have often deteriorated and are in a catabolic phase. The most common procedure is to bypass the obstruction with a side-to-side anastomosis or a proximal stoma and approximately 60% of these patients will be discharged from the hospital (Lau & Lorentz 1993). However, a second 'curative' procedure is possible in only very few patients (Gwin et al 1993, Lau & Lorentz 1993, Quentmeier et al 1990, Stulc et al 1986, Willett et al 1984). It is important to emphasize that the incidence of a benign cause of bowel obstruction is high, indicating that surgery is important and the rationale not to operate must be based on firm evidence of disseminated disease (Walsh & Schofield 1984).

'Second look' surgery based upon an increased serum CEA level or another tumour marker has been discussed earlier in this chapter. 'Second look' based on other criteria is a policy in some units. The rationale is, if possible, to give the patient a second chance with a 'curative' resection. The first report of 'second look' surgery by Wangensteen et al (1951) was enthusiastic. With new technology probably more patients will be found with asymptomatic recurrences due to different follow-up regimens. When surgeons are following their patients in a specific surveillance programme it is mandatory to accept the consequences and explore the abdominal cavity if no imaging techniques have found the recurrence and there is an obvious sign of metastatic disease. The value of 'second look' surgery is claimed to be good but the results have to be evaluated with caution, since a comparison with historical controls is always doubtful. No randomized trials have been carried out within this field, apart from the CEA 'second look' procedure mentioned previously (Northover & Slack 1984). With immunoscintigraphy (Collier et al 1992, Corman et al 1994, Petersen et al 1993, Winzelberg et al 1992) combined with radioimmunoguided surgery (Arnold et al 1992, Cohen et al 1991, Martin & Carey 1991) the results after a 'second look' operation might be better, but this new technology has to be evaluated more thoroughly before it can be recommended as a standard technique.

Local recurrence after 'curative' surgery for rectal cancer is difficult to treat and is often accompanied by pain and much suffering for the patient. It can not be emphasized enough that a local recurrence after rectal cancer surgery has to be prevented (Abulafi & Williams 1994). The use of adjuvant radiotherapy is widespread today and the local recurrence rate can be reduced by approximately 50% (Påhlman & Glimelius 1992) if the dose level is high enough (see Ch. 9). Education and training of surgeons is mandatory and in several countries there is today an ongoing discussion whether rectal cancer surgery should be performed by specifically trained colorectal surgeons or by general surgeons (Påhlman 1993).

When a recurrence has occurred it is rarely possible to perform a second 'curative' operation. Most suture-line tumours are pelvic recurrences growing from the pelvic wall into the lumen, indicating that very few patients can be 'cured' with a minor procedure. However, in the case of an anastomotic recurrence it is worthwhile giving prolonged preoperative radiotherapy combined with chemotherapy and after a recovery period of 3–4 weeks, trying to resect the tumour. With this approach some patients will survive but unfortunately the majority will not, although the quality of life may be improved without pelvic pain.

Surgery for a local recurrence after an abdominoperineal excision is not so successful. The most encouraging results have been reported by Wanebo & Margrove (1981) using an abdominosacral approach with an en bloc resection of the recurrent tumour and distal part of the sacrum. Simular enthusiastic results have been reported from Schiessel et al (1986) and Polk & Spratt (1979). However, only a small number (<5%) of the patients will survive more than 3 years and their quality of life, not always taken into account in the presentations, is probably impaired due to morbidity after such extensive surgery.

Palliative treatment

Unfortunately almost all patients with recurrent colorectal cancer have tumour spread which is incurable. Except in a small proportion of patients with localized hepatic and lung secondaries, no curative treatment is possible once distant spread has occurred. The median survival time after diagnosis is in the order of 6 months (Berge et al 1973, Moertel 1975). The need for palliative support is important since during this period many patients will suffer from anxiety, fatigue and pain.

Radiotherapy

Radiotherapy in the palliative treatment of colorectal cancer has mainly been used for pelvic recurrence and bone metastases.

The use of irradiation in pelvic recurrence has had two different aims. If the aim is to control the pain, a low dose has been used (20–30 Gy) and if pain recurs the treatment has been repeated (Griffith et al 1988, Herzog et al 1988, Overgaard et al 1984). The period of pain relief is approximately 6–8 months (Overgaard et al 1984). If the aim is to 'cure' the patients, a much higher dose has to be used (60–65 Gy). There are anecdotal cases reported where patients have been cured with radiotherapy (Overgaard et al 1984). The effect is even better when radiotherapy is combined with chemotherapy (5-Fu), but the toxicity will increase substantially with chemoradiotherapy (Wong et al 1991). The widespread use of adjuvant radiotherapy (both pre- and postoperative) will probably diminish the use of palliative radiotherapy, since the risk of damage to the surrounding tissue is obvious if the total cumulative dose of 65–70 Gy is exceeded.

In the treatment of bone metastases, mainly in the vertebrae and pelvic bones, radiotherapy will give excellent pain relief (Herzog et al 1988). Pain relief has also been demonstrated using radiotherapy when hepatic metastases are present (Lightdale et al 1979, Sherman et al 1978). Radiotherapy has also been used for brain metastases. However, due to the irradiation-induced oedema, these patients must be treated with corticosteroids.

Chemotherapy

Although colorectal cancer has traditionally been considered to be resistant to cytotoxic drugs, chemotherapy has been widely used in palliative treatment. It has no curative potential and the main endpoint in most trials has been objective tumour response. Criteria for assessment of responses have been defined by the UICC (Hayward & Rubens 1977) and criteria to assess drug-related toxicity by the WHO (Miller et al 1981).

It is difficult to interpret the results from different chemotherapy trials due to the heterogeneity of the patients in the trials arms. For example, bedridden and severely debilitated patients can expect a shorter survival compared with those fully capable of work. A common way to grade the general condition of cancer patients is according to a performance scale, such as the Karnofsky performance status (Karnofsky et al 1948) or the ECOG scale (Zubrod et al 1960). The performance status, white blood cell count and liver function tests are important prognostic factors for survival in advanced colorectal cancer (Edler et al 1986, Kemeny & Braun 1983). Performance status is one of the most important characteristics in patients with advanced colorectal cancer from a prognostic viewpoint. However, disease-free interval and the proportion of symptomatic patients may also affect the results of a clinical trial and a possible effect of these variables may wrongly be attributed to therapy (Graf et al 1991).

For many years the antimetabolite 5-fluorouracil (5-Fu) was the treatment of choice in advanced colorectal cancer with a reported objective tumour regression in about 20%, but no proven effect on survival (Cohen et al 1989). Due to the limited activity of 5-Fu alone, combinations have been used in order to biochemically modulate the 5-Fu effect. In an experimental model it was shown that administration of methotrexate before 5-Fu will improve the antitumoural effect (Bertino et al 1977) and in the Nordic randomized trial the combination of 5-Fu leucovorin and methotrexate was superior to 5-Fu alone (Nordic Gastrointestinal Tumor Adjuvant Therapy Group 1989). The findings that the effect of 5-Fu might be improved with the addition of folinic acid (leucovorin) reported by Waxman et al (1978) and Ullman et al (1978) have been substantiated in several clinical trials (Advanced Colorectal Cancer Meta-analysis Project 1992). However, there is no consensus on the optimal dose and schedule of 5-Fu and leucovorin (Erlichman 1991). The combination of 5-Fu and levamisole (Laurie et al 1989, Moertel at al 1990), the standard adjuvant treatment in most countries today, has not been tested in advanced cancer.

In general practice today, surgeons should be more aware of the good effects and not only the adverse effects of using palliative chemotherapy (Cunningham & Findlay 1993, Moertel 1994). If 5-Fu is combined with methotrexate and leucovorin the effect on symptom relief is approximately 50% (Nordic Gastrointestinal Tumor Adjuvant Therapy Group 1989). Since the toxicity with leucovorin is mainly gastrointestinal and lethal toxicity may occur if methotrexate is given to patients with impaired kidney function, it is advisable to use 5-Fu combined with leucovorin.

The question is when should this treatment be started? Should we wait until patients have developed symptoms or should the treatment be started as soon as possible after diagnosis of disseminated disease? Only one trial has studied the effect of palliative chemotherapy versus no treatment (Nordic Gastrointestinal Tumor Adjuvant Therapy Group 1992). In this trial patients with asymptomatic generalized colorectal cancer were randomized either to on expectant regime or early chemotherapy (5-Fu, methotrexate + leucovorin rescue). The group of patients who started chemotherapy immediately survived 6–8 months longer than the expectancy group, but no patient was cured with this regimen. According to these data, early commencement of chemotherapy can be justified. However, it is important to inform the patient about the adverse effects and to evaluate the effect of the treatment after 4–5 courses (approximately 4 months). If no response has occurred, treatment should be stopped. Since no good 'second line' therapy is available in colorectal cancer, patients who do not respond to the above combination should be followed with the best supportive care.

New technology

Immunotherapy is another promising approach in the treatment of patients with disseminated colorectal cancer. The median objective response rate with a combination of 5-Fu and interferon-α is 35% (Dahhauser et al 1993, Diaz-Rubio et al 1992, Wadler et al 1989, Weh et al 1992). The effect is of the same magnitude as for 5-Fu combined with leucovorin. In general practice the use of 5-Fu and leucovorin is probably better, since the toxicity is worse using 5-Fu and interferon (fatigue and treatment-induced fever).

Other mechanisms in immunotherapy have been used, such as interleukin 2 (IL-2) and lymphokine activated killer (LAK) cells. Promising results have been achieved in melanoma and renal cancer, but the results in colorectal cancer are not impressive (Johnson et al 1989, Rosenberg et al 1987). Monoclonal antibodies have also been used in the treatment of advanced colorectal cancer. The results are not as good as for chemotherapy and the treatment is more expensive. This form of therapy, however, is still recognized as experimental. Also, monoclonal antibodies attached to cancericidal agents have been used but only in animal models (Hyams et al 1987) and clinical trials are awaited.

Another approach which has recently been described is the use of intraoperative photodynamic therapy. The purpose with this type of treatment is to destroy residual recurrent tumour after surgical excision. A photosensitizing drug, haematoporphyrin derivate, is given preoperatively and the area of residual tumour is irradiated with a special dye laser. Singlet oxygen is released from the haematoporphyrin derivate which is cytotoxic (Allardice et al 1992). So far no deleterious effects have been shown with this treatment but it is too early to evaluate the effect on tumours.

Conclusion

Adenocarcinoma of the colon and rectum is one of the most common malignant tumours in the Western world with a peak incidence occurring at the age of 70–80 years. Roughly two-thirds of the patients will have 'curative' surgery (Berge et al 1973, Davis et al 1987, Påhlman et al 1985) and only half of these will survive for 5 years (Habib et al 1983, Öhman 1982). In spite of efforts aimed at early detection and modifications of the surgical technique, the survival prospects have only been moderately improved (Enblad et al 1988, Öhman 1982).

If a patient presents with residual or recurrent colorectal cancer, 'curative' treatment options are rare. New drugs or combinations of drugs or new treatment modalities should become available in the future. It is important to evaluate these modalities in a scientific way using randomized trials to explore their efficacy. The nihilistic approach from some quarters regarding chemotherapy and other non-surgical treatment modalities has to be changed. After providing full information, most patients want some type of treatment to obtain relief of symptoms and/or the possibility of a prolonged life. A good collaboration with medical oncologists and radiotherapists is necessary to provide acceptable palliation to this huge group of patients.

References

Abulafi AM, Williams NS 1994 Local recurrence of colorectal cancer: the problem, mechanisms, management and adjuvant therapy. British Journal of Surgery 81: 7–19

Adalsteinsson B, Påhlman L, Hemmingsson A, Glimelius B, Graffman S 1987 Computed tomography in early diagnosis of local recurrence of rectal carcinoma. Acta Radiologica Diagnosis 28: 41–47

Advanced Colorectal Cancer Meta-analysis Project 1992 Modulation of fluorouracil by leucovorin in patients with advanced colorectal cancer: evidence in terms of response rate. Journal of Clinical Oncology 10: 896–903

Agrez MV, Ready R, Ilstrup D, Beart RW 1982 Metachronous colorectal malignancies. Diseases of the Colon and Rectum 25: 569–574

Allardice JT, Grahn MF, Rowland AC et al 1992 Safety studies for intraoperative photodynamic therapy. Lasers in Medical Science 7: 133–142

Anzano MA, Rieman D, Prichett W, Bowen-Poe DF, Grieg R 1989 Growth factor production by human colon carcinoma cell lines. Cancer Research 49: 2898–2904

Armitage NC, Ballantyne KC, Evans DF, Clarke P, Sheffield J, Hardcastle JD 1985 The influence of tumour cell DNA content on survival in colorectal cancer. A detailed analysis. British Journal of Cancer 62: 852–856

Arnold MW, Schneebaum S, Berens A, Mojzisik C, Hinkle G, Martin EW 1992 Radioimmunoguided surgery challenges traditional decision making in patients with primary colorectal cancer. Surgery 112: 624–630

Atkin WS, Morson BC, Cuzick J 1992 Long-term risk of colorectal cancer after excision of rectosigmoid adenomas. New England Journal of Medicine 326: 658–662

Attiyeh EF, Stearns MW 1981 Second look laparotomy based on CEA elevations in colo-rectal cancer. Cancer 47: 1229–1234

Ballantyne GH, Modlin IM 1988 Postoperative follow-up for colorectal cancer: who are we kidding? Journal of Clinical Gastroenterology 10: 359–364

Regent R, Rustin GJS 1989 Tumour markers: from carcinoembryonic antigen to products of hybridoma technology. Cancer Surveys 2: 107–121

Benyon J 1989 An evaluation of the role of rectal endosonography in rectal cancer. Annals of the Royal College of Surgeons of England 71: 131–139

Berge T, Ekelund G, Mellner C, Pihl B, Wenckert A 1973 Carcinoma of the colon and rectum in a defined population. Acta Chirurgica Scandinavica (suppl) 438(1)

Bertino JR, Sawicki WL, Lindquist CA, Gupta VS 1977 Schedule-dependent antitumour effects of methotrexate and 5-fluorouracil. Cancer Research 37: 327–328

Böhm B, Schwenk W, Hucke HP, Stock W 1993 Does methodic long-term follow-up affect survival after curative resection of colorectal cancer? Diseases of the Colon and Rectum 36: 280–286

Brister SJ, Varennes BD, Gordon PH, Sheiner WM, Pym J 1988 Contemporary operative management of pulmonary metastases of colorectal origin. Diseases of the Colon and Rectum 31: 786–792

Bussey HJ, Wallace MH, Morson BC 1967 Metachronous carcinoma of the large intestine and intestinal polyps. Journal of the Royal Society of Medicine 60: 208–210

Cali RK, Pitsch RM, Thorson AG, Watson P, Tapia P, Blatchford GJ, Christensen MA 1993 Cumulative incidence of metachronous colorectal cancer. Diseases of the Colon and Rectum 36: 388–393

Chapuis PH, Dent OF, Fisher R, Newland RC, Pheils MT, Smyth E, Colquhoun K 1985 A multivariate analysis of clinical and pathological variables in prognosis after resection of large bowel cancer. British Journal of Surgery 72: 698–702

Cohen AM, Shank B, Friedman MA 1989 Colorectal cancer. In: DeVita VT, Hellman S, Rosenberg SA (eds). Cancer principles and practice of oncology, 3rd edn. J.B. Lippincott, Philadelphia, p 895–964

Cohen AM, Martin EW, Lavery I et al 1991 Radioimmuno-guided surgery using iodine-125 B72.3 in patients with colorectal cancer. Archives of Surgery 126: 349–352

Collier BD, Abdel-Nabi H, Doerr RJ et al 1992 Immunoscintigraphy performed with In-111-labeled CYT-103 in the management of colorectal cancer: comparison with CT. Radiology 185: 179–186

Corman ML, Galandiuk S, Block GE et al 1994 Immunoscintigraphy with ^{111}In-Satumomab Pendetide in patients with colorectal adenocarcinoma: performance and impact on clinical management. Diseases of the Colon and Rectum 37: 129–137

Cunliffe WJ, Hasleton PS, Tweedle DE, Schofield PF 1984 Incidence of synchronous and metachronous colorectal carcinoma. British Journal of Surgery 71: 941–943

Cunningham D, Findlay M 1993 The chemotherapy of colon cancer can no longer be ignored. European Journal of Cancer 29A: 2077–2079

Dahhauser LL, Freiman JH, Gilchrist TL, Gutterman JU, Hunter CY, Yeomans AC, Markowitz AB 1993 Phase I and pharmacokinetic study of infusional fluorouracil combined with recombinant interferon alfa-2b in patients with advanced cancer. Journal of Clinical Oncology 11: 751–761

Davis NC, Evans EB, Cohen JR, Theile DE, Job DM 1987 Colorectal cancer: a large unselected Australian series. Australasian and New Zealand Journal of Surgery 57: 153–159

Diaz-Rubio E, Jimeno J, Camps C et al 1992 Treatment of advanced colorectal cancer with recombinant interferon alpha and fluorouracil: activity in liver metastases. Clinical Investigation 10: 259–264

Dukes CE, Bussey HJR 1958 The spread of rectal cancer and its effects on prognosis. British Journal of Cancer 12: 309–320

Edler L, Heim ME, Quintero C, Brummer T, Queisser W 1986 Prognostic factors of advanced colorectal cancer patients. European Journal of Cancer Clinics and Oncology 22: 1231–1237

Enblad P, Adami HO, Bergström R, Glimelius B, Krusemo U, Påhlman L 1988 Improved survival of patients with cancers of the colon and rectum? Journal of the National Cancer Institute 80: 586–591

Enblad P, Glimelius B, Bengtsson A, Pontén J, Påhlman L 1985 DNA content in the carcinoma of the rectum and rectosigmoid. Acta Pathologica Microbiologica Immunologica Scandinavica 93: 277–284

Enker WE, Kramer RG 1982 The follow-up of patients after definitive resection for large bowel cancer. World Journal of Surgery 6: 578–584

Erlichman C 1991 Clinical experience in the treatment of colon and rectal cancer with fluorouracil and folinic acid. In: Adad A (ed) Medical treatment of colorectal cancer. Graficas Monterreina, Madrid, p 93–105

Gilbert JM, Feffrey I, Evans M, Kark AE 1984 Sites of recurrent tumour after 'curative' colorectal surgery: implications for adjuvant therapy. British Journal of Surgery 71: 203–205

Gilbertson VA, Nelms JM 1978 The prevention of invasive cancer of the rectum. Cancer 41: 1137–1139

Goya T, Miyazawa N, Kondo H, Tsuchiya R, Naruke T, Suemasu K 1989 Surgical resection of pulmonary metastases from colorectal cancer: 10-year follow-up. Cancer 64: 1418–1421

Graf W, Glimelius B, Påhlman L, Bergström R 1991 Determinants of prognosis in advanced colorectal cancer. European Journal of Cancer 27: 1119–1123

Griffith CDM, Ballantyne KC, Pollard S et al 1988 Radiotherapy for palliation of residual and recurrent rectal cancer. Journal of the Royal College of Surgeons of Edinburgh 33: 25–27

Gromberg JS, Friedman AC, Radecki PD, Grumbach K, Caroline DF 1986 MRI differentiation of recurrent colorectal carcinoma from postoperative fibrosis. Gastrointestinal Radiology 11: 361–363

Gunderson LL, Sosin H 1974 Areas of failure found at reoperation (second or symptomatic look) following 'curative surgery' for adenocarcinoma of the rectum. Clinicopathologic correlation and implications for adjuvant treatment. Cancer 34: 1278–1292

Gunderson LL, Sosin H, Levitt S 1985 Extrapelvic colon–areas of failure in a reoperation series: implications for adjuvant therapy. International Journal of Radiation, Oncology, Biology and Physics 11: 731–741

Gwin JL, Hoffman JP, Eisenberg BL 1993 Surgical management of nonhepatic intra-abdominal recurrence of carcinoma of the colon. Diseases of the Colon and Rectum 36: 540–544

Habib NA, Peck MA, Sawyer CN, Blaxland JW, Luck RJ 1983 An analysis of the outcome of 301 malignant colorectal tumors. Diseases of the Colon and Rectum 26: 601–605

Halvorsen TB, Seim E 1988 Degree of differentiation in colorectal adenocarcinoma: a multivariate analysis of the influence on survival. Journal of Clinical Pathology 41: 532–537

Hayward JL, Rubens RD 1977 Assessment of response to therapy in advanced breast cancer. British Journal of Cancer 35: 292–298

Heald RJ, Bussey HJR 1975 Clinical experiences at St. Marks's Hospital with multiple synchronous cancer of the colon. Diseases of the Colon and Rectum 18: 6–10

Heald RJ, Lockhart-Mummery HE 1972 The lesion of the second cancer of the large bowel. British Journal of Surgery 59: 16–19

Herzog J, Schmidt B, Fassbender T, Hübener K-H 1988 Die Stellung der Stralentherapie in der Behandlung von Lokalrezidiven bei Rehtumkarzinomen. Stralentherapie und Onkologie 164: 121–128

Hyams DM, Esteban JM, Lollo CP, Beatty BG, Beatty JD 1987 Therapy of peritoneal carcinomatosis of colon cancer xenografts and yttrium-90 labelled anti carcinoembryonic antigen antibody ZCE025. Archives of Surgery 122: 1333–1337

Jahn H, Joergensen OD, Kronborg O, Fenger C 1992 Can Hemoccult-II™ replace colonoscopy in surveillance after radical surgery for colorectal cancer and after polypectomy? Diseases of the Colon and Rectum 35: 253–256

Jass JR, Atkin WS, Cuzick J, Bussey HJR, Morson BC, Northover JMA, Todd IP 1986 The grading of rectal cancer: historical perspectives and a multivariate analysis of 447 cases. Histopathology 10: 437–459

Johnson DH, Williams NS, Newland AC et al 1989 Intraperitoneal production and systematic transfer of lymphokine activated killer (LAK) cells for treatment of disseminated gastrointestinal adenocarcinoma. British Journal of Surgery 76: 626–630

Karnofsky DA, Abelman WH, Craver LF, Burchenal JH 1948 The use of the nitrogen mustards in palliative treatment of carcinoma. Cancer 1: 634–656

Kemeny N, Braun DW 1983 Prognostic factors in advanced colorectal carcinoma. Importance of lactic dehydrogenase level, performance status and white blood cell count. American Journal of Medicine 74: 786–794

Kranjia ND, Schache DJ, North WR, Heald RJ 1990 'Close shave' in anterior resection. British Journal of Surgery 63: 673–677

Kronborg O 1986 Controversies in follow-up after colorectal carcinoma. Theoretical Surgery 1: 40–46

Kronborg O, Hage E, Deichgraeber E 1983 The remaining colon after radical surgery for colorectal cancer. The first three years of a prospective study. Diseases of the Colon and Rectum 26: 172–176

Kronborg O, Fenger C, Deichgraeber E, Hansen L 1988 Follow-up after radical surgery for colorectal cancer: design of a randomized study. Scandinavian Journal of Gastroenterology 23: 159–162

Langevin JM, Nivatvongs S 1984 The true incidence of synchronous cancer of the large bowel. A prospective study. American Journal of Surgery 147: 330–333

Lau PWK, Lorentz TG 1993 Results of surgery for malignant bowel obstruction in advanced, unresectable, recurrent colorectal cancer. Diseases of the Colon and Rectum 36: 61–64

Laurie JA, Moertel CG, Fleming TR et al 1989 Surgical adjuvant therapy of large bowel carcinoma: an evaluation of levamisole and the combination of levamisole and fluorouracil. Journal of Clinical Oncology 7: 1447–1456

Lavin P, Mittelman A, Douglass H, Engström P, Klaassen D 1980 Survival and response to chemotherapy for advanced colorectal adenocarcinoma. Cancer 46: 1536–1543

Levy AT, Cioce V, Sobel ME, Gabrisa S, Grigioni WF, Liotta LA, Settler-Stevenson WG 1991 Increased expression of the M_r 72,000 Type VI collagenase in human colonic adenocarcinoma. Cancer Research 51: 439–444

Lightdale CJ, Wasser J, Coleman M 1979 Anticoagulation and high dose liver radiation. A preliminary report. Cancer 43: 174–179

Lindmark G 1992 Perioperative predictors of tumour stage and prognosis in colorectal cancer. Doctoral thesis, Acta Universtatis Upsaliensis 375

Lindmark G, Glimelius B, Påhlman L, Enblad E 1991 Heterogeneity in ploidy and S-phase fraction in colorectal adenocarcinomas. International Journal of Colorectal Diseases 6: 115–120

Lindmark G, Gerdin B, Påhlman L, Glimelius B, Gehlsen K, Rubin K 1993 Interconnection of integrins 2 and 3 and structure of the basal membrane in colorectal cancer; relation to survival. European Journal of Surgical Oncology 19: 50–60

Lindmark G, Gerdin B, Påhlman L, Bergström R, Glimelius B 1994 Prognostic predictors in colorectal cancer. Diseases of the Colon and Rectum 37: 1219–1227

Luchtefeld MA, Ross DS, Zander JD, Folse JR 1987 Late development of metachronous colorectal cancer. Diseases of the Colon and Rectum 30: 180–184

Lunde OCH, Havig O 1982 Clinical significance of carcinoembryonic antigen (CEA) in patients with adenocarcinoma in colon and rectum. Acta Chirurgica Scandinavica 148: 189–193

Mansel JK, Zinmeister AR, Pairolero PC, Jett JR 1986 Pulmonary resection of metastatic colorectal adenocarcinoma: a ten-year experience. Chest 89: 109–112

Martin EW, Carey LC 1991 Second-look surgery for colorectal cancer. The second time around. Annals of Surgery 214: 321–327

Martin EW, Minton JP, Carey LC 1985 CEA directed second look surgery in the asymptomatic patients after primary resection of colorectal cancer. Annals of Surgery 202: 310–317

McCormack PM, Attiyeh FF 1979 Resected pulmonary metastases from colorectal cancer. Diseases of the Colon and Rectum 22: 553–556

Miller AB, Hoogstraten B, Staquet M, Winkler A 1981 Reporting results of cancer treatment. Cancer 47: 207–214

Moertel CG 1975 Clinical management of advanced gastrointestinal cancer. Cancer 36: 675–682

Moertel CG 1994 Chemotherapy for colorectal cancer. New England Journal of Medicine 330: 1136–1142

Moertel CG, Schutt AJ, Go VLM 1978 Carcinoembryonic antigen test for recurrent colorectal carcinoma. Inadequacy for early detection. Journal of the American Medical Association 239: 1065–1066

Moertel CG, Fleming TR, Macdonald JS et al 1990

Levamisole and fluorouracil for adjuvant therapy of resected colon carcinoma. New England Journal of Medicine 322: 352–358

Moertel CG, O'Fallon JR, Go VLM, O'Connell MJ, Thynne GS 1986 The preoperative carcinoembryonic antigen test in the diagnosis, staging and prognosis of colorectal cancer. Cancer 58: 603–610

Moore M, Jones DJ, Schofield PF, Harnden DG 1989 Current status of tumour markers in large bowel cancer. World Journal of Surgery 13: 52–59

Morson BC, Vaughan EG, Bussey HJR 1963 Pelvic recurrence after excision of rectum for carcinoma. British Medical Journal ii: 13–18

Nathanson SD, Schultz L, Tilley B, Kambrouris A 1986 Carcinoma of the colon and rectum. A comparison of staging classifications. American Surgeon 52: 428–433

Nathanson SD, Linden MD, Tender P, Zarbo RJ, Jacobsen G, Nelson LT 1994 Relationship among p53, stage, and prognosis of large bowel cancer. Diseases of the Colon and Rectum 37: 527–534

Northover JMA 1986 Carcinoembryonic antigen and recurrent colo-rectal cancer. Gut 27: 117–122

Northover JMA, Slack WW 1984 A randomized controlled trial of CEA prompted second look surgery in recurrent colo-rectal cancer: a preliminary report. Diseases of the Colon and Rectum 27: 576–581

Nordic Gastrointestinal Tumor Adjuvant Therapy Group 1989 Superiority of sequential methotrexate, fluorouracil, and leucovorin to fluorouracil alone in advanced symptomatic colorectal carcinoma: a randomized trial. Journal of Clinical Oncology 7: 1437–1446

Nordic Gastrointestinal Tumor Adjuvant Therapy Group 1992 Expectancy or primary chemotherapy in patients with advanced asymptomatic colorectal cancer: a randomized trial. Journal of Clinical Oncology 10: 904–911

Offerhaus GJA, Giardiello FM, Bruijin JA, Stinjen T, Molyvas EN, Fleuren GJ 1991 The value of immunohistochemistry for collagen IV expression in colorectal carcinomas. Cancer 67: 99–105

Öhman U 1982 Colorectal carcinoma – trends and results over a 30-year period. Diseases of the Colon and Rectum 25: 431–440

Overgaard M, Overgaard J, Sell A 1984 Dose–response relationship for radiation therapy of recurrent, residual and primarily inoperable colorectal cancer. Radiotherapy and Oncology 1: 217–225

Pagana TJ, Ledesma EJ, Mittelman A, Nava HR 1984 The use of colonoscopy in the study of synchronous colorectal neoplasms. Cancer 53: 356–359

Påhlman L 1993 Kvalitetsutredning om rectalcancerkirurgi. Ökad specialisering nödvändig. Läkartidningen 90: 2853–2855

Påhlman L, Glimelius B 1984 Local recurrences after surgical treatment for rectal carcinoma. Acta Chirurgica Scandinavica 150: 331–335

Påhlman L, Glimelius B 1992 Pre-operative and post-operative radiotherapy and rectal cancer. World Journal of Surgery 16: 858–865

Påhlman L, Glimelius B, Enblad P 1985 Clinical characteristics and their relation to surgical curability in adenocarcinoma of the rectum and rectosigmoid. Acta Chirurgica Scandinavica 151: 685–693

Petersen BM, Bass BL, Bates HR, Chandeysson PL, Harmon JW 1993 Use of the radiolabeled murine monoclonal antibody ^{111}In-CYT-103, in the management of colon cancer. American Journal of Surgery 165: 137–143

Phillips RKS, Hittinger R, Blesovsky L, Fry JS, Fielding LP 1984 Local recurrence following 'curative' surgery for large bowel cancer: II. The rectum and rectosigmoid. British Journal of Surgery 71: 17–20

Polk HC, Spratt JS 1979 The results of treatment of perineal recurrence of cancer of the rectum. Cancer 43: 952–955

Rosenberg SA, Lotze MT, Muyl LM et al 1987 A progress report on treatment of 157 patients with advanced cancer using lymphokine activated killer cells and interleukin 2 or high dose interleukin 2 alone. New England Journal of Medicine 316: 889–897

Quentmeier A, Schlag P, Smok M, Herfath C 1990 Reoperation for recurrent colorectal cancer: the importance of early diagnosis for resectability and survival. European Journal of Surgical Oncology 16: 319–325

Quirke P, Dixon MF, Clayden AD, Durdey P, Dyson JED, Williams NS, Bird CC 1987 Prognostic significance of DNA aneuploidy and cell proliferation in rectal adenocarcinomas. Journal of Pathology 151: 285–291

Safi F, Link KH, Beger HG 1993 Is follow-up of colorectal cancer patients worthwhile? Diseases of the Colon and Rectum 36: 636–644

Sauter EU, Bolton JS, Willis GW, Farr GH, Sardi A 1990 Improved survival after pulmonary resection of metastatic colorectal carcinoma. Journal of Surgical Oncology 43: 135–138

Schiessel R, Wunderlich M, Herbst F 1986 Local recurrence of colorectal cancer: effect of early detection and aggressive surgery. British Journal of Surgery 73: 342–344

Schlag P, Lehner B, Strauss LG, Georgi P, Herfarth C 1989 Scar or recurrent rectal cancer; PET is more helpful for diagnosis than immunoscintigraphy. Archives of Surgery 124: 197–200

Selby JV, Friedman GD, Quesenberry CJ, Weiss NS 1992 A case-control study of screening sigmoidoscopy and mortality from colorectal cancer. New England Journal of Medicine 326: 653–657

Sherman DM, Weichselbaum R, Order SE 1978 Palliation of hepatic metastases. Cancer 41: 2013–2016

Staab HJ, Andere FA, Stumpf E, Fisher R 1978 Slope analysis of the postoperative CEA time course and its possible application as an aid in diagnosis of disease progression in gastrointesinal cancer. American Journal of Surgery 136: 322–327

Ståhle E, Glimelius B, Bergström R, Påhlman L 1988a Preoperative clinical and pathological variables in prognostic evaluation of patients with rectal cancer: a prospective study of 327 consecutive patients. Acta Chirurgica Scandinavica 154: 792–797

Ståhle E, Glimelius B, Bergström R, Påhlman L 1988b Preoperative serum markers in carcinoma of the rectum and rectosigmoid. II. Prediction of prognosis. European Journal of Surgical Oncology 14: 287–296

Ståhle E, Glimelius B, Bergström R, Påhlman L 1989 Preoperative prediction of late cancer-specific deaths in patients with rectal and rectosigmoid carcinoma. International Journal of Colorectal Disease 4: 182–187

Stulc JP, Petrelli NJ, Herrera L, Mittelman A 1986 Anastomotic recurrence of adenocarcinoma of the colon. Archives of Surgery 121: 1077–1080

Törnqvist A, Ekelund G, Leandoer L 1982 The value of intensive follow-up after curative resection for colorectal carcinoma. British Journal of Surgery 69: 725–728

Ullman B, Lee M, Martin DW, Santi D V 1978 Cytotoxicity of 5-fluoro-2'-deoxyuridine: requirement for reduced folate cofactors and antagonism by methotrexate. Proceedings of the National Academy of Science USA 75: 980–983

Umpleby HC, Fremor B, Symes MO, Williamson RCN 1984 Viability of exfoliated colorectal carcinoma cells. British Journal of Surgery 71: 659–663

Vernava III AM, Longo WE, Vigro KS, Coplin MA, Wade TP, Johnson FE 1994 Current follow-up strategies after resection of colon cancer. Results of a survey of members of the American Society of Colon and Rectal Surgeons. Diseases of the Colon and Rectum 37: 573–583

Wadler S, Schwartz EL, Goldman M et al 1989 Fluorouracil and recombinant alpha-2a-interferon: an active regimen against advanced colorectal carcinoma. Journal of Clinical Oncology 7: 1769–1775

Waizer A, Powsner E, Russo I et al 1991 Prospective comparative study of magnetic resonance imaging versus transrectal ultrasound for preoperative staging and follow-up of rectal cancer. Diseases of the Colon and Rectum 34: 1068–1072

Walsh HP, Schofield PF 1984 Is laparotomy for small bowel obstruction justified in patients with previously treated malignancy? British Journal of Surgery 71: 933–935

Wanebo HH, Margrove RC 1981 Abdominal sacral resection of locally recurrent rectal cancer. Annals of Surgery 194: 458–465

Wangensteen OH, Lewis FJ, Tongen LA 1951 The 'second-look' in cancer surgery. Lancet 71: 303–307

Waxman S, Bruckner H, Wagle A, Schreiber C 1978 Potentiation of 5-fluorouracil effect by leucovorin. Proceedings of the American Association of Cancer Research 19: 149–153

Weh HJ, Platz D, Braumann D et al 1992 Phase II trial of 5-fluorouracil and recombinant interferon alfa-2b in metastatic colorectal carcinoma. European Journal of Cancer 28A: 1820–1823

Weidner N, Semple JP, Weich WR, Folkman J 1991 Tumour angiogenesis and metastasis-correlation in invasive breast carcinoma. New England Journal of Medicine 324: 1–8

Willett CG, Tepper JE, Cohen AM, Orlow E, Welch CE 1984 Failure patterns following curative resection of colonic carcinoma. Annals of Surgery 200: 685–690

Winzelberg GG, Grossman SJ, Rizk S et al 1992 Indium-111 monoclonal antibody B72.3 scintigraphy in colorectal cancer. Cancer 69: 1656–1663

Wong CS, Cummings BJ, Keane TJ et al 1991 Combined radiation therapy, mitomycin C, and 5-fluorouracil for locally recurrent rectal carcinoma: results of a pilot study. International Journal of Radiation, Oncology, Biology and Physics 21: 1291–1296

Zeng Z, Cohen AM, Urmacher C 1993 Usefulness of carcinoembryonic antigen monitoring despite normal preoperative values in node-positive colon cancer patients. Diseases of the Colon and Rectum 36: 1063–1068

Zubrod CG, Schneiderman M, Frei E, Brindley C 1960 Appraisal of methods for the study of chemotherapy of cancer in man: comparative therapeutic trial of nitrogen mustard and triethylene thiophosphoramide. Journal of Chronical Diseases 11: 7–23

12 Treatment of colorectal liver metastases

T. J. BABINEAU   G. STEELE, Jr

Introduction

Although virtually any solid tumour has the propensity to metastasize to the liver, only carcinomas of the colon and rectum produce metastatic lesions amenable (10–15% of the time) to curative surgical resection. This chapter deals with the biological characteristics of these metastatic lesions and the clinical characteristics of the patient one must select before embarking on hepatic resection for isolated recurrent colorectal carcinoma.

The liver has always been viewed with caution by surgeons. Although long known to be a common site for metastases, the liver's size and redundant blood supply had, until the last three decades, rendered it 'off limits' when considering major surgical resection of metastatic or primary tumours. However, with our enhanced understanding of the liver's anatomy and function (largely through advances in hepatic transplant surgery) selected primary and metastatic tumours of the liver may now be approached with a reasonable expectation for good outcome, occasionally even cure. More recent refinements in understanding the segmental anatomy of the liver, better perioperative care and improved anaesthetic and surgical techniques including complete vascular isolation, improved blood salvage and modifications of 'finger fracture' technique, along with a better appreciation of the biological limitations of metastatic tumour resection or cryoablation, have all made hepatic surgery a realistic treatment option for selected patients with isolated colorectal cancer metastases.

Our interest in regional therapy for colorectal carcinoma metastatic to the liver began during the resurgence of the Cady and Oberfeld approach of hepatic arterial infusion using either 5-fluorouracil (5-FU) or fluorodeoxyuridine (FUDR) (Steele 1991). Although the early experience (in the late 1960s and early 1970s) resulted in greater response rates than when patients were treated with systemic or oral 5-FU, the complications associated with this therapy were significant. The major reason for renewed interest in hepatic arterial infusion treatment was the introduction of the Infusaid^{TM} pump plus updated pharmacokinetic studies showing efficient hepatic extraction of FUDR, implying greater tumour effect and less systemic toxicity. Initial single institution studies of hepatic arterial FUDR infusion were quite varied in their results, probably because patients treated were highly selected and the definition of 'success' unclear (Weiss et al 1983).

A number of well-done national and international prospective studies have now been completed in which a clearcut increased probability of tumour response was found when FUDR was given via the hepatic arterial route compared to systemic treatment (Garnick et al 1983, Kemeny et al 1994, Weiss et al 1983). However, improvement in response rate is mitigated by three factors:

1 no significant increase in survival
2 the 'toxicity' of having to undergo a laparotomy for implantation of the pump
3 chemotherapy-related toxicity including a sclerosing cholangitis-type dose-related effect and bleeding gastritis/duodenitis due to back flow of chemotherapy from catheter tip malposition.

Taken together, these data lead us to recommend that except for a small minority of patients who have symptomatic liver-only (unresectable) disease, there is no justification for the use of hepatic arterial FUDR outside a formal trial setting. Thus, our group's continuing rationale for attempting to expand the surgical indications in treating hepatic metastases was (and remains) the lack of effective alternative treatments with curative potential.

Perspectives on the problem and background

The presentation of liver metastases from colorectal cancer is variable but usually takes one of three forms:

1. discovered at initial laparotomy for primary cancer resection
2. diagnosed later as part of a work-up for an elevated serum CEA
3. as a cause of symptoms (Saenz et al 1989).

If liver metastases are discovered at the time of initial laparotomy for colorectal cancer (synchronous disease occurs in 8–25% of patients), the primary tumour should be resected and followed by intraoperative staging of the liver with ultrasound, biopsy of the metastatic lesion and postoperative evaluation to determine the absence of additional extraabdominal disease recurrence. An exception to this occurs in any patient found to have a single liver metastasis when the operation for the primary colon or rectum cancer has gone smoothly and when the hepatic resection represents a relatively minor additional procedure (i.e. 'wedge' resection). Even in this setting, however, intraoperative ultrasonographic staging of the liver should be performed before embarking on resection to rule out any other unsuspected metastatic deposits within the liver (Stone et al 1994). Intraoperative ultrasound sensitivity is better than visual or palpation examination. Lesions as small as a 3–5 mm in diameter can be detected even in the depths of the right, left or caudate lobes.

It was estimated that 153 000 new cases of colorectal carcinoma was diagnosed in North America in 1994 and although the death rate from this disease has been decreasing, there will still be at least 58 000 deaths (Boring et al 1993). The predominant pattern of failure includes the liver as either the first or major site of distant disease spread (Ballantyne & Quin 1993, Steele 1994a) and 70–80% of patients who die from colorectal cancer will have liver involvement. However, although liver metastasis is often the primary determinant of patient survival, it is most often seen in the setting of diffuse disseminated disease, which makes surgical treatment irrelevant (Goslin et al 1982, Pestana et al 1964).

Only 9000 patients per year (less than 20% of patients in North America who experience recurrence after primary colon or rectum cancer resection) will be diagnosed with liver as the *only* site of failure, thus representing an extraordinarily biologically select subset (GITSG 1984, GITSG 1985, Steele 1994b). Taking this several steps further, of these 9000 patients, approximately 1000 to 1500 would be excluded from attempts at surgical resection due to comorbid disease and an additional 30–50% would be found at laparotomy to be ineligible for resection due to previously unsuspected extrahepatic or profuse intrahepatic disease. Of the 5000 remaining candidates for resection, assuming a 5% operative mortality (i.e. 250 perioperative deaths) and a 20–25% 5–10 year disease-free survival, no more than 1000 patients will be cured of their recurrent colorectal carcinoma by hepatic resection each year in North America. Finally, there is still some doubt that even these 1000 patients are cured, despite being so rigorously 'selected' since recent updated follow-up of the only prospective multiinstitutional liver resection trial has shown that there may be no plateau in the survival curve, even among the patients who had 'curative' resections (Steele 1995b). Such analysis puts the problem into the proper clinical perspective.

Any liver resection undertaken for isolated colorectal carcinoma recurrence must have cure, rather than palliation, as the goal. This important distinction is based on the fact that the great majority of patients who present with liver metastases do so with no symptoms. They are most often diagnosed by routine radiological studies prompted by a serial rise in serum CEA. This was clearly demonstrated in the Gastrointestinal Tumor Study Group (GITSG) 156-patient, 15 institution trial (GITSG 6584). Ninety percent of these patients were in the so-called 'zero' ECOG (Eastern Cooperative Oncology Group) performance group (i.e. no symptoms). Finally, for regional therapy of any kind (including liver resection) to be considered, there must be no extraregional disease.

The answer to the question 'Which patients with recurrent colorectal cancer should be candidates for a curative liver resection?' is best answered by reviewing the available single institution experiences with liver metastasis resection and the Hughes and Sugarbaker retrospective hepatic metastasis registry data (Hughes et al 1986, Hughes et al 1988, Steele & Ravikumar 1989) and expanding on reviews by Adson (1987) and Foster (Foster & Berman 1977). From these works (spanning an approximate 20-year period), it is apparent that there exists a highly select subset of patients who are theoretically curable of their recurrent (liver only) colorectal carcinoma. Whether the apparent cure rate is in fact a function of the surgery itself or whether surgery is functioning as a biological selection mechanism remains unclear. Nonetheless, a plateau in survival of 20–25%, 5–10 years following hepatic resection surgery for recurrent colorectal carcinoma has been implied.

Obviously, as one becomes more strict in excluding patients with multiple liver lesions or with disease outside the liver, the results from metastectomy will appear better. In addition, if one selects patients with more indolent disease (i.e. slow-growing lesions), results from resection will also seem better, but this success may well be attributable to lead time bias. Such selection biases may explain, in part, the differences observed among many single institution experiences after hepatic metastasis resection.

Since surgically staged, non-treatment controls cannot easily become a part of any prospective study of liver metastasis resection, one must rely on historical non-treated controls to gauge the efficacy of surgery. However, the historical controls must be carefully chosen to avoid artificially biasing in favour of whatever regional therapy is performed. It has become clear that most patients presenting to tertiary referral centres may already represent a biologically select group with relatively indolent tumour growth and consequently good survival expectations. The natural history studies of liver metastases are listed in Table 12.1. A number have characterized survival among selected patient subsets quite similar to those reported

Table 12.1 Liver metastases from colorectal cancer: natural history series (reprinted with permission from Steele & Ravikumar 1989)

Authors	Journal
Pestana C, Reitemeier RJ, Moertel CG et al	Am J Surg 1964; 108: 826–9
Jaffe BM, Donegan WL, Watson F et al	Surg Gynecol Obstet 1968; 127: 1–11
Bengmark S, Hafstrom L	Cancer 1969; 23: 198–202
Oxley FM, Ellis H	Br J Surg 1969; 56: 149–52
Cady B, Monson DO, Swinton NW	Surg Gynecol Obstet 1970; 131: 697–700
Abrams MS, Lerner HJ	Dis Colon Rectum 1971; 14: 431–4
Neilson J, Balsley I, Jensen H-E	Acta Chir Scand 1971; 137: 463–5
Baden H, Anderson B	Scand J Gastroenterol 1975; 10: 221–3
Wood CB, Gillis CR, Blumgart LH	Clin Onc 1976; 2: 285–9
Welch JP, Donaldson GA	Am J Surg 1978; 135: 505–11
Bengsson G, Calrsson G, Hafstrom L et al	Am J Surg 1981; 141: 586–9
Goslin R, Steele G Jr, Zamcheck N et al	Dis Colon Rectum 1982; 25: 749–54
Levin AN, Donegan WL, Irwin M	JAMA 1982; 247; 2809–10
Cady B	Semin Oncol 1983; 10: 127–33
Lahr CJ, Scong S-J, Cloud G et al	J Clin Oncol 1983; 1: 720–6
Wagner JS, Adson MA, van Heerden JA et al	Ann Surg 1984; 199: 502–7
Wood CB. In: van de Velde CJH, Sugarbaker P (eds)	Dordrecht: Martinus Nijhoff 1984; 47–54
Finan PJ, Marshall RJ, Cooper EH et al	Br J Surg 1985; 72: 373–7
Fujimoto S, Miyazaki M, Kitsukawa Y et al	Dis Colon Rectum 1985; 28: 588–91
Finlay IG, McArdle CS	Br J Surg 1986; 73: 732–5

176 Colorectal cancer

in the aforementioned hepatic resection series. Any surgical therapy, therefore, should be evaluated by comparison to these 'special' historical non-treated controls.

To date, there has been only one prospective multiinstitutional treatment plan which was undertaken to examine the efficacy of liver resection for patients with isolated metastatic disease from colorectal carcinoma. The study, begun in 1984, was the last trial performed by the Gastrointestinal Tumor Study Group (GITSG 6584) and was obviously compromised since randomization of patients to resection versus no resection after surgical staging was deemed both unethical and impractical. Despite this drawback, the trial managed to address a number of important questions:

1 How many patients were found to have unsuspected extrahepatic or diffuse intrahepatic disease at the time of exploration not allowing attempted resection for cure?
2 What was the surgical morbidity and mortality after resection?
3 What was the survival among patients resected for cure versus those who were found at surgery to have unresectable disease?
4 Were there any prognostic criteria that could be employed to exclude patients for whom surgery was ineffective?

In answering these questions the GITSG 6584 trial defined as the control group those patients who were found to have extrahepatic disease or unresectable disease within the liver at the time of laparotomy and did not undergo liver resection. The patients who did undergo resection were divided into two groups. The first were those patients that both the surgeon and the pathologist confirmed to be free of tumour at the margin of resection ('curative'). The second were patients found by the pathologist to have tumour at or near (i.e. <1cm) the resection margin ('non-curative resection').

The key endpoints of disease-free and overall survival have been analysed with a minimum follow-up of over 7 years. A total of 115 deaths have been reported to date. Forty four of the 69 patients who underwent curative resection have died. Fourteen of the 18 patients who underwent non-curative resection have died and 57 of the 63 in the non-resected group have died. Median survival times for patients receiving curative and non-curative resections and those receiving no resection at all are estimated to be 35.7, 21.2 and 16.5 months, respectively (Fig. 12.1). There was no significant difference in the survival distribution between the patients in the non-curative versus the non-resected treatment groups. However, survival among the curatively resected patients was significantly ($p=0.01$) superior to the distribution of non-curatively resected and non-resected patients. Among the 25 surviving patients who underwent curative resection, 16 remain free of disease. Six patients are alive more than 5 years from surgery and two of these six are disease-free. An estimate of 5-year survival probability for patients undergoing curative resection is currently approximately 23%, although the slope of the survival curve continues on a downward trend. Finally, no preoperative factors were identified that were predictive of resectability. Conventional CT scanning underestimated the number of lobes involved in one-third of the patients and overestimated involvement in 4%. Extrahepatic disease was discovered in 12% of patients with a

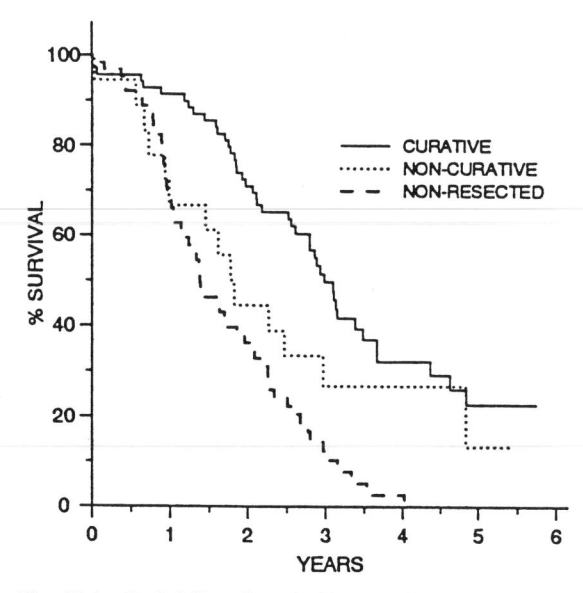

Fig. 12.1 Probability of survival by resection type. (Reprinted with permission from Steele 1994c.)

negative preoperative CT scan. Arteriography was performed in 82% of patients but was not helpful and is no longer recommended as part of preoperative staging.

Combining the recent update of the GITSG prospective data with the retrospective Hughes data, one soon realizes that most patients who undergo liver resection from isolated liver metastases will *not* be cured of their disease. Nonetheless, when resection is feasible, the chance for a 'complete response' remains higher than with any group of patients who undergo either systemic or regional (hepatic arterial) chemotherapy (Tables 12.2, 12.3 and 12.4). Inevitably, however, the high likelihood of recurrence either in the residual liver or outside the liver following resection makes the testing of effective regional or systemic therapy a compelling adjuvant question to be included in the patient's treatment regimen following resection (Kemeny et al 1993).

Preoperative staging of colorectal liver metastases

Given the rare chance of cure among even a biologically fortunate subset of patients, it becomes critically important to exclude those who can obviously not be helped by surgery. The past two decades have seen the development of

Table 12.2 Randomized trials evaluating intrahepatic arterial therapy (Infusaid) vs systemic 5-Fu (or 5-FUDR) in patients with metastatic colorectal cancer. Hepatic response (reprinted with permission from Steele 1993)

	Intraarterial	Systemic	Statistical significance
Memorial Sloan–Kettering	24/48 (50%)	10/51 (20%)	p=0.001
Northern California Oncology Group	21/50 (42%)	6/65 (10%)	p=0.0001
National Cancer Institute	13/21 (62%)	5/29 (17%)	p=0.003
North Central Cancer Treatment Group	14/26 (54%)	6/29 (21%)	p=0.01
French Cooperative Group*	34/70 (49%)	6/41 (14%)	NA

*Treatment given to 41/82 (50%) patients in systemic and 70/81 (86%) patients in intraarterial groups

Table 12.3 Randomized trials evaluating intrahepatic arterial therapy (Infusaid) vs systemic 5-Fu (or 5-FUDR) in patients with metastatic colon cancer. Median survival (months) (reprinted with permission from Steele 1993)

	Intra-arterial	Systemic	? Statistical significance
Memorial Sloan–Kettering*	17	12	No
Northern California Oncology Group*	17	16	No
National Cancer Institute	17	11	No
North Central Cancer Treatment Group	13	11	No
French Cooperative Group	14	10	p=0.02

*Crossover design

Table 12.4 Randomized trials evaluating intrahepatic arterial therapy (Infusaid) vs systemic 5-Fu (or 5-FUDR) in patients with metastatic colon cancer. Toxicity from intraarterial therapy (% patients treated) (reprinted with permission from Steele 1993)

	Gastritis/ulcer	Chemical hepatitis	Jaundice
Memorial Sloan–Kettering	17%	42%	8%
Northern California Oncology Group	NA	32%	16%
National Cancer Institute	38%	79%	21%
North Central Cancer Treatment Group	13%	NA	26%
French Cooperative Group	NA	63%	35%

178 Colorectal cancer

computed tomography (CT) scanning, magnetic resonance imaging (MRI), conventional (external) and intraoperative ultrasonography (US) and, most recently, laparoscopy and translaparoscopic ultrasonography, all of which have revolutionized the way in which the liver is imaged for the detection of primary or metastatic lesions.

Once a colorectal metastasis to the liver is suspected, staging is often best performed by CT scanning with or without vascular enhancement (Karl et al 1993). However, despite the results achieved by the most technologically advanced CT scan, ultrasonography is often the first rational diagnostic test in the radiological evaluation of a suspected liver metastasis. It is safe, relatively inexpensive and non-invasive (Ravikumar et al 1991a, 1991b).

Approximately one-third to one-half of all patients suspected of having liver-only or liver-predominant colorectal cancer metastases staged by conventional non-invasive diagnostic tests will be found at surgery to have extrahepatic disease or metastases within the liver too diffuse to allow surgical resection (Babineau et al 1994, Steele et al 1991, Vaughn & Haller 1993). During the past several years, laparoscopy and intraoperative ultrasonography have claimed a role in the surgical management of hepatic malignancies. These two diagnostic modalities can be used together to determine the resectability of a metastatic hepatic malignancy with minimal morbidity for the patient. Although neither of these can be used as 'screening' tests, both are capable of detecting lesions not appreciated preoperatively or, in the case of intraoperative ultrasonography, either visually or through palpation. This is particularly true for satellite lesions smaller than 1–1.5 cm in diameter or lesions located deep within the liver parenchyma. Since the resectability of metastatic hepatic lesions is dependent upon the surgeon's ability to make the liver 'disease free', intraoperative ultrasonography may demonstrate occult lesions or unfortunately positioned lesions that should preclude resection. Laparoscopy is also quite useful in demonstrating cirrhosis not suspected preoperatively (seen most often in the setting of hepatocellular carcinoma), identifying satellite tumour deposits in the liver and revealing previously unsuspected extrahepatic metastases.

All of these situations obviate any real benefit to the patient of major liver resection. If such high resolution staging can be done without the need for a full laparotomy, attempted resection should lead to a higher curative yield, with significantly less physiological toxicity.

Important considerations for hepatic resection

As the largest organ in the body (weighing approximately 1200–1500 g), the liver's gross and microscopic anatomy have been well characterized in most textbooks of surgery, yet the liver remains architecturally 'mysterious' to many surgeons. Its complex functions, dual blood supply, variable biliary and vascular anatomy and relative surgical inaccessibility make many general surgeons apprehensive when contemplating complex (or even straightforward!) hepatic surgery.

In 1957, Couinaud divided the liver into eight segments based primarily on the vascular supply as demonstrated by model casts produced by injections of the hepatic artery, portal vein and the bile ducts. The right lobe contains segments 5–8, while the left lobe contains segments 1–4 (Figs 12.2–5). Although extraordinarily elegant, these anatomic subdivisions are quite variable due to the extensive arborization of the intrahepatic vasculature. Hepatic resection primarily

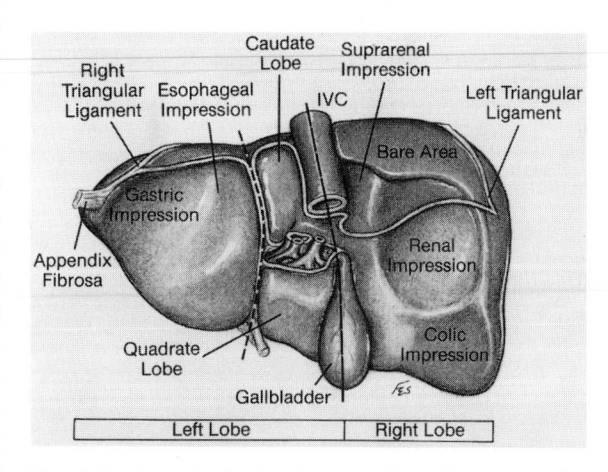

Fig. 12.2 Posterior landmarks of the liver. (Reprinted with permission by Warren et al 1991.)

Treatment of colorectal liver metastases 179

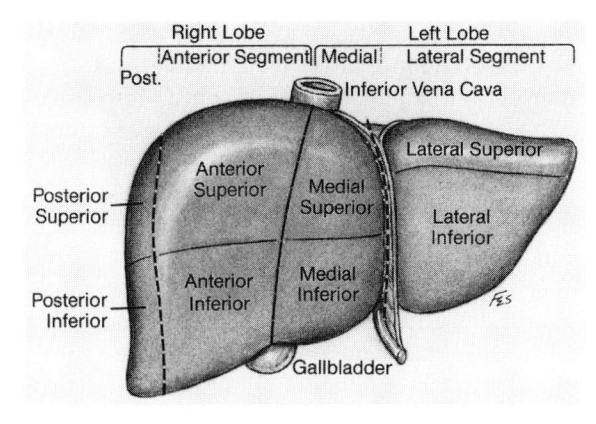

Fig. 12.3 Anterior surgical divisions of the liver. (Reprinted with permission by Warren et al 1991.)

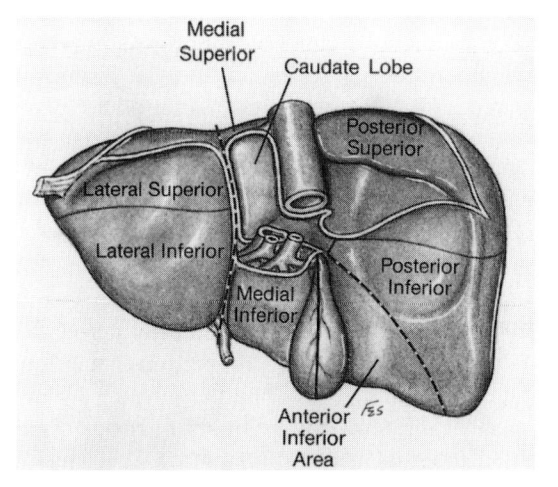

Fig. 12.4 Inferior landmarks of the liver. (Reprinted with permission by Warren et al 1991.)

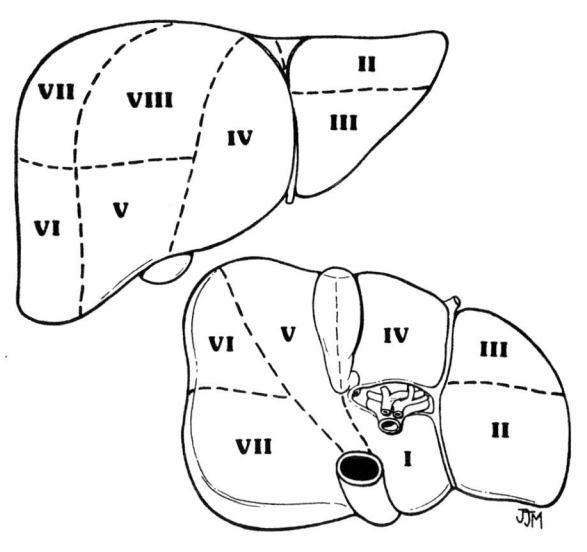

Fig. 12.5 Liver divided into segmental anatomy. (Reprinted with permission by Warren et al 1991.)

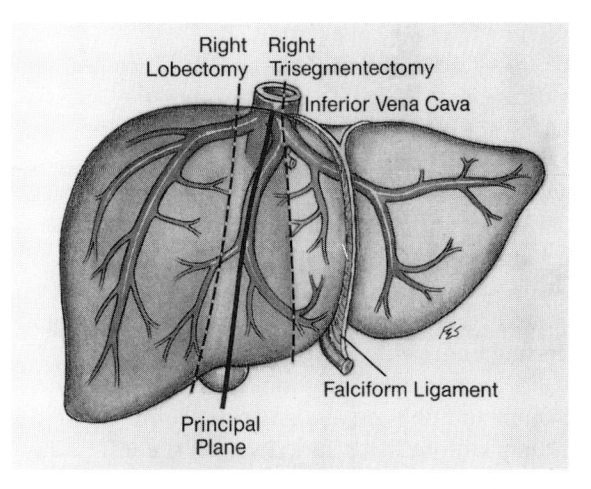

Fig. 12.6 Hepatic venous anatomy and the options for right lobectomy. (Reprinted with permission by Warren et al 1991.)

involves four distinct segments: the anatomic right lobe, the anatomic left lobe, the medial segment of the left lobe in conjunction with the right lobe (a right trisegmentectomy) and the lateral segment of the left lobe (Figs 12.6 and 12.7). Surgery that attempts to divide the liver along other planes increases the hazard and the blood loss. The required type of hepatic resection is determined by the precise anatomic location of the lesion(s). Heroic attempts to extend resections beyond normal anatomic boundaries (as in the case of advanced metastatic disease) are not justified and usually result in poor outcome because of the biology, even if the patient survives the immediate technical challenge.

Improvements in surgical techniques, perioperative management and anaesthetic monitoring have allowed hepatic resections for metastatic colorectal cancer to be performed with low mortality in many major centres. For hepatic surgery to be successful, however, the surgeon must adequately assess and prepare the patient preoperatively, pay meticulous attention to detail intraoperatively and be capable of managing the potential complications postoperatively. A complete understanding of the liver's anatomy, as well

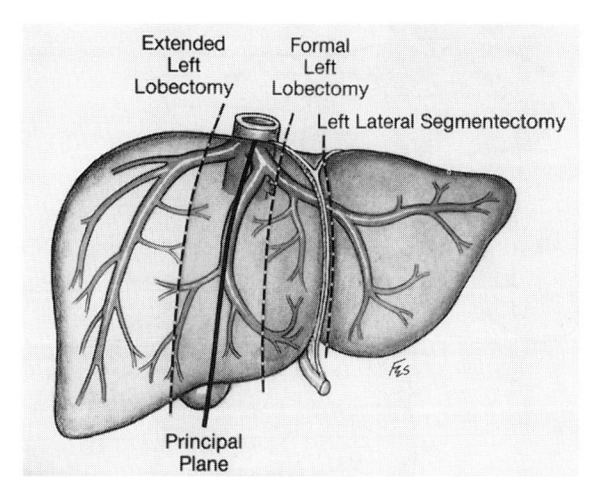

Fig. 12.7 Hepatic venous anatomy and the options for left lobectomy. (Reprinted with permission by Warren et al 1991.)

as its many variations, is a prerequisite for performing any resection or using newer techniques such as cryosurgical ablation.

Advanced age is not an absolute contraindication to hepatic surgery; often the 'physiologic' age and performance status of the patient are better measures of operability. Most surgeons would agree that cirrhosis is a contraindication to major hepatic resection due to the decreased regenerative capacity of the cirrhotic liver. A recent study, however, demonstrated that colorectal cancer rarely metastasizes to the cirrhotic liver, a finding not readily explained (Uetsuji et al 1992).

Preoperative testing should include a complete history and physical examination, complete blood count, routine liver function tests, chest X-ray, electrocardiogram and coagulation studies. Any coagulation defect should be corrected preoperatively with vitamin K or fresh frozen plasma or both. Particular attention should be focused on the nutritional status of the patient, since preoperative nutritional support may decrease postoperative complications in severely malnourished patients.

Laparoscopy may help stage the patient prior to a laparotomy. We recently reported a series in which laparoscopy demonstrated evidence of unresectability in 48% (14 of 29) of patients about to undergo a planned laparotomy for hepatic malignancy (Babineau et al 1994). Patients determined laparoscopically to be unresectable had a significantly shorter (1.2 days) hospital length of stay as compared with historical controls found to be unresectable by formal laparotomy (6.7 days). If deemed resectable, most patients are explored through a right upper quadrant or midline incision. Occasionally, with large tumours involving the right hepatic lobe, an extension of the incision into the right chest may be necessary to adequately obtain control of the superior vena cava and hepatic veins. After ruling out extrahepatic metastases, the liver is mobilized by dividing its ligamentous attachments. Intraoperative ultrasonography should then be performed to determine the presence of unsuspected lesions deep within the liver which would preclude a curative resection.

After completing the ultrasonographic, tactile and visual assessment, the appropriate type of resection necessary to encompass the lesion(s) is selected. The key technical factor is to obtain 1–2 cm of tumour-free margins, no matter what type of resection is required. The porta hepatis is dissected to isolate the hepatic artery, portal vein and bile duct. After the inflow to the liver is isolated, control of the hepatic venous anatomy takes priority. Gaining access to the three hepatic veins constitutes the most technically demanding part of the operation and the various techniques for control are well described elsewhere (Warren et al 1991). Following the hepatic venous dissection, the actual transection of the liver may be performed in a number of ways, but most surgeons still prefer the 'finger fracture' technique. The liver capsule is incised with cautery and the parenchyma fractured away by the fingers, exposing the veins, ducts and arteries which are subsequently ligated. Following transection of the liver fragment, haemostasis is meticulously obtained and multiple closed suction devices are left in place for 3–7 days postoperatively.

If severe haemorrhage occurs intraoperatively from a technical misadventure the liver can be completely isolated by applying a vascular clamp across the porta hepatis (Pringle's manoeuvre) and the vena cava compressed above and below the liver. Warm ischaemia will be tolerated by the liver for up to 1 hour. This vascular isolation technique often gives the surgeon time to define the extent of the technical problem and effect a repair. If the patient has not already exsanguinated, cardiac index remains remarkably stable in most patients despite this complete vascular exclusion of the liver. Ideally, if vascular isolation is required to perform a resection, it should be evident before the parenchymal dissection and can be undertaken in an orderly fashion. Tumour in the caudate lobe or near the vene cava may best be resected in this way.

Intraoperative management is a coordinated effort between anaesthesiologist and surgeon. Most major hepatic resections require arterial and central venous monitoring. Excessive bleeding is the most common and lethal intraoperative complication, still occurring in approximately 3–5% of patients. Improved intraoperative blood salvage techniques (including the use of the 'cell-saver' even in tumour resections), along with preoperative autologous blood banking, have decreased the amount of banked blood a patient should require during or after hepatic resection. In fact, most current hepatic resection series report a mean transfusion requirement of only 0–2 units per patient! This may be biologically important since many recent studies have claimed a poorer prognosis among patients with higher perioperative transfusion requirements (Okuno et al 1994, Rosen et al 1992). Of course, the postoperative course of a patient is often directly correlated with the amount of intraoperative blood loss which may be biological selection as much as causal.

Postoperatively, patients may have massive 'third space' requirements with major extracellular fluid sequestration. Metabolic alkalosis may occur when large amounts of blood products are given and can be corrected (if significant) with the central venous administration of 0.1 N hydrochloric acid. The most common postoperative complication following liver resection is sepsis involving either wound, lungs or abdomen. Bleeding, bile leak and hepatic failure are the other major serious complications. There is usually a transient rise in the serum bilirubin and other liver function tests postoperatively but these should return to baseline within 7–10 days. A persistently elevated bilirubin suggests biliary obstruction with or without a leak and warrants diagnostic evaluation. Persistent elevation in liver enzymes suggests an infectious complication or vascular injury. Serum albumin levels will transiently fall but there is no beneficial effect of supplemental albumin administration.

The proper technique of resection is characterized by the single goal of removing all metastatic disease with a minimum of a 1–1.5 cm margin of surrounding normal hepatic parenchyma. Anatomically defined lobectomy is not necessary if segmentectomy or 'wedge' resection completely removes all metastatic deposits. Although the size of a solitary lesion or the amount of hepatic tissue resected has not been shown to be a prognostic indicator following hepatic resection, the number of metastases resected does appear to be significant (Cady & McDermott 1985, Hughes et al 1988). Patients with more than three lesions have a shorter survival and some authors consider the presence of more than three separate metastases a contraindication to resection.

Finally, some lesions may be adequately treated with cryosurgical ablation which is the in situ destruction of tumour using subzero temperatures. This technique involves ultrasonographic localization of the hepatic lesion, placement of an encased liquid nitrogen probe within the lesion and lowering the tissue temperature to approximately −35°C for several minutes followed by slow rewarming. This cycle is repeated two to three times. The real-time monitoring of adequate freeze margins has allowed several groups to define extraordinarily low morbidity and effective ablation of liver tumour in over 200 patients (Steele 1995a). For patients with relatively small lesions in the depths of the right or left hepatic lobes, the avoidance of having to perform a right or left hepatic lobectomy decreases the morbidity and mortality with no noticeable change in either pattern of recurrence or overall survival (Fig. 12.8). Thus if the metastatic lesion is not contiguous to a major blood vessel (which creates a heat sink that militates against cryosurgical destruction of all tumour) *and* when there are no technical impediments to defining a 1–2 cm circumferential margin ultrasonographically, the chances for long-term and disease-free survival are comparable with the abovementioned retrospective and prospective liver resection data (Steele 1994c).

Follow-up for patients who have undergone either surgical resection or cryosurgical ablation of their isolated liver metastases is predicated on

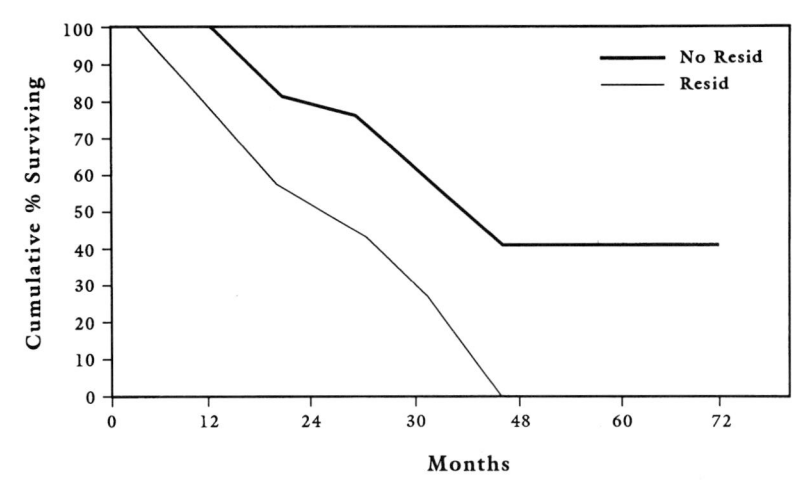

Fig. 12.8 Cryosurgical treatment of metastatic colorectal carcinoma: impact of residual disease. (Reprinted with permission from Steele 1994a.)

the fact that a small subset of these already biologically select patients may, in fact, be candidates for re-resection or recryosurgical ablation. Recent reports have described survivors at 5 years following re-resection (Fowler et al 1993, Que & Nagorney 1994). However, the majority of patients who recur will do so not only within the liver but outside the liver as well and thus require systemic therapy (Asbun & Hughes 1993, Curley et al 1993). Since current systemic therapy is non-curative and since non-curative systemic therapy in the absence of symptoms is not justifiable, close follow-up is less critical than if curative systemic treatment options were available. Nonetheless, we obtain a baseline CT scan within 1 week after liver resection or cryoablation and follow serial CEA levels quarterly for the first 2–3 years. Concurrently, periodic colonoscopic surveillance is performed to rule out the development of metachronous colorectal cancers or precancers.

Summary

Colorectal carcinoma metastatic to the liver is potentially curable. Given the lack of effective systemic therapy, surgical resection should be considered the treatment of choice for appropriate lesions. Although the number of patients who will ultimately present with liver-only metastases amenable to curative resection is relatively small, the chance of cure justifies an aggressive diagnostic work-up and surgical approach.

References

Adson MA 1987 Resection of liver metastases – when is it worthwhile? World Journal of Surgery 11(4): 511–520

Asbun HJ, Hughes KS 1993 Management of recurrent and metastatic colorectal carcinoma. Surgical Clinics of North America 73(1): 145–166

Babineau TJ, Lewis WD, Jenkins RL, Bleday R, Steele GD Jr, Forse RA 1994 Role of staging laparosopy in the treatment of hepatic malignancy. American Journal of Surgery 167(1): 151–155

Ballantyne GH, Quin J 1993 Surgical treatment of liver metastases in patients with colorectal cancer. Cancer 71 (suppl 12): 4252–4266

Boring CC, Squires TS, Tong T 1993 Cancer statistics, 1993. CA: A Cancer Journal for Clinicians 43(1): 7–26

Cady B, McDermott WV 1985 Major hepatic resection for metachronous metastases from colon cancer. Annals of Surgery 201(2): 204–209

Curley SA, Roh MS, Chase JL, Hohn DC 1993 Adjuvant hepatic arterial infusion chemotherapy after curative resection of colorectal liver metastases. American Journal of Surgery 166(6): 743–748

Foster JH, Berman MM 1977 Solid liver tumors. In: Major problems in clinical surgery. W. B. Saunders, Philadelphia, p 1–342

Fowler WC, Hoffman JP, Eisenberg BL 1993 Redo hepatic resection for metastatic colorectal carcinoma. World Journal of Surgery 17(5): 658–662

Garnick MB, Weiss GR, Steele GD Jr, Israel M, Schade D, Sack MJ, Frei E III 1983 Clinical evaluation of long-term, continuous-infusion doxorubicin. Cancer Treatment Reports 67: 133–142

Gastrointestinal Tumor Study Group 1984 Adjuvant therapy of colon cancer – results of a prospectively randomized trial. New England Journal of Medicine 310: 737–743

Gastrointestinal Tumor Study Group 1985 A controlled trial

of adjuvant chemotherapy, radiation therapy or combined chemoradiation therapy following curative resection for rectal carcinoma. New England Journal of Medicine 312: 1465–1472

Goslin R, Steele G Jr, Zamcheck N, Mayer R, MacIntyre J 1982 Factors influencing survival in patients with hepatic metastases from adenocarcinoma of the colon or rectum. Diseases of the Colon and Rectum 25: 749–754

Hughes KS, Simon R, Songhorabodi S et al 1986 Resection of the liver for colorectal carcinoma metastases: a multi-institutional study of patterns of recurrence. Surgery 100: 278–284

Hughes KS, Simon R, Songhorabodi S et al 1988 Resection of the liver for colorectal carcinoma metastases: a multi-institutional study of long term survivors. Diseases of the Colon and Rectum 31: 1–4

Karl RC, Morse SS, Halper RD, Clark RA 1993 Preoperative evaluation of patients for liver resection. Appropriate CT imaging. Annals of Surgery 217(3): 226–232

Kemeny N, Conti JA, Sigurdson E et al 1993 A pilot study of hepatic artery floxuridine combined with systemic 5-fluorouracil and leucovorin. A potential adjuvant program after resection of colorectal hepatic metastases. Cancer 71(6): 1964–1971

Kemeny N, Seiter K, Conti JA et al 1994 Hepatic arterial floxuridine and leucovorin for unresectable liver metastases from colorectal carcinoma. New dose schedules and survival update. Cancer 73(4): 1134–1142

Okuno J, Ozaki M, Shigeoka H et al 1994 Effect of packed red cell and whole blood transfusion on liver-associated immune function. American Journal of Surgery 168: 340–343

Pestana C, Reitemeier RJ, Moertel CG et al 1964 The natural history of carcinoma of the colon and rectum. American Journal of Surgery 108: 826–829

Que FG, Nagorney DM 1994 Resection of 'recurrent' colorectal metastases to the liver. British Journal of Surgery 81(2): 255–258

Ravikumar TS, Kane R, Cady B, Jenkins R, Clouse M, Steele G Jr 1991a A five year study of cryosurgery in the treatment of liver tumors. Archives of Surgery 126(12): 1520–1524

Ravikumar TS, Steele G Jr, Kane R, King V 1991b Experimental and clinical observations on hepatic cryosurgery for colorectal metastases. Cancer Research 51(23 Pt 1): 6323–6327

Rosen CB, Nagorney DM, Taswell HF, Helgeson SL, Ilstrup DM, van Heerden JA, Adson MA 1992 Perioperative blood transfusion and determinants of survival after liver resection for metastatic colorectal carcinoma. Annals of Surgery 216(4): 493–505

Saenz NC, Cady B, McDermott WV, Steele GD Jr 1989 Experience with colorectal carcinoma metastatic to the liver. Surgical Clinics of North America 69(2): 361–370

Steele G Jr 1991 Regional treatment of hepatic metastases from colorectal carcinoma – is hepatic arterial infusion using implantable devices worthwhile? Perspectives in General Surgery 2: 89–96

Steele G Jr 1993 Standard postoperative monitoring of patients after primary resection of colon and rectum cancer. Cancer 71(12): 4225–4335

Steele G Jr 1994a Advances in the treatment of early to late stage colorectal cancer: twenty years of progress. Annals of Surgical Oncology 2: 77–88

Steele G Jr 1994b Colorectal cancer. In: McKenna RJ Sr, Murphy GP (eds) Cancer surgery. J. B. Lippincott, Philadelphia, p 125–184

Steele G Jr 1994c Cryoablation in hepatic surgery. Seminars in Liver Disease 14(2): 120–125

Steele G Jr 1995a Hepatic metastases: results. In: Morris DL, McArde CS, Onik G (eds) Hepatic metastases: diagnosis and management. Butterworth-Heinemann, Oxford (in press)

Steele G Jr 1995b The management of colorectal cancer metastatic to the liver. In: Cameron JL (ed) Current surgical therapy, 5th edn. Mosby Yearbook, St Louis

Steele G Jr, Ravikumar TS 1989 Resection of hepatic metastases from colorectal cancer. Biological perspectives. Annals of Surgery 210: 127–138

Steele G, Bleday R, Mayer RJ, Lindblad A, Petrelli N, Weaver D 1991 A prospective evaluation of hepatic resection for colorectal carcinoma metastases to the liver: Gastrointestinal Tumor Study Group Protocol 6584. Journal of Clinical Oncology 9(7): 1105–1112

Stone MD, Kane R, Bothe A Jr, Jessup JM, Cady B, Steele GD Jr 1994 Intraoperative ultrasound imaging of the liver at the time of colorectal cancer resection. Archives of Surgery 129(4): 431–435

Uetsuji S, Yamamura M, Yamamichi K, Okuda Y, Takada H, Hioki K 1992 Absence of colorectal cancer metastasis to the cirrhotic liver. American Journal of Surgery 164(2): 176–177

Vaughn DJ, Haller DG 1993 Nonsurgical management of recurrent colorectal cancer. Cancer 71 (suppl 12): 4278–4292

Warren KW, Jenkins RL, Steele GD Jr 1991 Atlas of surgery of the liver, pancreas and biliary tract. Appleton & Lange, Norwalk, p 236–290

Weiss GR, Garnick MB, Osteen RT et al 1983 Long-term hepatic arterial infusion of 5-fluorodeoxyuridine for liver metastases using an implantable pump. Journal of Clinical Oncology 1: 337

Index

Abdominoperineal excision of rectum (APER), 69–76, 166
Active specific immunotherapy, 155
Adenoma-carcinoma pathway, 2, 41–43
Adenomas
  aetiology, 41–43
  benign, management, 44–46
  biopsy, 43
  diagnosis, 43
  dysplasia, 39
  familial *see* Familial adenomatous polyposis
  flat, 45
  with invasive carcinoma, management, 46–47
  local excision, 93
  lymph node metastasis, 46–47
  management, 44–47
  National Polyp Study, 40
  natural history, 47
  pedunculated, 44
  prophylactic removal, 43
  rectal, 45–46
  sessile, 44
  sigmoidoscopy, 30–33
  sporadic, 39–47
  surveillance, 34
  tubular, 39
  tubulovillous, 39
  villous, 39
Adenomatous polyposis coli (APC) gene, 2
  mutations, 11, 13, 23, 42, 47, 48
Adherens junctions, 2
Adjuvant therapies *see* Chemotherapy; Immunotherapy; Radiotherapy
Albumin, faecal, 30
Allele loss assays, 9–10
American Joint Committee for Cancer (AJCC), 58
Anal sphincter
  manometric studies, 76–77
  neosphincters, 81–84
Anoplasty, 87
Anorectal reconstruction, 81–88
Ascites, 163
Astler–Coller staging, 57
Australian clinico-pathological staging (ACPS), 59

Barium enema, 43
BCG organisms, 155
Blind stoma, 131

Bone metastases, 163
  radiotherapy, 166
Brain metastases, 47, 163
  radiotherapy, 166–167

Caecostomy tube, 131
Cancer family syndrome (Lynch syndrome II), 1, 23
Carcinoembryonic antigen (CEA), 30, 157–158, 161, 163
Cartilaginous exostoses, 47
Chemotherapy, 151–158
  palliation, 167–168
  and radiotherapy, 142–143, 146–147
Cimetidine, 155
Coloanal anastomosis, 69, 77–79
Colonic conduit, 87
Colonic pouch, 87
Colonic pouch-anal anastomosis, 79–81
Colonoscopy, 33
  polypectomy, 44–46
  preoperative, 160
  screening, 33
  surveillance, 161–162
Coloperineal anastomosis, 85
Colorectal anastomosis, 69, 76–77
Colostomy, 131, 159
Concord Hospital staging system, 59, 62–67
Congenital hypertrophy of the retinal pigment epithelium (CHRPE), 23, 47
Cowden's disease, 52
Cronkhite–Canada syndrome, 51–52
Cryosurgical ablation, 181
CT scan
  liver metastases, 178
  obstruction, 125–126
  recurrences, 164
Cyclin dependent kinases (cdks), 6
Cyclooxygenase inhibition, 49
Cytokines, 154
Cytosine deaminase (CD), 157–158

Deleted in colorectal cancer (DCC) gene, 7, 14
Digital examination, 147
Diverticulitis, 126
DNA methylation, 11, 15, 42
DNA ploidy, 11, 15
  and chemotherapy, 152
DNA repair genes, 10, 14
Dukes' staging, 56–57, 60–61
Dysplasia-carcinoma pathway, 2

Endometrial carcinoma, 1
Epidermoid cysts, 47
Erlangen magnetic ring, 82

Faecal occult blood tests, 25, 26–30
  surveillance, 162
Familial adenomatous polyposis (FAP), 1, 47–50
  attenuated, 23
  diagnosis, 48
  gene *see* Adenomatous polyposis coli (APC) gene
  genetic counselling, 48
  management, 48–50
  osteomas, 23, 47
  screening, 16, 23, 48–49
  sulindac therapy, 49
  surgery, 49
  upper gastrointestinal tract lesions, 49–50
Familial juvenile polyposis coli, 51
Family history, 24
5-Flucytosine, 158
Fluorodeoxyuridine (FUDR), 173–174
5-Fluorouracil, 153–154
  and folinic acid (leucovorin), 154, 156, 167, 168
  hepatic artery infusion, 173
  and interferon, 168
  and levamisole, 155–156, 167
  palliation, 167
  portal venous infusion, 156–157
  and radiotherapy (adjuvant X-ray infusion), 142–143, 146–147, 156
  side effects, 153–154
  studies, 155–157
  tumour resistance, 151
Folinic acid, 154, 156, 167, 168
fos gene, 4

GADD45 gene, 7
Gardner's syndrome, 1, 47
  genetic alterations, 11
Gastric polyps, 49
Gastrografin enema, 125
Gastrointestinal Tumor Study Group (GITSG), 61, 175, 176–177
Gene therapy, 157–158
Genetic counselling, 48
Genetics, 2–16
Gracilis muscle neosphincter, 83–84
Growth factor receptors, 8
Growth factors, 8

Index

GTP-ase activating protein (GAP), 3–4
Guaiac tests, 25, 26–27
Guanine nucleotide exchange factor (GEF), 4
Guanosine diphosphate (GDP), 3–4
Guanosine triphosphate (GTP), 3

Haematoporphyrin derivative (HpD), 74, 168
Haemoccult, 25, 26–30
  surveillance, 162
HaemoccultSENSA, 26–27
HaemoQuant, 26–27
Haem-porphyrin assays, 25
Hamartomas, 50–52
HemeSelect, 26–27
Hereditary non-polyposis colorectal cancer (HNPCC), 1–2
  Amsterdam criteria, 1
  genetic alterations, 11–12
  Lynch types, 1, 23
  screening, 16, 23–24
Hereditary site-specific colon cancer (Lynch syndrome I), 1, 23
High-risk groups, 23–24
hMLH1 gene, 7–8, 11, 24
hMSH2 gene, 7–8, 11, 23–24

Ileostomy, 131
Immunological tests, 25, 26
Immunotherapy, 151–158
  recurrences, 168
Implantable sphincter prosthesis, 81–82
Infusaid pump, 173
Interferon, 154, 168
Interleukin-2 (IL-2), 154, 168
International comprehensive anatomical terminology (ICAT), 62
International documentation system (IDS), 62
Intussusception, 51

Japanese Research Society staging, 59
jun gene, 4
Juvenile polyps, 50–51

K-ras oncogene
  mutations, 12–13, 15
  stool tests, 30

Laparoscopic surgery, 103–117
  bowel anastomosis, 104–105, 108–109
  bowel mobilization, 107
  Cleveland Clinic, Florida, 109–111
  controversies, 111–117
  conversion to laparotomy, 106
  cosmesis, 107
  costs, 113
  indications, 105
  learning/operating problems, 103–105
  lesion location, 104, 107–108
  ligation of vessels, 104, 108
  liver metastases, 178, 180
  lymph node resection, 114–115
  morbidity, 111–112
  patient positioning, 106
  port placement, 106–107
  procedures, 105–106
  recurrence, 115–117
  training, 105
Leucovorin, 154, 156, 167, 168
Levamisole, 154–155
  and, 5-fluorouracil, 155–156, 167
Liver
  cirrhosis, 180
  divisions, 178–179
  intraoperative ultrasonographic staging, 174, 178
  laparoscopy, 178, 180
  metastases, 160, 163, 173–182
  cryosurgical ablation, 181
  laparoscopic staging, 178, 180
  preoperative staging, 177–178
  presentation, 174
  radiotherapy, 166
  surgery, 165
  synchronous disease, 174
  resection, 174–182
Lung secondaries, 163
  surgery, 165
Lymph nodes
  metastases, 46–47
  resection, 114–115
Lymphokine activated killer cells, 155, 168
Lynch syndromes, 1, 23

Magnetic resonance imaging (MRI), 164
MDM2 gene, 7
Metastases
  bone *see* Bone metastases
  brain *see* Brain metastases
  follow-up, 159–160
  liver *see* Liver: metastases
  lung *see* Lung metastases
  lymph node, 46–47
  preoperative screening, 160
Metastasis genes, 10, 15
Methotrexate
  palliation, 167
  tumour resistance, 151
Microsatellites, 9, 11–12, 14
Mitogen-activated protein kinase (MAPK) cascade, 4
Monoclonal antibodies
  therapy, 155, 168
  tumour markers, 161
Mortality, 21

MRI, 164
Mucosectomy, 96–97
Muir–Torre syndrome, 2, 12
Mutated in colorectal cancer gene (MCC), 2, 13
myc gene, 4, 13

Nasogastric tube, 126
National Polyp Study, 40
Neosphincters, 81–84
  electrically stimulated, 84–86
NF1 GAP protein, 14
NM23 genes, 7, 10, 15
NSABP Clinical Trial, 60
Nuclear factors, 8
Nucleoside diphosphate kinases (NDPKs), 7

Obstruction, 123–132
  anastomosis, 130
  decompression, 127
  diversion, 130–131
  endoscopic decompression, 126
  palliation, 128
  preoperative management, 126
  presentation/examination, 124
  resectability, 127–128
  resection, 129–130
  surgery, 126–132, 165
Oldfield's syndrome, 47
On-table lavage, 130
Oncogenes, 8
  sporadic colorectal cancer, 12–13
Osteomas, 23, 47

p53 gene, 7, 13–14, 15
Palliative treatment, 166–168
  obstruction/perforation, 128
Perforation, 123–132
  anastomosis, 130
  diagnostic evaluation, 125–126
  diversion, 130–131
  palliation, 128
  preoperative management, 126
  presentation/examination, 124–125
  rectal tumours, 73
  resectability, 127–128
  resection, 129–130
  surgery, 126–132
Performance status, 167
Periampullary carcinoma, 48, 49
Perineal pain, 163–164
Peritonitis, 124
Peutz–Jeghers syndrome, 51
Photodynamic therapy (PDT), 74, 168
Polypectomy, 44–47
Polyps
  hamartomatous, 50–52
  hyperplastic, 50
  inflammatory (pseudopolyps), 52
  juvenile, 50–51
  lymphoid, 52

Polyps (contd)
  neoplastic see Adenomas; Familial adenomatous polyposis
Population screening trials, 27–30
Pringle's manoeuvre, 180
Proctosigmoidoscopy (rigid sigmoidoscopy), 30–32
Proctotomy, transsphincteric posterior, 46
Prognosis prediction, 162–163
Prognostic indexes, 55, 61
Protein kinase C, 157
Protooncogenes, 8
Pseudopolyps, 52
pTNM staging system, 58

Radiation enteritis, 136–137, 140, 143, 144
Radioimmunoguided surgery, 74
Radiotherapy, 135–148
  and chemotherapy, 142–143, 146–147
  cost-effectiveness, 135–145
  and DNA repair, 143
  dose, 140–141, 145–146
  efficacy, 137–139
  enteritis, 136–137, 140, 143, 144
  field size/shape, 141
  liver metastases, 166
  local recurrence, 137, 166
  mobile tumours, 148
  palliative, 166–167
  postoperative, 142
  preoperative vs. postoperative, 144–145
  radiosensitivity, 139
  sexual potency, 139
  sphincter preservation, 139
  staging, 139, 147–148
  and surgery, 143–145
  survival, 137–139
  technique, 145–146
  tethered/fixed tumours, 148
Raf1 pathway, 4
ras gene, 2–4
Rectal cancer
  abdominoperineal excision of rectum (APER), 69–76, 166
  anorectal reconstruction, 81–88
  coloanal anastomosis, 69, 77–79
  colonic pouch-anal anastomosis, 79–81
  coning, 73
  local excision, 93–101
  local recurrence, 72–74
  low anterior resection (colorectal anastomosis), 69, 76–77
  photodynamic therapy (PDT), 74
  radioimmunoguided surgery, 74

sphincter-saving resection (SSR), 69–76
  staging, 61
  survival, 74–75
  transanal endoscopic microsurgery (TEM), 93–101
  tumour perforation, 73
  ultrasound examination, 96
Rectoscope, 94–95
Recurrence, 163–166
  anastomotic, 166
  diagnosis, 163–165
  immunotherapy, 168
  local, 163–165
  palliative treatment, 166–168
  surgical treatment, 165–166
Restriction fragment length polymorphisms (RFLPs), 9
Retinal pigment epithelium, congenital hypertrophy, 23, 47
Retinoblastoma, 1 (RB1) gene, 4–7, 14
Retractors, 94
Rho pathway, 4
Risk factors, 23–24

Schmidt procedure, 82–83
Screening, 21–35
  colonoscopy, 33
  compliance, 21
  cost-benefit analysis, 34–35
  effectiveness, 22
  familial adenomatous polyposis, 16, 23, 48–49
  hereditary non-polyposis colorectal cancer, 16, 23–24
  population screening trials, 27–30
  sensitivity, 21
  sigmoidoscopy, 30–33
  specificity, 21–22
  studies, 25–30
  surveillance, 34
  target population, 22–24
  tests, 25
  ulcerative colitis-associated cancer, 24
Sebaceous cysts, 47
Sebaceous gland tumours, 2
Second look surgery, 165–166
Sigmoidoscopy
  flexible, 32–33
  rigid (proctosigmoidoscopy), 30–32
Signal transducers, 8
Single strand conformation polymorphism (SSCP) assays, 9
Smooth muscle neosphincter, 82–83
Sphincter-saving resection (SSR), 69–76

Sporadic colorectal adenocarcinomas
  DNA repair genes, 14
  genetic changes, 12–15
  gross DNA changes, 15
  metastasis genes, 15
  oncogenes, 12–13
  tumour suppressor genes, 13–14
Staging, clinicopathological, 55–67
  and chemotherapy, 152
  liver metastases, 178, 180
  and radiotherapy, 139, 147–148
Stereoscopic optical instruments, 95
Stomas, 131, 159
Striated muscle neosphincter, 83–84
Sulindac, 49
Surveillance, 34, 159–163
  colonoscopic, 161–162
  follow-up programme, 160
  Haemoccult-II, 162
  patient selection, 159–160
  prognosis prediction, 162–163
Suture-line tumours, 166

Thymidylate synthetase inhibitors, 157
Tissue polypeptide antigen (TPA), 161
Tissue polypeptide specific antigen (TPS), 161
TNM staging system, 58
Topoisomerase-I, 157
Transanal endoscopic microsurgery (TEM), 93–101
Tube caecostomy, 131
Tubular adenomas, 39
Tubulovillous adenomas, 39
Tumour markers, 161
Tumour suppressor genes, 9–10
  sporadic colorectal cancer, 13–14
Turcot's syndrome, 1, 47
Tyrosine kinases, 157

Ulcerative colitis-associated cancer, 2
  genetic changes, 15
  screening, 24
Ultrasound examination, 96, 164
  intraoperative, 174, 178
Union International Contre le Cancer (UICC), 58

Villous adenomas, 39

WAF1/CIP1 gene, 7
Wound dehiscence, 99–100

Zanca's syndrome, 47